"A brilliant book . . . *Winning the War Against Asthma &*
Allergies **must be read by everyone**, the medical profes-
sionals and the public alike." *Devi Nambudripad, D.C., L.Ac.,*
O.M.D., Ph.D., President of Nambudripad Allergy Research
Foundation

"If you suffer from asthma or allergies this book offers the
help you need. Dr. Cutler is a **modern day healer who re-**
spects the body's innate ability to heal itself . . . I believe
it truly offers a ray of sunlight in a very misunderstood area of
affliction." *Howard F. Loomis, Jr., D.C.*

"Millions of Americans suffer from allergies. Dr. Ellen Cutler
has created a unique approach to the management and treatment of a wide variety of allergic disorders This easy to read
book will point you in the right direction. **It's a must read if**
you or a loved one suffers from allergies." *Alan H. Pressman,*
D.C., Ph.D., Author of The GSH Phenomenon *and* The Physician's Guide to Healing

"*Winning the War Against Asthma & Allergies* by Dr. Ellen
Cutler is **a veritable encyclopedia of solutions, a masterful**
work from an outstanding practitioner **which no asthmatic or**
allergy afflicted person can afford to miss reading." *Gary*
Wagner, Producer of Alternative Medicine Television Program

"After just a few treatments with NAET, I felt like someone let
me out of jail. Six months into my treatment program with Dr.
Cutler, I could eat any of my favorite foods again, enjoy wine,
play with my Saint Bernard, and resume all my athletic activities. **Dr. Cutler has changed my life by helping me over-**
come my asthma and allergies forever." *Claire Pogue,*
asthma sufferer

Winning the War Against Asthma & Allergies

This book is dedicated to the memory of my mother and father
Gloria and Leonard Wagner

Winning the War Against Asthma & Allergies

A Drug-Free Cure for Asthma and Allergy Sufferers

BY ELLEN W. CUTLER, D.C.

Delmar Publishers

I(T)P® International Thomson Publishing

Albany • Bonn • Boston • Cincinnati • Detroit • London • Madrid
Melbourne • Mexico City • New York • Pacific Grove • Paris • San Francisco
Singapore • Tokyo • Toronto • Washington

Cover Design: Brucie Rosch

Delmar Staff
Publisher: Bill Brottmiller
Editor: Greg Vis
Consulting Editor: Claire Pogue
Marketing Manager: Denise Davis
Art and Design Coordinator: Carol Keohane
Editorial Assistant: Diane Biondi
Author Photograph: Courtesy of German Herrera

Copyright© 1998
by Ellen W. Cutler, D.C.

a division of International Thomson Publishing Inc.
The ITP logo is a trademark under license.

Printed in the United States of America

For more information, contact:

Delmar Publishers
3 Columbia Circle, Box 15015
Albany, New York 12212-5015

International Thomson Editores
Campos Eliseos 385, Piso 7
Col Polanco
11560 Mexico D F Mexico

International Thomson Publishing—Europe
Berkshire House 168-173
High Holborn
London WC1V 7AA
England

International Thomson Publishing GmbH
Königswinterer Strasse 418
53227 Bonn
Germany

Thomas Nelson—Australia
102 Dodds Street
South Melbourne, 3205
Victoria, Australia

International Thomson Publishing—Asia
221 Henderson Road
#05-10 Henderson Building
Singapore 0315

Nelson Canada
1120 Birchmount Road
Scarborough, Ontario
Canada M1K 5G4

International Thomson Publishing—Japan
Hirakawacho Kyowa Building, 3F
2-2-1 Hirakawacho
Chiyoda-ku, Tokyo 102
Japan

Library of Congress Cataloging-in-Publication Data
Cutler, Ellen.
   Winning the war against asthma & allergies : a drug-free
cure for asthma and allergy sufferers / by Ellen Cutler.
      p.   cm.
   Includes bibliographical references and index.
   ISBN 0-8273-8622-2
   1. Asthma—Alternative treatment.   2. Naturopathy.   I. Title.
RC591.C88   1997
616.2'38—dc21

97-9404
CIP

TABLE OF CONTENTS

ACKNOWLEDGEMENTS

I would like to express my sincere gratitude to the people who were of invaluable assistance in the creation of this book.

The staff of Tamalpais Pain Clinic who were very helpful from the beginning to the end in researching and developing the specific diets for the many allergy treatments so they could be as accurate as possible.

The many people who helped to research, edit, and prepare this manuscript including Ariana Garfinkel, Debra Cutler, D.C., Sangeet Duchane, and Fran Massimino.

Stephan Bodian who masterfully edited the manuscript and whose attention to detail, unceasing patience, and talents for writing added immeasurably to this book.

Dr. Steve Bock for writing the foreword and whose material was innovative and vital to this manuscript.

All my patients—my extended family—with whom I've worked for many years. They gave me the opportunity to learn and research the many tools of healing and shared their hearts and souls with me so I could be of utmost service.

My son Aaron who watched me work many late hours at my office and home and always gave me encouragement and love. My daughter Gabrielle who enabled me to learn and discover new ways to treat children and acute illnesses, and who said to me after the manuscript was finished, "Mommy, I am so proud you wrote this." And a special acknowledgment to my wonderful, loving, patient husband who was always there for me, sacrificed a year and a half of many intimate moments for the writing of this book and who, in the end, helped me finish the final draft of the manuscript. Thank you Steven. I love you.

Devi Nambudripad, D.C., L.Ac., the founder of allergy elimination and the developer of NAET. She is an extraordinary woman who has enabled thousands of individuals to regain true and lasting health and unlimited energy. Dr. Devi's never ending dedication to her patients and students is a constant source of inspiration to my work. Her own healing, which led to the discovery of NAET, has given the world a wonderful breakthrough in the area of allergies and chronic illness. Asthmatics now have an alternative to their lifelong struggle and conventional treatment with drugs. Not a day goes by that I don't praise the work of Devi Nambudripad and thank her for what she has taught me. This book is my dedication to her work and my appreciation of her contribution to the healing profession. I believe she should win the Nobel Prize and be recognized as an exceptional human being.

Finally, Claire Lussier-Pogue, the woman who made this all possible. She always had vision, unceasing inspiration, motivation, and dedication. She has always been there for me, and without a shadow of a doubt, she is the sister I have always wanted. I dedicate the Winning the War series to Claire Pogue, and I thank her from my heart.

FOREWORD

It was my pleasure to review Dr. Cutler's book *Winning the War Against Asthma & Allergies.*

Our present health-care system has broken down; technology is becoming more and more extensive. Drug management with conventional medical methods are costing patients more and more, and even with all of this, patients are not feeling well. We are seeing an increased array of immune problems like cancer, autoimmune problems, allergies, chronic fatigue, asthma, etc.

The field of alternative medicine treats with various biological therapies such as diet manipulation, detoxification, nutritional pharmacology, enzyme therapy, homeopathy, Chinese medicine, acupuncture, chiropractic, and mind-body technique to name but a few. This is done by assessing all the factors that contribute to a person's overall balance or lack of balance (or dis-ease). There are various ways to assess a person's "terrain," that is, the soil or chemistry that makes us up and predisposes us to be susceptible to stresses, diseases, infections, chemical toxins, or allergies.

Dr. Cutler's approach for treating asthma adds a new dimension to the allergy dilemma. It not only identifies the offending substances, but also clears the body of its reactivity to the substance or substances. The patient then can go on with his or her life, including diet, in a more functioning manner.

She shows a very knowledgeable grasp of the field of clinical ecology. She gives you a picture of how to look at what you may be exposed to, in daily and everyday life, and how it may adversely affect your body, particularly your allergic and asthma symptoms.

Allergies can signify various states in each person. In one case, the allergy could be signaling a warning that there are too many substances to which the person is heavily exposed (this is common for all of us in our environment). In another case, it could be signaling that our body is on overload and our immune system is overflowing. In others, it can be that we have an emotional problem spilling over into physical symptoms.

Dr. Cutler blends the field of clinical ecology with kinesiologic and electroacupuncture testing, along with enzyme therapy, acupuncture, and body energetics to manage the allergic asthma patient. She emphasizes the role of chemicals and other substances in the environment and their effect on everyone.

A patient of mine had seen Dr. Cutler. Her asthma had been treated with various medications. She was allergic to various substances and still had severe asthma after undergoing treatment with numerous conventional antiasthma medications. She is in a much improved state of health, off most of her medications, able to eat foods that she has been unable to to eat, and can come into contact with other substances that she had heretofore been unable to eat. She has become better educated and empowered to deal with her allergies. I feel that Dr. Cutler's book is a tremendous addition to the healing arsenal. A biological therapy (working with nontoxic medicines) that taps into the healing energy of a person and functions as a continuing education process in a person's journey through life, is one that all complimentary physicians are constantly seeking. I welcome it.

—Steven Bock, M.D.

PREFACE

I see people every day in my office who are winning the war against asthma and allergies. Not only do they overcome their need to use asthma medication, but also say farewell to the disease permanently. The victory is sweet indeed.

"As an acute asthma sufferer," wrote one of my patients, "I've had to fight daily battles, using medication and avoidance. But with NAET and enzyme therapy I've been able to win not only the battles, but the war forever." The road to complete recovery is short and easy for some patients, long and arduous for others, but it is a journey that is well worth every challenge.

My work with allergies started almost 20 years ago and eventually led me to write this book. In my clinical experience with all types of chronically ill individuals, three contributing factors have repeatedly presented themselves: poor digestion, dietary stress, and allergies. Although this book focuses on the relationship between allergies and asthma, it can benefit all those who suffer from allergies or other chronic health problems.

Many asthmatics live with symptoms every day of their lives. They experience heaviness in their chest, breathing difficulties, perhaps some coughing or wheezing, and often find themselves struggling for oxygen, a problem normal individuals rarely ever think about. Asthmatics develop these symptoms in response to foods, molds, chemicals, or a variety of other substances, as well as to changes in temperature, humidity, or other environmental factors. These reactions happen in seconds and can be life threatening.

There is little doubt that asthma is an allergic disease. Asthmatics are affected by many allergens such as formaldehyde in perfumes, new clothing, carpets, and plastics; chlorine and fluoride in the water supply; hydrocarbons in car exhaust; trichloroethylene in dry-cleaned garments; natural substances such as textiles, pollens, milk, feathers, yeast and fungi; mercury amalgams in teeth; viruses; bacteria; and even emotions.

This book is divided into six main sections: Part I—Allergies, Part II—Asthma, Part III—Nambudripad Allergy Elimination Technique (NAET) Therapy, Part IV—Adjunctive Therapy, Part V—Case Studies, and Part VI—Resource Guide. Chapter 11 offers case histories documenting the result of NAET treatment and enzyme therapy. I suggest that you read it before Chapter 1 because it complements this introduction and helps you appreciate why the information this book presents is a must-read for all asthma and allergy sufferers.

Chapters 1–3 explain the types, origins, and causes of allergies and summarize the various allergy testing and treatment approaches including NAET. It also features a detailed self-help emergency treatment and a muscle response allergy test that could save your life.

Chapters 4–7 review the symptoms of asthma and the numerous allergens that can trigger an asthma sufferer. These allergens include food, hormones, glands, vitamins, fungi, viruses, bacteria, cold, humidity, mold, pollen, dust, animals, salicylates, chemicals, metabolic imbalances, genetic factors, aspirin, birth control pills, vaccines, and the corticosteroids asthmatics inhale. Once the allergens are pinpointed by an NAET practitioner, the allergies they cause can be eliminated and will no longer pose a problem.

Chapter 8 is a complete guide to creating an allergy-free environment for asthma sufferers. Once people have completed NAET treatment, many of these suggestions no longer need be followed. But until the allergies are eliminated, this chapter can be extremely helpful to all allergy sufferers, especially asthmatics.

Chapters 9 to 11 describe in detail this revolutionary allergy elimination technique which has so transformed the lives of many asthmatics. Imagine for a moment that your son or daughter is triggered, without warning, into a life-threatening attack that can leave them unable to breathe or call out for help. Childhood asthma can be a living nightmare for parents. Yet every day I see children who suffer from chronic asthma symptoms undergoing treatment that eventually transform them into normal, healthy, asthma-free kids. Watching as their own lives and the lives of their children are turned around, these parents often ask me why NAET is not the mainstream approach to treating allergies and asthma.

These three chapters delineate the most common treatment protocols for the many different asthmatics, including children and infants.

Chapter 12 discusses stamina and the effects of NAET treatment on exercise, energy levels, sleep habits, and mental health.

In addition to breathing problems, most asthmatics appear to suffer from poor digestion, including constipation, diarrhea, bloating, and irritable bowel syndrome. Many are sugar and starch intolerant and are deficient in critical, life-supporting enzymes that are needed for every chemical reaction in our bodies. These enzymes work to build our bodies from proteins, fats and carbohydrates; no vitamin or mineral can function without their support. Of the more than 5,000 enzymes that have been discovered, four are food enzymes found in raw food, and 22 are digestive enzymes made by the pancreas. The rest are metabolic enzymes, that involve all the different systems of the body and help maintain a healthy immune system.

I learned about enzymes from Dr. Howard Loomis, who, along with Edward Howell, is one of the foremost pioneers in enzyme therapy. Their research has initiated an exciting new phase in the study of nutrition and its implications for asthma and other chronic health problems. According to Loomis, all asthmatics suffer enzyme deficiency as a result of poor digestion, which eventually compromises immune system function. Chapter 13 is a complete overview of enzyme therapy, including how it is used, why it is important for asthmatics, and why proper digestion and utilization of foods is paramount in health and vitality.

Chapter 14 presents a series of case studies that show how NAET treatments cured a variety of afflictions.

Chapter 15 is a resource guide, and covers all the necessary ingredients for proper NAET treatments, food guides for the allergens, diets for the different enzyme deficiencies and food intolerances, a glossary of terms, a list of NAET practitioners, and other important resources for both health practitioners and asthma sufferers. Glossary terms are printed in bold type the first time they appear in the book. This book also has an on-line companion on our Internet site (http://www.allergy2000.com) which features new research findings, an "Ask the Experts" column, an updated list of trained NAET professionals, and more.

The knowledge this book provides can reduce your risk of death from asthma by helping you identify and eliminate its true causes. It can enable you to see yourself not as an average asthma or allergy sufferer but as an individual with your own unique biochemical makeup, allergies, and needs. Most asthmatics have been told that asthma is a chronic problem they will have to contend with for the rest of their lives. This book shows that asthma can be cured, not miraculously and instantaneously but inevitably and permanently, once the allergies that cause it have been eliminated.

Every asthmatic should be able to lead a normal, drug-free life. If you're an asthma sufferer who wants to overcome your condition and prevent your children and loved ones from developing it themselves, read this book and discover how you can secure optimal health and win the war against disease. If you're a health practitioner dealing with the asthma and allergies of your patients, this book will introduce you to a new approach that may revolutionize your practice.

As we approach the twenty-first century, the growing incidence of asthma reflects an increase of chemical pollutants in our environment and food, a decline in adequate nutrition caused in large measure by poor absorption of vitamins, minerals, and other nutrients, and an exponential rise in the use of pharmaceutical drugs that weaken and suppress the immune system. At the same time, the dawn of the new century heralds a new awakening to drug-free alternative approaches to chronic health problems. People are disillusioned with the medical establishment and are demanding remedies that enliven their bodies and minds and encourage rather than suppress their own healing force. We all need a chance to reclaim control and responsibility for our health. This book offers new understanding of the symptoms and causes of asthma and empowers everyone with an alternative approach of overcoming it, now and forever.

I ALLERGIES: TYPES, CAUSES, SYMPTOMS, TESTING, AND TREATMENTS

1 | DEFINING ALLERGIES

BROAD DEFINITION OF ALLERGIES

In this book I explore the relationship between allergies and asthma and I would like to begin by defining the term allergy. An **allergy** is an abnormal, adverse physical reaction of the body to certain substances known as **allergens** (or **antigens**). These substances can be toxic (exhaust fumes or other petrochemicals) or nontoxic (pollens or food) and allergy sufferers will react to quantities that are harmless to most people.

When exposed to allergens, allergic individuals develop an excess of an **antibody** called **immunoglobulin E (IgE)**. The IgE antibodies react with allergens to release **histamines** and other chemicals from cell tissues that produce various allergic symptoms. In other words, the **immune system** mistakenly identifies harmless substances as dangerous invaders and activates antibodies to defend the body. The development of an allergy begins with sensitization to the substance on first contact, usually without symptoms. A second exposure to the substance, however, allows the previously created antibodies to become active and produce symptoms.

Although a person can develop allergies to practically any substance, the most common allergens include pollen, dust, **dust mites**, animal dander (skin, saliva, hair, or fur), feathers, cosmetics, mold, insect venom, certain chemicals, drugs, medicines (especially penicillin), and foods. The most troublesome foods are usually peanuts, other tree nuts, shellfish, milk, eggs, wheat, and soy. Allergens may cause a reaction following inhalation, injection, ingestion, or contact with the skin. Allergic reactions can involve any part of the body, but most frequently affect the nose, chest, skin, and eyes. The rarest and most dangerous type of allergy is called **anaphylactic shock**. It can affect many organs at once and is evidenced by rapid decreases in blood pressure, rash or hives, breathing difficulties, abdominal pain, swollen tongue or throat, diarrhea, fainting, asphyxiation and, too often, death.

It is estimated that between 35 and 50 million people in the United States suffer from allergies. Allergies can emerge suddenly at any age without prior warning. Many studies have shown conclusively that parents with allergies tend to have children with allergies. Some research suggests that the tendency to develop an allergy of some kind is inherited, although not the tendency to a particular allergy. However, I have repeatedly seen in my practice that a child's allergic tendencies are often related to those of his or her parents, and I often have treated parents and their children for the same allergies. Some people tend toward allergic reactions (these individuals are known as atopic). Once a person develops one allergy, others commonly follow.

Part of the difficulty in determining the number of allergy sufferers lies in how broadly or narrowly one defines the term. Medical doctors and scientists often support a narrow definition, asserting that the only true allergies result from the activation of IgE antibodies. Millions of people, however, experience allergic symptoms without the antibody reaction. These people are said to have an intolerance or a **hypersensitivity** to particular substances. Although the causes may differ, the diagnosis and treatment of allergy and intolerance often overlap. As a result, allergy research and information benefits more people than those with traditional allergies alone.

In my clinical work I have found that the measurements and treatments for allergies and intolerances are exactly the same and I use the terms interchangeably. For example, many asthmatics are *intolerant* to sugars and *allergic* to animal dander. **Muscle response testing** with these two substances yields identical results, and I treat them in the same way.

Allergies can cause a predisposition to colds and the flu by compromising the immune system and lowering resistance. Once the body becomes host to viruses and bacteria, it is difficult to distinguish a cold from an allergic reaction, especially since the two often occur simultaneously. Allergies don't generally cause fever, however, and colds, unlike allergies that refuse to go away, do not linger for more than a week or two.

In this book, I take the wider view of an allergy as any negative or abnormal response in the immune system. For example, I believe there is no such thing as a simple cold. A cold is the response of a challenged immune system, whether it is to a food, a pollen, or a virus. Because a virus is also an allergen, I treat a cold like an allergy, and experience excellent results.

TYPES OF ALLERGIES

Allergies can be classified according to the causative substance or the resulting symptoms. There are also active (acute) allergies and hidden (chronic) allergies.

The first category includes the following subtypes:

- ingestants, also referred to as food allergy

- inhalants such as dust

- contactants such as latex or chemicals

- injectants such as drugs

- infectants such as viruses or bacteria

- physical agents such as cold or heat

- organs

- autoimmune allergies such as those to hormones that can include thyroid, estrogen, testosterone, cholesterol, and adrenaline

- insect allergies

Allergies defined by symptoms include:

- hay fever

- **asthma**

- skin conditions (**eczema**, hives, rashes)

- headaches and migraines

- stomach upset

- chronic fatigue

- depression

- chronic pain

- conjunctivitis

- anaphylactic shock

- the most widespread allergy-related diseases.

Active or acute allergies can be of the "immediate type" in which symptoms appear within seconds of contact after every exposure (for example, hives, itching, vomiting, coughing, wheezing) and usually subside within an hour. Or they can be of the "delayed type" in which the reaction occurs hours or days after contact because the allergen is not the food itself, but instead a chemical by-product of digestion.

Hidden or chronic allergies can cause severe developmental and functional problems, deficiencies, or chemical imbalances. For example, an allergy to B vitamins can cause B vitamin deficiencies and result in chronic health problems such as **chronic fatigue syndrome, attention deficit disorder (ADD)**, depression, digestive problems, asthma, and headaches. The diagnosis and treatment of chronic allergies is the focus of this book.

Food Allergy

A food allergy is the immune system's response to a certain food during which IgE-mediated chemicals trigger an allergic reaction. After ingesting foods to which he or she is allergic, a person may experience vomiting, stomach pain, swelling and bloating, diarrhea, constipation, eczema or hives, an asthmatic attack, breathing difficulties, joint pain, migraines and, on occasion, anaphylaxis. In extreme cases, an individual can have an allergic reaction to minute amounts of the allergen such as skin contact with the food, or kissing someone who has eaten the food. The eight foods that cause ninety percent of all allergic reactions are milk, eggs, wheat, peanuts, soy, tree nuts, fish, and shellfish. Peanuts, nuts, fish, and shellfish commonly cause the most severe and dangerous reactions.

Conventional medicine has no cure for food allergies, except strict avoidance of the allergens. The **Nambudripad Allergy Elimination Technique (NAET)** approach described in this book is an efficient, effective, and permanent method of allergy desensitization. People can determine which foods they are allergic to through

an elimination diet, skin or blood testing, and muscle response testing (refer to the section on muscle testing in
Chapter 2).

Children and adults with food allergies experience a
wide variety of symptoms including abdominal pain,
headaches, runny noses, asthma, chronic coughing, attention problems, and behavioral problems. Many feel these
allergies disappear as a child matures to adulthood, but in
reality they do not. Often, some of the acute symptoms
lessen over time, but the allergy becomes chronic or hidden, and has the potential of causing developmental or
functional problems and persistent maladies.

Twenty-five percent of adults believe they have food
allergies but conventional medicine claims that only one
or two percent are actual allergy sufferers. Those who do
not have allergies, according to the limited definition of
mainstream medicine, have what is usually called a food
intolerance, which can be equally uncomfortable. The
difference is that a genuine food allergy is caused by antibodies that can be identified by blood testing, whereas
food intolerance is a broader term encompassing many
illnesses caused by food. Food intolerance does not register on conventional allergy tests although it can be
measured using muscle response testing.

Some causes of food intolerance are chemicals such
as caffeine and food colorings (tartrazine) that do not
produce adverse effects in the majority of the population,
but do trigger allergic symptoms in some people. A deficiency of enzymes (the chemicals that help digestion)
can cause problems as well. If a person lacks one or
more enzymes, he or she can experience digestive problems such as diarrhea and stomach pain after consuming
the food the missing enzyme digests. For example, people who have difficulty drinking milk have frequently lost
the enzyme that digests lactose, the sugar in milk. In my
clinical practice, I have found that people who are "lactose intolerant" are essentially allergic to lactose. When

we treat patients for lactose intolerance, they are fully able to tolerate milk with no side effects. In fact, a complete clinical study on milk allergy showed that the NAET method is ninety-nine percent effective.

Finally, studies indicate that taking antibiotics can increase the chances of food intolerance in some people. The antibiotics apparently kill some types of bacteria in the large intestine and allow others to flourish, causing an abnormal reaction during digestion that produces various unpleasant chemical by-products and associated symptoms. Antibiotics can also cause an abnormal amount of yeast, or Candida, in the intestines that leads to an imbalance of other healthy intestinal flora or microorganisms. I have had successful results in treating Candida and other abnormal **pathogens** with NAET.

Drug Allergy

A severe, even life-threatening reaction to certain drugs and chemical additives, particularly penicillin, occurs in a small percentage of people. Other problematic drugs include aspirin, vaccines, insulin, and illegal drugs. Most often, the allergic reaction appears as a skin condition such as itching, hives, rashes, swelling, or peeling skin. Other symptoms can include incontinence, headache, dizziness, high blood pressure, moodiness, depression, agitation, edema, insomnia, hyperactivity, heart palpitations, bloating, constipation, diarrhea, blurred vision, hot flashes and, of course, drug dependence and addiction. For example, 5,000 men and women who participated in Operation Desert Storm experienced severe side effects, probably allergic reactions, to a drug they were instructed to take every day called pyristigimide bromide. This medication was supposed to protect them from harmful exposure to nerve gas. These men and women developed numerous health problems from tearing eyes and runny noses to chronic fatigue, twitches, cramps, blurred vision, incontinence, diarrhea, and other serious maladies. Even now, five years later, they continue to experience these symptoms and show signs of suppressed immune systems and long-term muscle damage. This drug was developed in 1955 for myasthenia gravis and was approved only for investigative use.

Insect Allergy

In general, the normal toxic reaction and discomfort that follow an insect sting is not considered an allergy. However, many people have severe allergic reactions to bee and wasp stings that can sometimes be fatal. These IgE-mediated reactions induce rashes, runny noses and eyes, swelling of the throat, asthma attacks, and anaphylactic shock.

Occupational Allergy

This term refers to allergies that develop in people as a result of working with industrial dusts, vapors, gases, fumes, nickel, chromium, rubber, dyes, formaldehyde, glues, in heat, and the like. Symptoms can manifest themselves within weeks, or take years of repeated exposure before they appear. The least protected parts of the body (hands, arms, face) are affected most frequently. Protective masks, gloves, and clothing can help prevent a reaction and even save a life. For example, bakers who handle different foods can prevent reactions by wearing gloves and masks if necessary.

Latex Allergy

Often categorized as an occupational allergy because it is frequently found among health-care workers, latex allergy is surfacing in increasing numbers among the general population as well. The offending material can be found in balloons, gloves used for washing dishes or handling food, dental and medical gloves, condoms, clothing and shoes, carpets, rain slickers, pacifiers, baby-bottle nipples, and air pollution. Symptoms include swelling, welts, itchiness and hives after contact, sneezing and nasal congestion, watery and itchy eyes, chronic fatigue, and occasionally anaphylactic shock. Generally, the people with the highest risk of developing latex allergy are those with high levels of exposure to latex, a history of allergies, multiple surgeries as children, or food allergies. Studies have shown also that people with allergies to certain fruits and vegetables—particularly bananas, kiwis, raw potatoes, tomatoes, celery, carrots, stone fruits, figs, avocados, papayas, passion fruit, hazelnuts and water chestnuts—are more likely to develop latex allergy.

Skin Conditions

The most common skin condition, eczema, is a rash or irritation that can be either wet or dry, occasionally chapped, and most often accompanied by severe itching. Although the cause isn't always clear, the condition often appears in children of families with a history of allergic disease. Milk and woolen clothes are possible contributors to the condition. Eczema usually begins in the first year of life as a facial rash and is often a precursor of asthma. Later in life it can appear on the insides of the elbows, the backs of the knees, the neck, ankles, wrists, and the backs of the hands.

Contact eczema has similar symptoms to common eczema, but can be traced to direct contact with a variety of substances including nickel found in coins, stainless steel, chromium found in cement and leather, rubber found in gloves and boots, and preservatives found in creams, ointments, and cosmetics.

Hives, or urticaria, is evidenced by a warming of the skin with redness and itching, or white raised wheals. It can appear very suddenly and may last for hours or a whole day.

NAET is quite effective in treating eczema and other skin conditions in all age groups. I usually find that eczema in children is caused by an allergy to wheat, corn and B vitamins. In adults, the allergens can range from foods, clothing, animals, chemicals, and creams to fungus, yeast, and bacteria. Acne also responds, sometimes dramatically, to treatment of those basic allergies and then the bacteria in the system.

Conjunctivitis

The main symptoms of conjunctivitis include redness of the eyes and itchiness. It most often affects adults. Treating environmental allergies early with NAET can help prevent this condition.

Anaphylaxis

The most severe and life-threatening allergic reaction, anaphylactic shock, is usually a sudden response of the immune system to foods, insect stings, or medication. Symptoms can include any combination of the following: swelling, difficulty breathing, hives, vomiting, diarrhea, cramps, and a drop in blood pressure. An anaphylactic reaction can occur in as little as five to 15 minutes and medical attention is needed immediately. When waiting for medical assistance, stimulation of the respiratory acupuncture points can provide some relief of the symptoms and improve breathing (refer to the emergency treatment procedures in Chapter 9).

Hay Fever (Allergic Rhinitis)

Hay fever is a condition that afflicts millions of Americans. Symptoms range from runny or stuffy nose, sneezing, swelling of mucous membranes, and itchiness of the throat, palate, and eyes to loss of smell and taste. Primary causes are airborne inhalants such as grass, weeds, tree pollens, and mold spores. Hay fever can be seasonal or intermittent. NAET has been extremely successful in handling these type of allergies. In our clinic I have seen symptoms reverse immediately after NAET treatment for ragweed or other pollens, and these results have been replicated by other practitioners.

Asthma

During an asthma attack, an individual's bronchial tubes swell periodically and the muscles surrounding the tubules go into spasm. This obstructs the flow of air to the lungs, leading to wheezing, coughing, and difficult, labored breathing. Asthma may begin at any age and has the potential to recur and become chronic. It is an allergic disease that is always triggered by allergens. These allergens include not only foods, pollens, and environmental factors such as perfume, animal dander, and chemicals but also bacteria, climactic conditions, and emotions. When these allergies are active from birth, asthma can be diagnosed early in life, even in infancy. When the allergies are hidden and chronic, they can cause other chronic functional and developmental problems such as fatigue, coughing, or headaches. Tissues break down slowly with chronic allergies, with minimal secretion of immune mediators that cause minor muscle contraction, swelling, and increased mucus secretion. When other stressful factors are added to the system—menopause, emotional stress, medication, or gastritis—the allergic load is increased and late-onset asthma can occur.

ORIGINS AND CAUSES OF ALLERGIES

An allergic reaction can be IgE mediated or non-IgE mediated. An IgE-mediated allergy is the traditional type recognized by most medical doctors in which immunoglobulin E antibodies are produced in response to environmental allergens and foods. Typical symptoms are hay fever and some forms of eczema. A non-IgE-mediated allergy, not always recognized as an allergy by conventional physicians, is a negative change in the immune system that can cause a variety of symptoms. Allergens that are non-IgE mediated may affect the sympathetic and parasympathetic nervous systems. Take, for example, an asthma case. Irritation of the lungs from allergies to dust, smoke, perfume, or bacteria may stimulate the parasympathetic nervous system to secrete acetylcholine. Acetylcholine constricts bronchial muscles and increases mucus production, thereby triggering an asthma attack.

Allergens such as bacteria, viruses, or certain foods seem to create antigen-antibody complexes by combining with T and **B cells**, the adaptive defenses of the body produced in bone marrow. These antigen-antibody complexes lodge themselves in certain tissues of the body (for example, in the lungs or bronchioles of asthmatics). When trying to destroy these complexes, the immune system brings about an **autoimmune reaction** that inflames and destroys healthy tissue. This inflammation triggers the asthma attack and creates a chronic condition until the allergens and complexes are removed.

The most common cause of allergies is genetic. The probability of a child developing an allergy is increased if one or both parents suffer from any type of allergic condition, and is the strongest factor for predicting future allergies. If one parent suffers from allergies, the child will develop allergies seventy-five percent of the time. If both parents have allergies, the child will develop allergies one hundred percent of the time.

The second most common cause of allergies is poor digestion. If a food is not properly digested, it will eventually trigger an allergic reaction.

Chemotherapeutic drugs, excessive antibiotics, steroids, or exposure to toxic chemicals or radiation are also important factors in the development of allergies or depressed immune reaction. For example, when antibiotics and steroids are used concurrently over a long period of time, as is often the case with asthmatics, the antibiotics destroy the good microflora of the intestines, and strengthen and increase the longevity of bad microflora or yeast. This leads to **candidiasis**. A suppressed immune system is unable to destroy these yeast cells that can eventually scar the intestinal villi. This allows toxins, undigested food, and yeast to enter the bloodstream through the intestine and leads to a systemic yeast problem, which, in turn, stimulates the creation of **circulating immune complexes (CICs)** and autoimmune reactions.

When an expectant mother is exposed to various toxins such as chemicals or radiation, or suffers an illness such as a flu or an infection, allergies will often occur in the child. Altered cells do not carry over the genetic codes and do not undergo normal development. As a result, organs and tissues may develop nonfunctional sensory nerve receptors that are unable to conduct messages to and from the spinal cord and brain. In some people these nerve receptors become hyposensitive toward certain items; in other people they become hypersensitive. When hyposensitive fibers predominate, few allergic reactions are seen but poor growth, chronic fatigue, and poor functioning of body and mind are evident also. Active, acute allergies result from hypersensitivity, whereas hidden or chronic allergies result from hyposensitivity.

Finally, chronic or severe malnutrition can also cause allergies. If the body is deficient in protein, vitamins, and minerals, enzymatic and metabolic processes cannot occur. This results in undigested food and an increase in the production of toxic metabolites that can eventually lead to allergies. These vitamins and minerals are also needed for effective immune function to protect the body when fighting off infections.

ALLERGIC LOAD PHENOMENON

In my estimation, over ninety percent of the population has allergies or intolerances, most of which are genetic in origin. However, in the majority of people, these allergies are hidden or inactive. It is the allergic load phenomenon that activates these allergies in certain people. If, over a period of time, one confronts other, more active, or acute allergens, and one is physically, mentally, or emotionally stressed—lacks sufficient sleep or eats poorly—these chronic hidden allergies become pronounced and the body falls prey to other problems. Resistance breaks down, the immune system cannot keep these allergies in check, and chronic emotional, functional, or developmental problems arise. Then, for the first time, one can experience asthma, arthritis, swelling, chronic pain, headaches, or chronic fatigue.

For example, last week a woman came into my office complaining of asthma and chronic sinusitis. She had experienced a stuffy nose from time to time but she had never been diagnosed with asthma. About two years ago, when the asthma began, she had a bad case of the flu that put her out of work for a month. Around the same time, her mother died of cancer and she was beginning to develop premenopausal symptoms. After a complete examination I began some allergy testing. I found she was very allergic to hormones, flu viruses, certain environmental and chemical substances, sugar, dairy products, grains, and many other foods. She was particularly intolerant of sugars and carbohydrates and was unable to absorb these foods.

It soon became apparent that she was experiencing the allergic load phenomenon. She was living on pasta and breads, and had never fully recovered from the flu virus to which she was also allergic. The death of her mother added to her stress, and her premenopausal state caused hormonal fluctuations. With her immune system compromised, certain hidden allergies manifested themselves, her system became overly sensitive, and she developed asthma. It didn't happen overnight, however; in fact, most of the allergies were there from the beginning.

ILLNESSES AND CHRONIC DISEASES RELATED TO ALLERGIES

We don't usually imagine that allergic reactions can play a role in seemingly unrelated medical conditions. Many experts, however, are drawing connections between a history of allergies and numerous other chronic conditions from alcoholism to obesity. Allergies also are considered partially responsible for some types of behavioral or emotional problems. We have had excellent results in cases of obesity, as well as those of depression and exhaustion, of seeing the problem as rooted in allergies and using NAET to clear the allergies.

Alcoholism

The concept of alcoholism is that alcoholics might be allergic to the ingredients in alcoholic beverages. This causes deficiencies of those ingredients and leads to strong cravings for such beverages. The substances people are usually allergic to are B vitamins, sugar, grapes, brewer's yeast, malt, or corn and become addicted to an alcoholic beverage that contains any or all of the allergens.

I have treated alcoholics successfully with NAET. Eilleen, an alcoholic in her early thirties, was referred to me by her parents, both of whom had excellent results with the method (her father with hay fever and her mother with menopausal symptoms). Their daughter had been an alcoholic for ten years. During this time she suffered some near-fatal car accidents and financial disasters because of her drinking, and she had tried a number of treatment facilities and therapists with no success. People usually crave the foods to which they are allergic, and Eilleen hoped that I might be able to help her with her intense craving for alcohol which then would enable her to make better use of traditional treatments.

I performed a full examination that included a complete enzyme evaluation and allergy testing protocol. Like most alcoholics, she was especially allergic to all the B vitamins, all sugars, and alcohol. I prescribed an enzyme for sugar digestion and began to treat her for the basic allergies, including the B vitamins and sugars. Then I treated her for alcohol. Six hours after the treatment, she called to tell me she was drunk. I immediately felt disappointed. But then she added that she was drunk not because of the alcohol or sugar, but simply as a result of the process of clearing the allergy. The difference was that this time she was completely cognizant of everything that was happening which was never the case when she was actually drunk. I imagine that she was detoxifying the alcohol. She also noted how good she felt.

The next day, when I retested her, she was no longer allergic to alcohol. She then attended a three-week alcohol treatment program, and I didn't hear from her again until three years later when she called to tell me how grateful she was. She said she hadn't had a single drink since the allergy clearing which was a breakthrough for her.

Obesity

Similar to alcoholics, people who struggle with excessive weight may be allergic to their favorite foods and unable to resist indulging their intense cravings. Additionally, some people have noticed that hunger can be a symptom of an allergic reaction. For example, when sufferers of a wheat allergy eat a wheat-heavy meal, they may feel strong cravings to eat again within a short period of time, even though they no longer need the nutrition.

Arthritis

Arthritis has been attributed partially to an allergic reaction in the joints to common foods. When some arthritic patients avoid certain foods or environmental allergens, their symptoms diminish. Acid foods seem to be especially troublesome, as are the nightshades which include tomatoes, white potatoes, eggplant, peppers, and tobacco (refer to Part 6). I have also found arthritic patients to be allergic to bacteria and parasites that can trigger the autoimmune reaction.

I have had many successes with arthritis sufferers. A woman with severe arthritis in her sacroiliac and hips came to me seeking help with her extreme chronic pain and migraine headaches. Unfortunately she was a housekeeper and cook. This caused her to be on her feet most of the day and to be very active. When I performed a full examination and allergy testing I found her to be highly allergic to all the basic allergens, acid-forming foods, the nightshade family, and fifteen different bacteria. She was unable to digest proteins and fats, yet she was eating large amounts of protein because she was trying to lose weight. The uric acid content in her urine sediment was quite high, generally an indicator of high protein consumption. I recommended an **enzyme** to help her digest fats and proteins, and I prescribed a diet lower in protein and fats and higher in complex carbohydrates. I treated her with NAET for all the basic allergies, acid foods, and all the bacteria. After all the bacteria were cleared, her hip and sacroiliac pain almost completely subsided and her flexibility improved by seventy-five percent. In addition to being able to take care of her household responsibilities, she now walks three miles a day and has lost thirty pounds. She also smiles a lot when I see her.

Migraines and Headaches

Allergies are a common culprit in recurring headaches. Research has found again and again that some migraine sufferers can eliminate their symptoms by avoiding certain triggering foods, particularly milk, eggs, wheat, aged cheese, MSG, chocolate, oranges, tea, coffee, beef, corn, cane sugar, yeast, and alcoholic beverages.

A sensitivity to extreme weather, smoke, exercise, pollen, chemical fumes, and stress can also cause chronic headaches. The woman with arthritis experienced headaches daily and migraines weekly. No remedy worked for her headaches. While treating for the arthritis, I also treated her with NAET for female hormones, estrogen, progesterone, thyroid hormones T_3 and T_4, and adrenaline. I had to treat her for progesterone three times before it completely cleared. I even had her treat herself at home for this allergen because it was so severe. After completing the hormone clearing, her headaches disappeared and never returned.

Psychological and Behavioral Conditions

Perhaps some of the least recognized but most interesting effects of allergies are psychological conditions. Evidence is mounting that in some people certain allergens can actually result in, or aggravate, emotional and behavioral problems including depression, hyperactivity, learning difficulties, anxiety, irritability, and schizophrenia. NAET practitioners have had excellent results with attention deficit disorder (ADD), hyperactivity, and other behavioral problems in children and adults. Children with attention deficit disorder are treated for the following:

- the basic allergies

- possibly mercury and fluoride

- thyroid and thyroid hormones

- yeast or Candida

- foods such as wheat, dairy, sugar, artificial sweeteners, food additives, food coloring, and chocolate

- environmental allergies such as radiation, dust, chemicals, mold, and pollution

- emotional traumas

I also supplement these children with enzymes and minerals and make strong dietary recommendations based on an individual evaluation. Treating children with NAET is fulfilling and rewarding because the changes in their physical and emotional health are immediate and profound.

2 | ALLERGY TESTING

In addition to self-assessment questionnaires that help determine whether or not a person has the symptoms commonly associated with allergies, there are a number of frequently used allergy tests administered by qualified health professionals. These include skin reaction tests, blood tests, pulse test, muscle response test, and electronic test.

SELF-ASSESSMENT QUESTIONNAIRES

The following self-assessment questionnaire helps determine the presence of symptoms that commonly raise suspicion of allergies. A significant number of "yes" answers to the following questions would indicate further testing and/or consultation with a doctor.

1. Do any blood relatives suffer from allergy syndromes (hay fever, asthma, skin rashes, severe reactions to drugs or insect stings), food allergies, addictive disorders (alcohol or drug abuse, compulsive eating), diabetes or low blood sugar,

arthritis, headaches, or digestive disorders? Were any blood relatives hyperactive, learning-disabled, or bed wetters as children?

2. Did your mother experience severe stress during her pregnancy with you? Was your birth difficult or complicated?

3. As an infant, did you have any problem tolerating bottle formula or breast milk? Did you have problems with weight gain, colic, or vomiting?

4. As an infant, did you suffer from frequent digestive, respiratory, or skin problems?

5. Were you "difficult" in infancy and/or childhood, often crying or irritable, overactive or underactive? Did you have problems sleeping, trouble learning, or paying attention at school?

6. As a child, were you often sick, plagued by ear infections, sore throats, swollen glands, colds, bronchitis, croup, stomach aches, constipation, diarrhea, or headaches?

7. As an adult, are you always tired even though you get enough sleep (six to eight hours)?

8. Do you frequently have puffy eyes? Wrinkles or dark circles under your eyes? Itchy, red, watery, burning, painful or light-sensitive eyes? Blurred vision? Baggy, swollen eyelids?

9. Do you often have a stuffy, watery, runny nose? Sneeze several times in a row? Rub nose upwards or wiggle nose? One cold after another, without feeling sick? Nosebleeds? Excessive mucus?

10. Do you have asthma or wheezing? Do you cough or wheeze with laughter, exercise, cold air, cold drinks, at night, or when it's damp outside?

11. Do you have skin rashes such as eczema or atopic dermatitis? Itchy rashes or hives, especially in arm or leg creases? Cracked toenails or fingernails? Acne? Dandruff? Loss of hair?

12. Do you have recurrent earaches? Fluid behind your eardrums? On and off hearing trouble? Ears popping or ringing? Flushed, red earlobes? Dizziness? Itchy ears? Drainage from ear?

13. Do you suffer from digestive problems? Swelling or soreness of face and lips? Itchy roof of mouth? Canker sores? Bleeding gums? Bad breath? Nausea and stomach aches? Excess gas, diarrhea, or constipation? Belching? Itchy rectal area? Ulcers? Colitis?

14. Do you have difficulty gaining or losing weight? Binge eating?

15. Do you have repeated bladder infections, difficulty urinating, or water retention?

16. Is your pulse or heartbeat irregular after eating?

17. Have you ever had seizures?

18. Do you have sinus problems, earaches, or sore throats? Headaches, dizziness, convulsion? Insomnia? Leg or muscle aches, back pain, swollen or stiff joints, arthritis? A constant low-grade fever, feeling flushed or chilled, excessive sweating, fainting spells?

19. Do you have dark circles under your eyes, a pale complexion, a bloated or puffy face?

20. Are you a picky eater? A binger?

21. Do you feel like you are high one moment, low the next, with depression appearing for no reason?

22. Do you have trouble concentrating, sometimes feeling confused and spacy? Are you hyperactive,

overly nervous, frequently anxious, quick to anger?

23. Does a change in your surroundings or the seasons change how you feel?

The following questionnaire helps us determine if an asthma sufferer is in control of his or her disease.

The questions, to be answered with a yes or no, are:

1. Have you visited your doctor one or more times in the past six months because of your asthma?

2. Have you visited a hospital emergency room one or more times in the past year for asthma treatment?

3. Have you missed one or more days of school or work in the past year because of your asthma?

4. Have you been awakened one or more times in the past month by coughing or wheezing?

5. Has your asthma prevented you from participating in particular exercises or sports?

6. Do you use more than one canister of your bronchoinhaler each month?

7. Do you use your bronchodilator more than three or four times each day?

8. Do you sometimes forget to take your prescribed asthma medication?

9. Do you sometimes choose not to take your prescribed asthma medication?

10. Would you like more information on how to use your inhaler properly?

The following questionnaire was developed by the American College of Allergy, Asthma, and Immunology for further assessment of asthma sufferers:

Activities

1. When I walk or do simple chores, I have trouble breathing or I cough.

   Yes   No

2. When I perform heavier work, such as walking up hills and stairs or doing chores that involve lifting, I have trouble breathing or I cough.

   Yes   No

3. Sometimes I avoid exercising or taking part in sports like jogging, swimming, tennis, or aerobics because I have trouble breathing or I cough.

   Yes   No

4. I have been unable to sleep through the night without coughing attacks or shortness of breath.

   Yes   No

Symptoms

5. Sometimes I can't catch a good, deep breath.

   Yes   No

6. Sometimes I make wheezing sounds in my chest.

   Yes   No

7. Sometimes my chest feels tight.

   Yes   No

8. Sometimes I cough a lot. *always*

   Yes   No

Triggers

9. Dust, pollen, and pets make my asthma, cough, or trouble breathing worse.

Yes   No

10. My asthma gets worse in cold weather.

Yes   No

11. My asthma gets worse when I'm around tobacco smoke, fumes, or strong odors.

Yes   No

12. When I catch a cold it often goes to my chest.

Yes   No

Hospital Visits

13. I made one or more emergency room visits because of asthma or breathing problems in the last year.

Yes   No

14. I had one or more overnight hospitalizations because of asthma or breathing problems in the last year.

Yes   No

Medication Problems

15. I feel like I use my asthma inhaler too often.

Yes   No

16. Sometimes I don't like the way my asthma medicine(s) make me feel.

Yes   No

17. My asthma medicine doesn't control my asthma.

Yes   No

Anxieties

18. My breathing problem or asthma controls my life more than I would like.

Yes   No

19. I feel tension or stress because of my breathing problem or asthma.

Yes   No

20. I worry that my breathing problem or asthma affects my health or may even shorten my life.

Yes   No

SCRATCH TEST OR SKIN REACTION TEST

Some tests for allergies involve provoking an allergic reaction on the skin by exposure to a minute amount of an allergen. Most commonly, this is accomplished by applying drops of an allergenic extract to the skin surface that has been pricked or scratched. Other possibilities include:

- introducing a small quantity of allergenic extract with a needle between the layers of skin (intradermal test)
- placing a piece of gauze soaked in a suspected allergen over the skin for a prolonged period of time (patch test)
- putting a drop of allergenic extract in the eye (conjunctival test, rarely used today)

If the test is positive, the site of the injection or exposure swells and the surrounding area becomes inflamed. This is generally not useful to determine food intolerance but is a simple method of detecting sensitivity to inhalant allergens. A reaction can occur after 15 minutes and up to 24 to 48 hours later.

RADIOALLERGOSORBENT TEST (RAST)

The radioallergosorbent test (RAST) is an initial laboratory test administered to a patient's blood sample to measure the amount of IgE antibodies in blood. The number of antibodies increase with the severity of the allergy. The blood sample is tested for specific IgE antibodies against likely allergens in the patient's environment.

PULSE TEST

Pulse testing for allergies measures the heart rate before and after exposure to a suspected allergen and is an effective method for determining allergic reactions to foods. Pulses can be felt at various points. The radial artery at the wrist is the most common and probably the simplest to locate. Three fingers are placed lightly over the artery on the inside of the wrist, slightly above the thumb. Other areas to read the pulse are located at the temporal region of the skull, the popliteal region in back of the knee, the pedal pulses behind the malleolus of the ankle, the carotid artery in the neck, and the femoral pulse in the groin area. A normal pulse should be even and forceful, at a regular rhythm, with no delays, interruptions, or other irregularities.

The pulse generally deviates from normal in allergic patients. It usually becomes faster and more forceful, but can also become slower and weaker. This test can be helpful in detecting a food allergy. Unfortunately, if one eats several foods at a time, which, of course, we all do, it is hard to determine exactly which food is causing the allergic reaction. Many of my patients come into my office already knowing they have food allergies because they used this method of diagnosing themselves.

MUSCLE RESPONSE TEST

Also known as applied **kinesiology**, this test was developed in 1964 by Dr. George Goodheart, a chiropractor, to diagnose or read certain blockages in the body. Muscle response testing is also a method of using the relative strength of the muscles to uncover allergies, nutritional imbalances, and structural misalignments in the body.

This method identifies blockages in the electromagnetic energy fields when one is exposed to, or in contact with, an allergen. Muscle testing bypasses the conscious and subconscious minds. When a suspected allergen is held in the hand, a strong muscle will weaken if an allergy to the substance is present.

The person to be tested generally lies down or sits up and extends an arm at a ninety-degree angle, thumb down, in front of him. The facilitator pushes against the arm to establish the strength of the testing muscle (indicator muscle) while the subject resists. When the person holds a food or other substance to which he or she is allergic, the indicator muscle will immediately and markedly weaken. People can learn to perform this technique on others, and can teach others to test them. Muscle testing procedures can detect both hidden and active or acute allergies and can indicate which substances should be avoided.

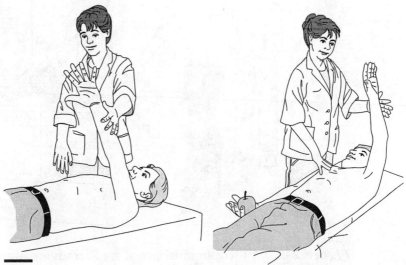

Figure 2–1   Muscle testing for identifying allergies.

SURROGATE MUSCLE TEST

This technique is used to determine allergies in infants, young children, and elderly, weak, or physically incapacitated adults. It utilizes energy conductivity to diagnose allergies in a person who otherwise could not be muscle tested. The surrogate touches the skin of the person being tested and the facilitator muscle tests the surrogate. When the one being tested holds a particular item, the surrogate's response indicates whether that person does or does not have an allergy to the item.

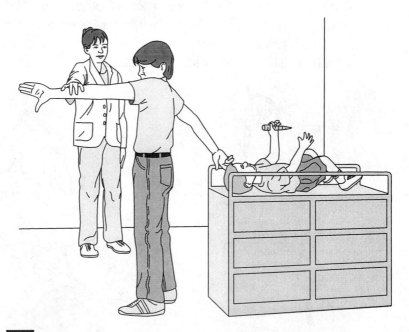

Figure 2–2   Surrogate muscle test for identifying allergies in infants, toddlers, or weak individuals.

O-RING TEST

People can be taught to test themselves using a method similar to muscle testing. The tester makes a circle by opposing his little finger and thumb on one hand. Then, with the other index finger, he or she tries to separate the two opposing fingers. They should be strong and inseparable. If they are not strong, there can be structural misalignment or carpal tunnel syndrome that renders the technique ineffective. If they are strong, the potential allergen is held in the hand being tested, with the fingertips touching the allergen. If the circle is strong, the person is not allergic to the substance. If the fingers weaken and the circle separates, they are allergic to the substance. This technique takes practice to learn, but it can be a survival tool for severely allergic individuals who can use it to test their foods before eating.

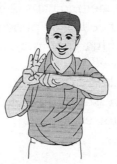

Figure 2–3 O-Ring test for self-testing allergies.

ELECTRONIC TEST

Electronic devices have been used for more than a century in the treatment and diagnosis of patients. Two German scientists, Voll and Werner, designed and built an instrument to chart and verify the relationship of acupuncture points to their corresponding organs and systems. This instrument can directly infer the functional status of these structures. Specific acupuncture points are charged with approximately one volt of direct current, resulting in measurements of resistance along particular meridians. A meter is used to show readings of irritation to the electromagnetic pathways or organ systems (for example, blockages in the flow of electromagnetic energy). Electronic devices work by reading the galvanic skin response, a measure of this flow. Because this process is still considered investigational, these meters have been approved for investigational use only by the Food and Drug Administration (FDA) in the United States.

Electronic devices such as the one developed by Voll and Werner are used for food and environmental allergy testing. Correlations with other test procedures have shown that the electro-acupuncture device (EAV) test is accurate in detecting sensitivities to foods, chemicals, pesticides, herbicides, environmental irritants, dental irritants, fungi, bacteria, and viruses as well as dysfunctions of organs and systems. The method causes little or no discomfort because there are no needles or puncturing of the skin. A low-level electric stimulus (not perceptible by the subject being tested) is passed through the body while the patient holds a brass handle in one hand and a metal probe is placed against acupressure points on the hands and feet. A reading is taken for each point and stored in the computer for future analysis.

3 TYPES OF ALLERGY TREATMENTS

The simplest and most effective approach to treating allergies is to avoid the allergenic substance entirely. When avoidance is difficult or even impossible, as with environmental allergens, a number of other treatments are available.

MEDICATION

Medication is probably the most commonly used treatment for allergies. There are **antihistamines** to relieve itching, hay fever, and irritation from airborne allergens; **bronchodilators** or inhalers for asthma symptoms; decongestants; steroids; **corticosteroids**; and cromolyn, taken orally before eating to prevent gastrointestinal (GI) symptoms. Used primarily to suppress symptoms, these medications can have many side effects including drowsiness, anxiety, frequent and painful urination, nausea, dry mouth, vomiting, loss of appetite, abdominal discomfort and cramps, constipation or diarrhea, headaches, loss of sexual libido, depression, and fatigue.

There are two main types of asthma medications designed to reverse the irritation and constriction of air pas-

sages in the lungs and bronchial tubes. Relievers or bronchodilators are designed to relax the muscles in the bronchial tubes and *provide* rapid relief of asthma symptoms.
Preventers are designed to reduce **inflammation** in the
airways and *prevent* asthma symptoms. The relievers include beta-2 medications, anticholinergics, and theo-
phyllines. The preventers are either steroids or nonsteroids.

The most widely used medications in the treatment
of asthma are the beta-2s which include salbutamol, or-
ciprenaline, fenoterol, terbutaline sulfate, and procaterol.
Although they are usually taken through an inhalant device known as a puffer, they can also be administered as
tablets or in syrups. The beta-2s provide immediate relief
that lasts up to four hours. The oral preparations provide
longer-lasting relief but can cause side effects, in particular, a fine tremor of the hands or slight heart palpitations.
Beta-2 medications are extremely effective in treating
acute asthma episodes.

Preventer medications work to reduce inflammation,
congestion, and "twitching" in the bronchial tubes. Steroids, the most powerful preventers available today, can
cause yeast infections that lead to soreness and white
spots in the mouth and throat. When taken for long periods of time, they suppress the body's natural production
of steroids, reduce growth rate, cause weight gain, diabetes, or cataracts, and weaken bones. Short courses of
steroid tablets (prednisone), however, are extremely effective in treating acute asthma episodes. There are three
nonsteroid preventers, each of which acts in a slightly different way. These medicines are safer but supposedly less
powerful than the inhaled steroids. They are more frequently used for children.

These asthma drugs have allowed many people, children as well as adults, to live relatively normal lives, and
they have saved thousands, if not millions of lives. But
they do not go to the root of the asthma and enable these
individuals to free themselves of their dependence on me-

dication. In contrast, NAET does go to the root of asthma by diagnosing and treating the allergies that cause it. By desensitizing the asthma sufferer to each of these allergies, NAET can reduce or completely eliminate the need for medication. In the chapter on asthma, I explain the many allergies that can trigger this condition and in Chapter 9, I describe an effective technique for clearing them.

ALLERGY SHOTS

Allergy shots, or immunotherapy, are another commonly used treatment approach. Allergy shots desensitize the person to the allergen by injecting a small amount of an extract of the substance under the skin's surface. The dose is gradually increased until a maintenance dose is obtained. After three years or the allergy has been eliminated, the injections are generally stopped.

Allergy shots are often effective in treating allergies to pollen, dust, and animal dander, but they have not proven useful for allergies to food. Additionally, food shots may cause side effects including sore arms, hives, throat spasms and, on occasion, even death. By controlling reactions to airborne allergens, however, shots can reduce the load effect and thereby reduce the allergic response to foods.

For many years, doctors have tried using allergy shots, primarily for pollens, to treat people who suffer asthma attacks. Studies have shown that while these people were receiving the shots they suffered fewer asthmatic symptoms, but the effects diminished over time and disappeared entirely after two years. In addition, the shots were extremely expensive.

ROTATION AND ELIMINATION DIETS

Elimination and **rotation diets**—also called exclusion or simplification diets—are widely used by physicians and individuals to diagnose and eliminate allergic reactions. These regimens remove all potential allergens from the diet and then reintroduce them one at a time at different intervals while observing their effects. Although they can be helpful in detecting hidden allergies, rotation diets are difficult to sustain and generally fail.

HOMEOPATHY

Homeopathic treatment appears to have a positive effect in treating allergic asthma and other disorders related to allergies. In one study of asthma sufferers, twenty-eight percent were randomly allocated to either a homeopathic remedy or a placebo in addition to their regular care. The rest received only their regular care. Patients kept diaries of their symptoms and doctors made an evaluation of respiratory function and bronchial reactivity after four weeks. Patients taking the homeopathic remedy experienced a reduction in the intensity of their symptoms after one week, an improvement that persisted for eight weeks. Eighty-two percent of the patients in the homeopathic group improved, compared with thirty-eight percent in the placebo group. The greatest response occurred among patients with the severest symptoms. Data from this trial were pooled with two others of similar design and a group analysis was performed. All trials showed similar benefits from homeopathic treatment.

ENZYME POTENTIATED DESENSITIZATION (EPD)

Enzyme potentiated desensitization (EPD) is a method of immunotherapy developed by Dr. Leonard McEwen of London in the mid 1960s. It involves desensitization using a series of injections containing a combination of mixed allergens and the enzyme beta-glucoronidase administered every two to three months at first and then less frequently over time. Because many allergens are treated at once, only nine or ten injections are required and the results are reportedly longer lasting than are conventional allergy shots. Beta-glucuronidase in combination with other allergens causes T-suppressor cells to multiply and differentiate and allows them to recognize the allergen originally injected. These T-cells then supposedly suppress any adverse reaction when the individual is then exposed to the allergens. I am not aware of how successful this approach has been in the treatment of asthma.

BEE POLLEN

An antiallergic product that has gained some popularity in recent years is bee pollen. The pollen is actually a mixture of bee digestive enzymes, nectar, and reproductive dust from the flowers visited by the bees. Because bee pollen contains some of the airborne grass and ragweed pollens to which people are most allergic, it can act the same as allergy shots to desensitize an individual with a small quantity of the substance to which he or she is allergic. But allergy shots deliver pollen in an undiluted form, whereas oral dosages are broken down by enzymes during the digestive process. The patient might have to take up to 10,000 times as much pollen orally as he or she would through injection to achieve the same results. The other disadvantage of taking bee pollen is that one never knows exactly what it contains because it varies from week to week and from beehive to beehive. Also, bee pollen in large dosages can cause unpleasant side effects or be contaminated with environmental pollutants.

CHIROPRACTIC CARE

Chiropractic care has been known to help strengthen the immune system by strengthening the nervous system. A healthy immune system means resistance to disease, allergies, and chronic illness, and one that is free of spinal musculoskeletal misalignments. "Chiropractic is able to hypothesize that skeletal disrelations, particularly in the complex spinal structures, can lead to the loss of nervous system integrity and, hence, to the loss of health elsewhere in the body" (*Essential Principles of Chiropractic* by Virgil V. Strang). Many studies have observed the effect of a healthy nervous system on immune system health. In one study, for example, people under chiropractic care for five years or more were found to have a two hundred percent greater immune system competence than people who had not received chiropractic care.

In particular, chiropractic care has proven effective in asthmatics by restoring nerve supply to the lungs and bronchioles and helping to feed and restore the respiratory system.

ACUPUNCTURE

Extensive research has shown that acupuncture helps people with a variety of conditions including pain, anxiety, arthritis, eczema, migraines, and allergies by promoting natural healing and improving bodily functions. Developed and practiced in China over the past 2,000 years, acupuncture treats the whole person rather than a particular disease, attempts to address the root cause of the problem rather than symptoms alone, and works to restore balance between the physical, emotional, and spiritual aspects of being. Instead of treating standard points for specific allergies, the acupuncturist treats each allergic individual differently depending on the diagnostic picture that emerges after examining the pulses, the tongue, and other indicators.

Acupuncture has proven successful in reducing the sensitivity of allergic individuals. In *The Journal of Tradi-*

tional Chinese Medicine 1993 (Dec. 13, [4]: 243–8), acupuncture and desensitization were compared in the treatment of 143 cases of type I allergies. The results proved that acupuncture therapy provided remarkable success against type I allergic reactions. The curative effect was higher in the acupuncture group with allergic asthma, allergic rhinitis, and chronic urticaria.

NAMBUDRIPAD ALLERGY ELIMINATION TECHNIQUE (NAET)

NAET was developed by Dr. Devi Nambudripad, a registered nurse, chiropractor, and acupuncturist who has done extensive research in the areas of allergies. NAET is a revolutionary new technique that utilizes chiropractic, acupuncture, and kinesiology to permanently desensitize a person to an allergen. Much of this book on allergies and asthma, as well as the upcoming books in this series, will focus on NAET. This approach is based on a thorough understanding of the body as bioenergy, and a recognition that the body consists not only of matter but also of electromagnetic pathways and currents. This concept, along with a detailed description of NAET, is presented in Chapter 9.

When an allergen is encountered by an allergic individual, it can cause certain blockages in the electromagnetic pathways or U currents. These blockages are connected to certain organs, cells, or systems and cause what we call allergic symptoms. For example, certain allergenic foods can cause blockages in the digestive system through energy pathways, and these blockages in turn create digestive symptoms such as bloating, flatulence, and pain. NAET clears these blockages by reprogramming the nervous system and neutralizing the body's immune mediators, thereby permanently desensitizing a person to the allergen. Any allergen can be treated in this way.

EMERGENCY TREATMENT

In the event of anaphylactic shock or other allergic emergencies, it is crucial that the patient receive first aid treatment within the first 10 to 15 minutes. People who are prone to severe allergic reactions should carry an allergy kit with antihistamines and a syringe containing the drug epinephrine (a bronchodilator that opens the airways and restores blood pressure to normal) for immediate emergency self-treatment. Applying a tourniquet above an insect sting will slow the circulation and absorption of blood, and placing ice on the sting area reduces swelling. The patient should lie on his or her side with the head turned to one side to avoid choking if vomiting occurs. If the person stops breathing, mouth-to-mouth resuscitation should be performed by someone who knows how to do it. As soon as possible, the person should be taken to a hospital emergency room or doctor's office.

In an emergency, the NAET treatment can help save the life of a patient who is waiting for medical assistance. It can be self-administered. By using the acupressure points of NAET, the symptoms can be reduced or eliminated almost immediately. Stimulation of the acupressure points while the subject holds the suspected allergen starts to reverse the allergic reaction and allows the immune system to recover. For example, if you eat a cookie that causes abdominal pain or wheezing and coughing, hold the cookie in your hand and treat yourself by using the acupressure points, preferably every ten minutes until symptoms subside or medical assistance is available. Refer to the Self-Treatment section of Chapter 5 for complete instructions on how to perform the NAET self-treatment.

ASTHMA: WARNING SIGNS, SYMPTOMS, CAUSES, RESPIRATORY DISEASES, AND PREVENTIVE MEASURES

4 | DEFINING ASTHMA AND ASTHMA SUFFERERS

The Incidence of Asthma: Claire's Story

My story begins several years ago, on a perfect fall afternoon, when I went for a walk after work with my St. Bernard puppy, Kim. For the past year or so, I had limited my exercise to excursions with Kim because I had been diagnosed with adult-onset asthma. On this particular day, however, I was feeling great. I called my husband at work to let him know that I would walk north on the country road where we lived, and he should pick me up on his way home. This gave me time for a fifteen- to twenty-minute walk, mostly downhill. As a routine precaution, I used my inhaler before embarking on my small journey.

I was enjoying the brisk walk, kicking up the leaves in my path and breathing in the moist smell of their decomposition. Kim and I strode side by side, eating peanuts together. As we approached the bottom of the hill, the sun dropped, and I could feel the cold, damp microclimate created by a nearby stream. Feeling a little tightness in my chest, I started to cough intermittently. I cut Kim loose so she could run down to the stream to drink some water while I caught my breath. A few minutes later, when we resumed our walk, my coughing was worse, and my throat had begun closing up. I reached for my inhaler but could not find it. Could I have forgotten it on the kitchen table? Should I backtrack and hurry home? No! There was no way I could make it up the steep half-mile hill while wheezing and coughing. I tried to remain calm and take small breaths, knowing that my husband would be coming down the road in five minutes or so. I sat down by the side of the road to wait.

Five minutes passed with no cars in sight, each second seeming like an eternity. Where could he be? By now, I was wheezing and coughing my heart out, struggling to breathe, drenched from head to toe with sweat, and caught in the grips of a full-blown asthma attack. Every burst of wind from the open fields sent chills through my body, and my mind was growing foggy from the lack of oxygen. It was dark now, and the only light in view came from a farmhouse half a mile down the road. I was panicked, and so was Kim. Why was Sandy taking so long to get home?

I decided to walk toward the light to seek help. Part of me wanted to give up and go to sleep, but my mind was waging yet another battle with this deadly disease. I could see my life pass in front of me. Every twenty yards or so, I collapsed, but Kim nudged me and barked at me, coaxing me on. I was crying hysterically from despair and the pain in my chest. By the time I made it to the farm house, I was about to faint.

I knocked hard on the glass door, and an old man let me in. As hard as I tried, I could not talk but could only wheeze and cough. Motioning for a piece of paper and a pen, I wrote, "A glass of hot water, please. And please call my husband Sandy," followed by the phone number. While the man's wife hurried back with some hot water, I saw Sandy's Jeep heading up the road. The water helped to soothe my throat and allowed me to speak a few words: "Tell him to hurry with my inhaler." With each passing second, I felt like my life was slipping away from me.

When Sandy finally arrived with my inhaler, I took several hits but got little relief. I pleaded with him to take me home where I would feel safe. As soon as he had finished driving me home and carrying me into the house, he called my asthma specialist, who immediately prescribed prednisone, accompanied by two puffs on my inhaler every ten minutes for the first hour. He said that if I did not improve within fifteen minutes, we should go to the emergency room. My heart was racing from the large dose of Albuterol I had inhaled. Tears rolled down my face as I gasped for air and wondered if these battles were worth the fight. Each battle seemed to be more difficult than the last. Reluctantly I took yet another dose of prednisone, knowing that it would send me on another emotional roller coaster ride. The drugs were only buying me time, I realized, and the quality of my life was rapidly declining. I wanted to win the war, not the battles!

How had I ended up like this? I had always been a natural athlete, with good stamina and no prior history of asthma. Then one day, while I was mountain biking with my husband in Colorado where we lived at the time, he remarked that I was wheezing when I told him I was out of breath after climbing a hill. He had grown up with an asthmatic father, but I had no idea what he was talking about and brushed it off, assuming it must be the cold spring air. I continued to wheeze and cough intermittently over the next six months, but the doctors I consulted only prescribed cough medicine. Then, during a visit with my sister and brother, who have had asthma since childhood, they told me that my constant coughing was asthma. Why me? I thought. Why now?

Once I was diagnosed with asthma, I tried every conventional and alternative treatment available. Conventional medicine saved my life but also deeply depressed my immune system with months of antibiotics, prednisone, inhalers, and sinus surgery. Prednisone alone sent me into a deep depression, including months of suicidal thoughts, that put my relationship with my husband to the test. The man is a rock of Gibraltar and the primary reason for my not giving up the fight. Over a period of ten months, alternative medicine, including dietary restrictions, chelation and oxidative therapy, and acupuncture, helped me to rebuild my immune system, eliminate the need for prednisone, and control my asthma to some extent. Given my high vulnerability and the life of restrictions I needed to abide by, however, I still found myself questioning the meaning of life. I felt like a prisoner of my own body: I was unable to resume my active lifestyle, I could not engage in sports, I had to avoid any environment with smoke, chemicals, or perfumes, I could not eat my favorite foods and wines, and I had to keep my beloved dog outside.

Three years after I first discovered I had asthma, an acquaintance who saw Dr. Ellen Cutler in San Francisco referred me to her sister-in-law, Dr. Debra Cutler in New York, for treatment with NAET (Nambudripad allergy elimination technique). Five days before my appointment, I was having yet another acute asthma episode. After my first five NAET treatments, I felt like someone had let me out of jail. For the first time in three years, I could go to bed without my inhaler, I stopped having my nocturnal asthma attacks (which typically lasted an hour and a half), and I ceased the constant daily coughing.

While visiting the Bay Area on business, I saw Dr. Ellen Cutler on several occasions for further testing and NAET treatments. After fifteen treatments, I went skiing in Colorado for a week and never used my inhaler. I had more energy and stamina than my husband, who had exercised regularly for the past three years! Smoke no longer had a devastating effect on me, and I was able to enjoy some of my favorite foods and wines and play with my dog, Kim. NAET is a powerful treatment in the long-term elimination of allergies that lead to asthma. With the help of NAET I finally knew that I could win the war against asthma.

Now, when I look back at the walking incident, I can see how I stacked the cards against myself: from the peanuts, the dog saliva, and the moldy leaves (all of which I was highly allergic to but did not know) to the abrupt changes in climactic conditions and the fact that I left my inhaler behind. I was really lucky. The odds were that I would end up as one of the many thousands of people who die of asthma each year. In fact, the death rate from asthma has more than doubled in the past decade despite advances in medication and treatment. With NAET this trend can now be reversed.

WHAT IS ASTHMA?

Asthma is a respiratory condition that affects more than ten million Americans and is one of the leading causes of school and work absences. In severe cases, asthma can be life threatening. Deaths occur more frequently in adults, with more than eighty percent of the 4,000 asthma-related deaths in 1985 occurring in adults over the age of forty-five.

Asthma is a respiratory condition in which the bronchial tubes overreact; therefore, it is also called wheezy bronchitis or bronchial asthma. An asthmatic's bronchial tubes are hypersensitive and hyperactive. When they are temporarily narrowed or blocked by mucus, breathing becomes difficult. During an asthma attack the muscles around the airways tighten, the linings of the airways become inflamed and swollen, and the glands produce an overabundance of thick mucus, further narrowing the airway passages.

The asthmatic has difficulty breathing, especially exhaling carbon dioxide. This indicates that the body has less oxygen available and that carbon dioxide has built up to dangerous levels. Once an asthma attack is triggered by some substance or condition, the airways in the lungs become sensitive to other triggers that results in chronic asthma.

Most people have heard of asthma but few realize how serious or life threatening it can be. One patient I had successfully treated for asthma with enzyme therapy and NAET had a forty-seven-year-old friend who was also an asthmatic. She frequently suggested that her friend come to see me but because of circumstances she did not.

The friend went to Las Vegas, and while in a casino started to have an asthma attack, probably triggered by smoke, alcohol, or food sensitivities. Unable to locate her inhaler, she collapsed and died. Because the security guard and the people around her did not realize what was happening to her, they could not help.

Asthma is a life-threatening disease but it can be prevented and cured with enzyme therapy and NAET.

WARNING SIGNS OF ASTHMA

People have many different warning signs of an impending asthma attack and it is important for them to tune into their own red flags. Most sufferers have one or more of the classic symptoms. The first is a wheezing and low or loud whistle that is heard when they breathe. The whistle can be hardly noticeable or quite loud. The second is a mild cough or a hack that simply will not stop. The next classic symptom is chest tightness, similar to a tight grip around the chest. The last is shortness of breath. People with this symptom cannot take a deep breath. They feel as if they are trying to breathe through a straw, or worse, like they are drowning. Breathing out is especially difficult.

Pulmonary function studies, such as those done with a spirometer, are breathing tests that accurately measure lung capacity. The person breathes into a closed tube connected to a machine that shows how much air a person can blow out and how much the lungs can hold. Asthmatics have difficulty exhaling because of obstructed bronchioles.

If a child has several bouts of wheezing, shortness of breath, or coughing, he or she probably has asthma, particularly if the symptoms come and go. The child may wake up frequently at night with coughing and wheezing because symptoms tend to worsen at night. In infants and young children, asthma is often difficult to distinguish from chest infections such as **bronchitis**, and doctors may prescribe antibiotics or cough syrups. Typically, the symptoms do not respond to those treatments. Depending on the child's age, the symptoms may interfere with feeding, exercise, and even speech, and the teacher might send the child home often because of frequent coughing that disrupts the class.

In young children, asthma is likely if recurrent head colds with coughs and wheezing occur several times a year and persist for several weeks. Many physicians will ask questions about symptoms and try to determine which factors—infection, exercise, or allergies—bring on symptoms. An allergy history is usually taken because it is clear that asthma is caused by allergies. Most people diagnosed with asthma are also diagnosed with allergies. It is important for a doctor to note whether a child responds to asthma medications or antibiotics.

Lung Function Tests

Because the main problem in asthma is the narrowing of the bronchial tubes, doctors have developed lung function tests to measure how much the tubes have been narrowed. These tests are used to diagnose asthma, are simple and painless, and can usually be done easily by children over five or six. They cannot be used on younger children, however.

The simplest of these is a *peak flow rate test*, measured with a device called, not surprisingly, a **peak flow meter**. The child is asked to breathe in deeply, then blow out as hard and fast as possible through the meter, as if blowing out a candle. The meter measures the maximum speed with which air can be forced out of the lungs. If the bronchial tubes are blocked, the child cannot achieve a normal speed. This is called a reduced flow rate. Asthma medication dilates the bronchial tubes to allow more air-flow. If a child responds well to this medication, the diagnosis of asthma is confirmed.

The *exercise test* is also quite simple. The child runs on a treadmill or rides a bicycle for six minutes, and the peak flow rate is measured before, during, and after exercise. Most children with asthma will show a drop in the peak flow after exercise.

The *challenge test* uses a chemical called methacholine that causes a slight narrowing of the bronchial tubes in children with asthma but has little or no effect on those who do not have it. In this test, lung function is measured. The child is asked to inhale a mist of methacholine and the lung function is measured again. The strength of methacholine is gradually increased and the lung function test repeated until the bronchial tubes narrow and lung function begins to fall slightly. This test gives a measure of the degree of sensitivity of the bronchial tubes and how much they are affected. The greater the sensitivity, the smaller the amount of chemical needed to cause narrowing of the airways in the lungs.

These challenge tests are safe and painless and the child is closely observed throughout. Because children under five are not able to do reliable breathing tests, diagnosis in that age group is usually based on symptoms and how patients respond to asthma medications and antibiotics.

In 1995, the American College of Allergy, Asthma, and Immunology announced a simple and inexpensive screening test to help with the early detection and management of exercise-induced asthma. Called the **free running asthma test (FRAST)**, it involves measuring the breathing of high school students, having them run for six or seven minutes nonstop, and then testing them again. Studies using this test have found a thirteen- to eighteen-percent incidence of exercise-induced asthma, including students who did not know they had asthma.

A major advantage of this kind of test is that it can be given by gym teachers or other school personnel to large groups of students. The objective is to make asthma screening tests as routine as hearing tests. A disadvantage of the FRAST is that some children might not be able to run for six or seven minutes. Also, the test must be repeated at different times of the year because results may vary depending on seasonal factors. Despite these limitations, the FRAST is one of the best methods available to diagnose subtle asthma in high school students and prevent it from becoming life threatening in the future.

PRECURSORS OF ASTHMA

People who develop asthma begin with eczema, an itchy skin condition, in early infancy. Eczema usually affects the cheeks of infants and the creases in the elbows and knees of older children. Children with eczema usually are allergic to B vitamins, that indicates, or may be a precursor to, a wheat allergy. When the B vitamins and wheat allergies are eliminated, eczema usually clears up readily and the later occurrence of asthma is prevented. I have found B vitamins to be the most important basic allergen of asthma, as well as for some other conditions. Eliminating B vitamin allergies is also necessary for eliminating sugar allergies, important for overall good health.

Eczema has been described as the "itch that rashes." It is characterized by an intense itching that provokes scratching and keeps the skin chapped. Sometimes it oozes and can become infected. Chronic scratching can lead to a dry, scaly, and thickened skin known as lichenification. Atopic dermatitis is usually caused by allergens that include foods, heat, wool or other clothing, animals, feathers, wheat, milk, eggs, soy, peanuts, and fish. Treating for the appropriate allergen with NAET can make atopic dermatitis or eczema disappear.

Some children with asthma, or with allergies that have the potential to develop into asthma, also have allergic rhinitis, an irritation of the lining of the nose and eyes that produces a runny nose, sneezing, and red, itchy, watery eyes. Asthma can be prevented in these children by eliminating the allergies causing the rhinitis.

SYMPTOM COMPLEXES OF ASTHMA

Asthma can develop at any age but approximately twenty-five percent of children with asthma develop symptoms in their first year. Asthma varies greatly from one person to the next in terms of how severe the symptoms are and how often they occur. Most people fit into one of four basic types: mild; moderate; severe; and coughing. Each type has particular treatment needs.

Mild Asthma

Fifty percent of individuals have mild asthma and may have symptoms only once or twice a year. Because symptoms clear up quickly with the use of bronchodilators, most people with mild asthma use medications only when needed. Mild cases are most commonly triggered by viruses and viral allergies. Some only have symptoms when pollens are present. These individuals' symptoms can be relieved almost entirely, and very quickly, by treating the few basic allergies. Children or adults who are just beginning to show signs of becoming asthmatic can be treated for the basic allergens with NAET and then treated for specific allergens such as pollens or viruses.

Moderate Asthma

Moderate asthmatics make up about forty percent of all asthmatics. They have symptoms about once a month and may require daily preventative medications. For example, they may be on inhaled corticosteroids as well as bronchodilators.

Severe Asthma

Five percent of the people with asthma are severe asthmatics. They require daily preventive medications and a bronchodilator three to four times a day to maintain reasonable control. They are admitted to the hospital frequently. Wheezing and coughing occur most of the time, and exercising or particitpating in sports is difficult. These people benefit from treatment for the basic allergies but they need NAET treatment for many other allergens as well (refer to Chapter 10). We have to do a thorough investigation with them to identify the allergen to which they are reacting. With the elimination of each allergy, there is more freedom and fewer asthma reactions being triggered. These people may require up to two years of treatment but with NAET, enzymes, and dietary recommendations, they can usually reduce their use of medications within the first eight months.

Coughing Asthma

Coughing asthmatics sometimes complain only of a chronic cough that comes and goes. The cough tends to be dry and typically gets worse at night. Patients may use asthma medications to control it. We have found that many of these asthma reactions are triggered by exercise, viral allergies, and bacterical (infective) allergies. Coughing is usually unrecognized as asthma but is common in people of all ages. Some of these people develop the more typical symptoms of asthma later in life although some do not.

Coughing asthmatics respond very well to NAET. This condition is usually caused by allergies, most commonly to inhalants, perfumes, chemicals, fabrics, and infections, especially if there is mucus in the chest or a loose cough. When mucus is not present, the cough is usually related to food allergies. Once I start treating these people with NAET, they become aware of how they cough after eating certain foods.

One woman coughed every time she ate chocolate. Apparently her family had eaten an excessive amount of chocolate when she was a child. After I treated her for chocolate, she never had the symptom again. Chocolate is a common asthma trigger, along with gas exhaust, gas heat, hormones, adrenaline, and atmospheric conditions.

A young boy who came to see me had a chronic cough from the age of two that was not related to any kind of infection. When he was treated for some of the basic allergens such as wheat, corn, certain fruits, bacteria, and vaccinations, the cough stopped and he no longer had trouble sleeping.

Another chronic cough, one that is involuntary or psychogenic, is now being studied by researchers. This cough usually has a "barking" or "honking" sound and can persist for months or years. The person may cough as often as every few seconds. This condition differs from asthma in that there is no shortness of breath, usually no difficulty conversing, and the cough disappears when the person is sleeping. Many of the tests are negative for any kind of pulmonary problem.

The "happy wheezer" is another person with potential problems. This occurs in a baby from three to twelve months who develops a wheeze that may persist for weeks or even months. These infants are active and not distressed. They eat well and gain weight. Sometimes they do not require treatment and their wheeze settles down in the second year of life. Usually it is related to certain allergens such as breast milk, fabric, or feathers.

It is important to be able to recognize the signs of an asthmatic episode in children. Adults usually know when they are having or are about to have an attack, but children may not. Their parents must be able to detect the danger signs and get treatment when necessary. Early signs include increased coughing at night or early in the morning, more breathlessness with exercise, increased need for bronchodilator medicine, and a decrease of twenty percent or more in peak flow readings below the child's personal best value.

There are four signs that tell a parent when a child is troubled with asthma. The first sign is a high-pitched whistling wheeze at night that is more pronounced as the child breathes out. As an asthma episode progresses the airways are blocked and the wheezing stops. This is a sign of a worsening condition. The second sign is retracting respirations where the soft tissue is sucked in as the child inhales. This is most obvious below the rib cage. Parents will also notice that the child uses the large muscles in the neck and abdomen to help breathe. The third sign of asthma is prolonged exhalation. Because the bronchial tubes are blocked in acute asthma, a child has difficulty getting air out of the lungs. As a result, exhalation becomes prolonged and labored. The fourth sign is shortness of breath. Because of this the child may have difficulty putting words together or be unable to sleep or exercise. Normal breathing rates will also increase.

CONDITIONS RELATED TO ASTHMA

Some conditions and their symptoms are frequently associated with asthma. A brief discussion of the more common ones follows.

Chronic Bronchitis

Chronic bronchitis and chronic sinusitis are respiratory diseases or problems associated with asthma. I have found that asthma sufferers usually have chronic bronchitis throughout the year, although it is more common in the colder, wetter months when they are more vulnerable to infection. These infections may be caused by infectants that are allergens themselves, or they may be linked to allergens (cold, dust, or some foods). When these other allergens are encountered, the infectants (bacteria, virus, or fungi) can surface and create an infection that may lead to bronchitis or chronic coughing. Asthmatics must be treated for these chronic infectant allergies with NAET and enzyme therapy to break this link and rid themselves of these infections. It is equally imperative for people with other chronic health problems to be treated for infectant allergies.

Allergic Rhinitis, Chronic Sinusitis, and Chronic Ear Problems

Allergic rhinitis produces an itchy, runny nose, sneezing, nasal congestion, itching eyes, tearing, and red eyes. Some asthmatics have seasonal rhinitis caused by pollens in the spring, late summer, and early fall. Others have chronic, year-round rhinitis that leads to headaches and chronic congestion. Often related to indoor allergens such as house dust, molds, and pets, chronic rhinitis is characterized by stuffiness, mucus discharge, and problems when exposed to air conditioning, heated houses with low humidity in the winter, weather changes, irritants, fumes, odors, or tobacco smoke.

When the allergens are linked to infectants, this condition can develop into chronic sinusitis as well as ear, nose, and throat (ENT) problems, enlarged tonsils and adenoids, snoring, otitis media, or middle ear disease. In children the condition might cause hearing problems later in life. Children with allergic nasal disease are often restless sleepers who wake up at night because of coughing, stuffy and runny nose, and sneezing. They have a thick nasal discharge, sometimes green. As the condition worsens they might suffer headaches and fever, eventually developing asthma, or causing their present asthma to worsen. Other complications of allergic rhinitis include loss of taste and smell that results in decreased appetite and weight loss, teeth deformities from breathing through the mouth (jaw problems), nose bleeds, and teeth grinding.

In treating allergic nasal disease, the first step is to eliminate the allergens from the environment and then eliminate the reaction to the allergens through NAET Treating for the basic food allergies (dust, mold, odors, smoke, insecticides, paint, feather pillows, fabrics, and other possible environmental allergens) is important. There are also enzymes that help to eliminate nasal congestion. I have found that working with allergies to bacteria and viruses is also effective in reducing chronic rhinitis.

Ear problems, chronic infections, and fluid in the ear can lead to hearing loss and a delay in speech development in children. Allergy is definitely the underlying cause for these problems. Many physicians use tubes in the ear for drainage but this involves some risk of injury as well as discomfort and inconvenience. Such invasive treatment is unnecessary because the chronic allergies related to ear infections and fluid in the ear can be eliminated with NAET.

Recent studies at Children's Hospital of Pittsburgh, Pennsylvania, have shown that eustachian tube obstruction can occur after exposure to allergens and may lead to the buildup of fluid in the ear. The eustachian tube serves many functions. It protects the middle ear cavity, drains secretions produced in the middle ear, and ventilates the middle ear. Obstruction of this tube is a significant problem among children. More studies are needed to establish the relationship between allergy, ear infection, and fluid buildup in the ear but there is enough information to determine that individuals with ear problems usually show signs of allergy. They have swelling of the nasal lining, nasal stuffiness, dark circles under the eyes, asthma, and eczema. Through my testing procedures I have found children with ear problems clearly allergic to many substances and foods. I have also found a higher incidence of ear infections and fluid in the ear among children who live in places with many allergens, especially in homes where tobacco is smoked.

Many over-the-counter drugs do not help with the prevention of ear infections or fluid in the ears but I have had excellent results with NAET. I have treated for dust, molds, animal dander, B vitamins, fungi, and foods, especially milk and sugar. Sugar is probably the most common food related to ear infections. Taking children off milk and sugar produces an immediate decline in the number and frequency of infections, and treating with a combination of NAET, chiropractic adjustments, enzyme therapy, and nutritional education eliminates these chronic ear infections almost entirely.

Up to fifty percent of all patients with asthma suffer from chronic sinusitis. This condition aggravates an asthma condition and produces asthma episodes. The symptoms of sinusitis are headache, tenderness of the sinus areas, nasal congestion, postnasal drip, and stuffiness. The nasal congestion might worsen at night when the individual is lying down and results in coughing. Other symptoms include pain and pressure in the teeth, cheeks, forehead, and behind the eyes, fever, sore throat, earaches, bad breath, and a decreased sense of smell. Many different allergens can cause chronic sinusitis including viruses, bacteria, inhalants, fabrics, pollen, dust, flowers, and perfume. Because people with chronic sinusitis end up with frequent earaches and chronic sinus infections, it is especially important to treat for bacterial and viral allergies. If the infections are treated with antibiotics only, they will keep occurring. With NAET they can be prevented.

Over the years I have had good results with a special cranial technique for people with chronic sinusitis. Called the "nasal specific," it involves inserting tiny latex balloons into the nasal passageways and inflating them, thereby opening the passages and allowing drainage. It also rebalances and frees up certain cranial structures.

One man came to me who was suffering from chronic, allergy-related sinus headaches he had experienced his whole life. He never had a sense of smell or taste and he was subject to ongoing sinus infections for which he was constantly taking antibiotics. He also complained of depression because of tiredness and irritability and because he was having difficulty breathing and unable to smell or taste. We treated him with NAET and enzyme therapy for a period of six to eight months for all the different basic allergies and foods such as wheat, grains, wine, alcohol, and viruses, and bacteria as well as grasses and trees. Because he worked in a furniture factory we treated him for dust, wood, and upholstery. Gradually he regained his sense of taste and smell, and his sinus headaches and chronic infections disappeared.

When he came for his last treatment for perfume, he said, "I never believed I could ever smell and taste. This has been a miracle. I have also seen incredible changes in my work. I have become more productive and successful. The people I work with say I am much easier to work with. I am happier and my business has been booming ever since. Besides saving my life as far as changing my way of living, this has changed my work and allowed me to climb to new levels in my profession."

Emphysema and Bronchiectasis

Emphysema is a disease characterized by distention and damage of bronchioles and alveoli, by breathlessness on exertion, and by wheezing. Bronchiectasis is a disease characterized by dilation of the **bronchi** with production of large amounts of sputum. There are recurrent fevers and episodes of pneumonia. This condition may develop from pneumonia or whooping cough. Both of these conditions can be characterized as bacterial allergies and treated for infectants as well as environmental toxins, inhalants, and food.

5 GENETIC AND ENVIRONMENTAL CAUSES OF ASTHMA

GENETICS

Extensive research is being done in several countries to determine whether asthma is genetically caused. No gene for asthma has yet been found, but a gene that may be responsible for allergies was discovered several years ago and it could spell good news for asthma sufferers. In my own practice, I have noticed that asthma often runs in families, and when both parents have asthma, my experience shows the child will probably develop it.

I have had good results in treating the familial tendency toward asthma with NAET (refer to the DNA and RNA section in Chapter 10). If we work with DNA or RNA as well as deal with the causes of asthma or asthmatic triggers, there is a strong possibility that we can prevent the genetic transmission of asthma in the future.

INFECTANTS

Infectants are at the root of severe asthma and often act as triggers for asthma attacks. As a result, most of my clinical research in recent years has been in the area of infectants as allergens. Allergies to these infectants including bacteria, viruses, fungi, and parasites are common and can be debilitating.

In a study that supports my theory of the link between infectants and asthma, David Hahn, M.D., Medical Director of the Dean Foundation for Health Research and Education in Madison, Wisconsin, found that antimicrobial therapy can cure asthma in some adults who are positive for the bacteria chlamydia pneumonia. He found that eighty-five to one hundred percent of the adult-onset asthmatics in the study tested positive for chlamydia pneumonia, compared to only fifty percent of the general population. Previous studies of antibiotic treatment might have been unsuccessful because they did not treat effectively for the organism. In my practice, I have found a high incidence of this bacterial allergy in asthmatics and have had success treating it with NAET and enzyme therapy. Dr. Hahn contends that, despite doubts expressed by some experts, there is a growing body of evidence that bacterial allergies do exist.

I also believe that many of the antibiotics and other drugs used to treat infectants only drive them deeper into the system, mask the symptoms, weaken the immune system, and toxify the body, especially the liver. When a person is not allergic or hypersensitive to an organism, the organism can be easily eliminated by the immune system or, in extreme cases, with antibiotics. An infectant that is an allergen can stay in the body and surface when the immune system is weak or overloaded. The overload might occur because of an overabundance of allergies, emotional stress, or a toxic system. This reemergence can produce cycles of chronic bronchitis, chronic ear infections, and chronic sinus infections.

An allergy to an infectant can be treated with NAET and enzyme therapy, thereby ending the cycle of infection. Asthmatics tend to store many bacteria and viruses in their systems as allergens that create excessive mucus, coughing, wheezing, sore throats, tightness in the chest, and difficulty breathing. I have found NAET to be dramatically successful in both children and adults for treating infections of viruses including flu and herpes, bacteria, parasites, and fungi including Candida.

Individuals can be successfully treated with their own saliva at the first sign of infection such as a runny nose, a cough, a slight fever, or tightness of the chest. This technique is particularly effective if they have already been cleared for many infectants. Keep in mind, however, that new infectants are always showing up. I discovered this treatment when a colleague became ill with a cough, fever, and runny nose. I called Dr. Nambudripad and asked for treatment suggestions so my friend would have more energy and stamina. She recommended that I treat him for his own saliva. To my amazement he began to improve, and after the second treatment was much better.

This incident began a research project in my practice and at home. As soon as one of my family members sneezed, coughed, or experienced any symptoms, I had them spit into a glass and did a muscle test on the saliva. If they showed any weakness I treated them with NAET. Invariably they improved immediately and their symptoms disappeared. Treating with NAET when symptoms first arise can cause an instantaneous reversal of symptoms and prevent an asthma attack or further progression of an infection.

Self-Treatment

Since immediate treatment is essential, I hold classes to teach people how to do this treatment on themselves or their family members at the first sign of symptoms. The symptomatic person holds a glass vial or jar containing the saliva, is given acupressure on the points indicated in the diagram beginning with the right hand and progressing around the body clockwise three times, then ending with the right hand. Light pressure is applied in a circular motion for seven seconds at each point (refer to Figure 5–1).

Performed at the onset of symptoms and every two to three hours thereafter, this treatment stimulates the body's immune mediators to fight the virus or bacteria and generally leads to an elimination of symptoms within twenty-four hours. Certain enzymes with natural antibiotic properties can also be helpful in bolstering the immune system, and other allergens may also be included in the NAET treatment if they are suspected of causing a susceptibility to infection.

When treating chronic illnesses such as asthma, it is important to check the saliva at the first signs of infection as well as treating all other possible infectants to prevent further allergies. I always perform another muscle test fifteen minutes after each treatment to ensure it was successful.

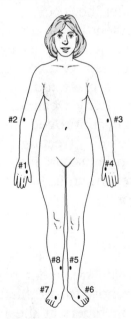

Figure 5–1   Self-treatment for runny nose, sore throat, fever, cold, viruses, and the flu at first onset of symptoms. This treatment can also be used for combinations of the above symptoms or emergencies.

To help prevent asthma attacks, I often treat asthmatics with their saliva on every visit (they hold both the allergen being treated on that visit and their saliva sample) in case they have been exposed to some new infectant. Many asthma patients bring in their saliva samples and ask to be tested because they know how effective this treatment is. This technique is also important for anyone with chronic health problems. Some of my patients used to become ill with some virus or bacteria every other week and were on antibiotics intermittently for years. After we began testing and treating for their saliva, they no longer became ill.

Antigen-Antibody Complexes

We have also found that infectants can link up with other allergens—food, environmental factors, inhalants, and even other infectants—by means of the antigen-antibody complexes. Exposure to linked allergens can result in chronic infections that act as triggers for asthmatics.

For example, a bacterial allergy in an asthmatic can be linked with a chocolate allergy, forming an antigen-antibody complex. When the asthmatic eats chocolate, an infectious reaction results—fever, excess mucus, bloating, sweating at night, sinus infections, ear infections, runny nose—and this reaction can trigger the asthma.

These antigen-antibody complexes, made up of T and B cells from the bone marrow, invade tissues or organs of the body and latch themselves onto the tissue cells. When the immune system tries to destroy these complexes, it destroys its own tissue cells (autoimmune or autoaggressive reaction). If the complexes inhabit the bronchial or lung tissue, inflammation and autoaggressive reactions occur. These reactions cause a destruction of tissue and trigger chronic asthma attacks. If the complexes lodge themselves in synovial fluid in the bone, they can cause arthritis or colitis in the colon. Infertility, chronic fatigue, migraines, Alzheimer's disease, and senility can also be caused by this autoimmune phenomenon.

After seeing how well these treatments worked, I began to research and experiment in my practice by clearing all bacteria, viruses, parasites, and fungi in patients suffering from chronic health problems such as candidiasis, asthma, chronic fatigue, chronic sinusitis, chronic ear infections, bronchitis, and eczema. With the help of muscle testing and other techniques, I began to treat chronically ill people with NAET for these infectant allergens with excellent results (refer to NAET Case Studies in Chapter 14).

Bacterial Allergies

I have found that people suffering from chronic bacterial allergies often suffer from arthritis and those with bacterial and parasitic allergies suffer from chronic gastrointestinal (GI) problems. People who have ulcers or gastritis are sometimes suspected of having Heliobacter pylori, a bacterium that seems to play a part in duodenal ulcers. It is also suspected of being involved in allergies and allergic reactions such as hay fever. Chronic viral allergies can result in chronic infections such as Epstein-Barr, mononucleosis, and herpes and people with infective allergies tend to have more frequent chronic fatigue.

Allergies to Parasites

Allergies to parasites such as malaria or Giardia can challenge and compromise an immune system. These parasites may live in the body for fifteen or twenty years and can be carried by children as well as adults. Asthmatics can have allergies to parasites that lodge in the lungs. Children should be taught to wash their hands after touching animals because animals carry many parasites that can be passed on to humans.

Fungal Allergies

Fungal allergies are another group that can cause chronic illness, particularly asthma and upper respiratory tract infections. Fungi include Candida, aflatoxin, Aspergillis, and many others. I rarely see an asthmatic who does not have large amounts of fungi in their system, including Candida. Candida is a systemic fungal infection that manifests itself in different parts of the body. It is sometimes found in the bronchi or lungs of asthmatics and can be a cause of emphysema. Candida is treated with NAET, enzymes, and a ten-day diet (refer to the section on Candida in Chapter 11).

Allergies to Vaccines or Immunizations

I include allergies to vaccines in the category of infectants because I have seen they can be a troublesome trigger for asthma and other chronic health problems. For example, people with chronic joint and nervous system problems do well when treated with NAET for polio. I have also treated many children suffering from side effects of the diphtheria-pertussus-tetanus (DPT) vaccine. When the DPT vaccine is given to people who are allergic to it, it can cause chronic immune suppression and can be involved in immune reactions. Children with these allergic reactions might develop asthma or chronic ear infections. I always teach parents how to use muscle testing to check their children for an allergic response to the vaccines before the children are inoculated. NAET can successfully treat for allergies to the vaccines, rendering the vaccination harmless.

Several studies have been done in the United States and abroad on anaphylactic reaction to the measles-mumps-rubella (MMR) vaccine to determine if the reaction is caused by an egg allergy. A recent study reported that 222 children with severe egg allergy were safely immunized, and the majority of the handful of children who had an anaphylactic reaction to the vaccine did not have a history of egg allergy. Researchers suspect that something else in the vaccine is causing the reaction. Perhaps the children are allergic to the vaccine itself, which is why muscle testing is recommended.

I receive questions from parents every week as to whether or not they should immunize their children. I always tell them I believe it is a personal decision that each parent has to make after careful study and research. There is so much written about it that I refer them to various sources and avoid giving my opinion. I do say that I would like to test the children for vaccines before they are immunized to avoid adverse reactions. I have seen adverse reactions to both the MMR and the DPT vaccines that can cause long-term health problems, especially for asthmatics.

Flu Vaccines

Adults should think about vaccinations also. Every year many Americans receive the flu vaccine. When people ask me if they should get the vaccination, I tell them I do not have an opinion either way, but I do ask them to be tested and treated with NAET to ensure they are not allergic to the vaccine before they use it. If people are allergic to the vaccine, they can suffer many side effects such as the flu, depression, sleeping problems, other central nervous system effects, muscle aches, fever, and flu-like symptoms. When we treat them for the flu virus with NAET, they rarely get the flu—and if they do, they only get a mild case.

The flu vaccine is produced from eggs and activated particles of influenza viruses. For this reason, people with a strong egg allergy could react severely and should consider alternatives. Unfortunately, many people are not aware of their egg allergies. One man with multiple food allergies did not know he was allergic to eggs. He had a flu vaccination and was sick for days. I finally treated him for his egg allergy and many of the symptoms cleared up. Now he is tested for the vaccine before he receives it.

If people are given a vaccine to which they are allergic, it will not be eliminated from the system and can contribute to autoimmune problems. The immune system forms antigen-antibody complexes with the vaccine which, in turn, creates more toxicity than the liver and the other organs of elimination can handle.

INGESTANTS

The following section contains discussions of some common ingestants to which people are allergic.

Drugs and Supplements

Drugs and supplements such as vitamins can also cause problems. Aspirin, for example, is a common trigger for asthmatics. An asthmatic person told me today that she was at a party recently and got a headache. Someone gave her an Excedrin® and she immediately began wheezing and had to use her inhaler. Chemical dyes such as tartrazine are used in some foods and drugs and can also cause reactions.

When new patients come to see me, I always make sure they bring any drugs they are taking, including antidepressants such as Prozac®, Zoloft®, and Wellbutrin®, and synthetic hormones such as Synthroid®. Many people are allergic to these drugs because they contain synthetic chemicals that are not produced naturally by the body. I treat for drug allergies with NAET. Frequently, drug allergies need to be treated again and again and checked every few months, perhaps because the companies change some of the materials or a new prescription is not the same as the last. This is particularly true of generic brands. With asthmatics, it is important to look at each drug as a potential allergen.

AMALGAMS

Modern silver amalgam is mixed with mercury. It has been used as a tooth restoring material for over 180 years, and accounts for seventy-five to eighty percent of all tooth restorations. Worldwide, hundreds of metric tons of mercury are placed in teeth each year. Some of this material makes its way into sewage and refuse systems.

Mercury is highly toxic to the human body and seems to vaporize continuously from dental fillings. The process is intensified by chewing, toothbrushing, and drinking hot liquids. After chewing or toothbrushing, it takes almost ninety minutes for the rate of vaporization to return to the previous rate. This process puts an individual on a roller coaster of mercury vapor exposure each day that peaks at breakfast, lunch, mid-afternoon coffee or tea, evening meals, and bedtime snacks. The larger the number of fillings and the larger the chewing surface, the greater the mercury exposure. It is estimated that the average individual with eight biting surfaces of silver amalgams is exposed to large amounts of mercury daily.

The release of mercury may be stimulated by other factors as well. One study placed amalgam in synthetic saliva and exposed it to a computer monitor for six hours. The amalgam was found to release two to five times as much mercury as that not exposed to a monitor. This may account for an increase in allergic reactions to electricity and some of the adverse health effects of exposure to computer monitors.

In Sweden, some researchers believe that the way to treat electrical allergies is to replace all amalgam with nonmetallic fillings. Despite autopsies showing that mercury levels in brain and kidney tissue are higher in people with mercury fillings, many dentists in the United States have resisted the conclusion that mercury is a health hazard. I have talked to many dentists, however, who say that amalgams should be replaced because as a person gets older, the mercury released causes more and more problems. If a person replaces mercury fillings, it is important to make sure he or she is not allergic to mercury because removal of the fillings will release mercury into the system and a reaction could cause serious health problems. More problems may result when silver fillings are replaced with gold because many people are allergic to gold as well. The best thing to do is to check all new filling material for allergic reactions.

One researcher claims that mercury is more toxic than lead, cadmium, or arsenic. He argues that no exposure to mercury can be considered harmless. One average size amalgam filling can release enough mercury to exceed the United States Environmental Protection Agency's (EPA) adult index standard for nondietary mercury for more than one hundred years. Mercury from amalgam passes rapidly into the system and accumulates in body tissues in the brain, kidneys, liver, fetus, and in breast milk. The amount of mercury in these tissues correlates to the number of amalgam fillings.

Mercury suppresses the immune system and causes antibiotic resistance at doses below amalgam exposure levels. Mercury can contribute to cardiovascular depression, kidney failure, reproductive disorders, and depression. I have seen mercury fillings cause allergic reactions and chronic sinusitis, and contribute to asthma attacks. With long-term exposure they are also a factor in ear infections, memory problems, ADD, hypersensitivity, fatigue, and other chronic health problems, all of which respond to NAET treatment for mercury. Because mercury is passed to fetuses and through breast milk, I also check children for mercury, even if they do not have fillings. Possible signs of mercury exposure in children are asthma, attention deficit problems, hyperactivity, and behavioral problems.

Other dental materials can cause problems as well. Cariophyllus or carnation oil, used to disinfect pulpitis, can be very damaging to kidneys. Phosphate cements, used to fill root canals, are toxic to the dentist as well as to the patient. Zincum Oxydatum, used for filling root canals and gum dressings, is also toxic, and acrylate, autoprylate, polyester, and vinylpolymerisate nonhardening thermoplastic can be irritating to the GI tract.

I have also noticed that dentists are adversely affected by mercury vapors. In one study, dentists and control subjects who had not suffered occupational exposure to mercury were tested on motor speed, visual scanning, visual motor coordination and concentration, verbal and visual memory, and visual motor coordination speed. The dentists scored thirteen and nine-tenths percent worse than the control subjects. They scored ten percent lower on trail making, digits span, logical memory, delayed recall, and on Bender Distal Time Test Scores. It would seem that mercury is harmful to both dentists and their patients.

An article from the International Dental Amalgam Mercury Syndrome (DAMS) Newsletter by Stephen O'Dell, D.D.S., sums up the mercury problem:

> There is a limit that we can tolerate and beyond that limit we reach the threshold of our body's ability to maintain health.
>
> Mercury is one of the worst environmental poisons. It is a strong protoplasmic poison that penetrates all living cells of the body.
>
> Toxic metals like mercury and lead are very difficult for our systems to eliminate. They affect the liver, the heart, the digestive system, the kidneys, the gallbladder, thyroid, pituitary, parathyroid, the hormone producing organs, etc. . . .

With heat and chewing the mercury leaches out of the filling and is absorbed into the body. The roots of absorption are through the tooth pulp, the surrounding tissue, the sinus, the lungs, and the digestive system.

Mercury is cytotoxic and in the intestinal tract kills normal bacteria. The normal bacteria that survive become mercury tolerant but lose their normal function. The result is a lack of intestinal function and yeast-like symptoms. In many cases yeast infections and yeast-like symptoms go hand in hand with mercury poisoning.

INHALANTS

The following categories contain examples of allergens that enter the body through inhalation.

Dust

The worst indoor allergen for asthmatics is house and office dust. There are many components of dust that provoke allergic reactions but the most important is dust mites. A dust mite is a microscopic insect-like creature related to the spider that lives in mattresses, pillows, blankets, carpets, upholstered furniture, and curtains and thrives in humid and warm conditions and at low altitudes. Its diet consists of shed scales of human skin. Female mites can lay twenty-five to fifty eggs and a new generation is produced every three weeks. Mattresses and other household items contain large numbers of living and dead mites. The waste products of these creatures are the main allergen in house dust and the one that causes the most problems for asthmatics. Each mite produces about twenty waste particles each day and these particles can continue to produce allergic reactions including runny nose, sneezing, watery eyes, coughing, and wheezing long after the mite is dead.

Several studies have shown that children exposed to dust mites are more likely to become asthmatics. The allergens produced by the mites are so hard on the lungs they can trigger asthma in some individuals. The level of exposure to house dust mite allergens and the severity of asthma in children are intricately linked. Dust mite allergy can be especially bad in homes where the indoor humidity is high or in houses located at low altitude. Carpeting laid over concrete tends to harbor dust mites.

House dust can also be produced indoors from fibers, plant and animal material in the home such as feathers, cotton, wool, jute, hemp, or animal hairs. Less appealing components of house dust include human skin scales, animal dander and saliva, molds, and cockroach droppings.

Jackie, an eight-year-old girl with asthma, coughed incessantly after lying down in bed every night. When we treated her for dust, her mattress, and the upholstery she no longer coughed at bedtime.

Cockroaches

Another environmental allergen comes from the cockroach. Tropical in origin, these common pests require a constant source of heat and tend to infest buildings that are continuously heated. In contrast to dust mites, cockroaches are not affected by changes in humidity and are able to search for water in taps, drains, toilets, even people's mouths. Since the two determinants of cockroach infestation are heat and food supply, it is not surprising that apartment houses and projects are particularly susceptible. In Chicago, Detroit, Philadelphia, New York, and Boston B. germanica (the German cockroach) might be the major source of indoor allergens associated with asthma.

Pets

A common source of allergens is domestic pets. I constantly treat people for allergies to animals and animal dander, including reactions to leather. Cat dander is the most potent, and controlling the dander can be difficult. A cat carries 60 to 130 milligrams of allergen on its coat and sheds it at the rate of about .1 milligram per day. As a result, carpets and upholstered furniture can accumulate large quantities of cat dander. Cat hair is not the trigger for an allergic reaction. Rather it is the allergy produced by proteins in the dander and saliva. The allergens become airborne as microscopic particles that, when inhaled into the nose and lungs, can produce asthma symptoms. Although individual cats may produce more or less allergen, there is no relationship between the pet's hair length and allergen production, and no such thing as a nonallergenic breed.

Individuals with animal allergies can react to proteins from the animal's dander, urine, or saliva that are spread throughout the house. The urine of small animals such as gerbils and mice also can produce allergic reactions and cause problems for asthmatics. Removal of the animal may be the most effective control measure, but the results will not be immediate. Allergens can remain in a house for months after the animal is removed.

Cat allergen can even be found in homes where cats have never lived and in office buildings or public places where animals are not allowed. This is because cat allergen is particularly sticky and is carried on clothing from places with cats to other locations. It is almost impossible not to be exposed to some level of cat allergen. Because more allergen is present in locations with cats, an allergic individual is more apt to have rapid onset of symptoms there. The amounts of airborne particles can be reduced by opening windows, using exhaust fans, and employing efficient air cleaners.

Carpets, upholstered furniture, and mattresses will hold cat allergen even after a cat is removed or banished from the bedroom. It can take up to twenty weeks for allergen levels in carpets to decrease to the level found in homes without cats and up to five years in mattresses.

Since cat allergen can also be found on vertical surfaces, walls should be cleaned as well when attempting to decrease allergen levels.

Since cat allergen is so potent and such a potential trigger for asthmatics, children can react from playing with other children who have cats because of the dander or saliva on them. As a result, I always treat asthmatics for cat allergen.

Carol was a patient with severe asthma, eczema, and chronic animal allergies, especially to cats. In her work environment she reacted dramatically to the cat dander carried on the clothes of coworkers who owned cats. It was the only allergen she could imagine that would cause such severe reactions. Her itching, pain, and wheezing were so severe that they almost disabled her.

After her basic allergies were cleared with NAET, her eczema subsided. Two days ago we treated her for cats and dogs, and to her own and her coworkers' amazement, she is allergy and symptom free. She can now continue working without disabilities

Feathers

Feathers can produce a variety of reactions. Many people sleep with down pillows and comforters, unaware that feathers may cause sinus problems and trigger asthma. One woman who came to me suffered from sinus problems most of her life. We treated her with NAET for feathers. After twenty-five hours I retested her. Her runny nose and other sinus symptoms were completely gone.

Synthetic Fibers

Synthetic fiber bedding is also a source of inhalant allergens. One researcher noted: "British researchers compared 486 children who had suffered wheezing attacks in the past year to a similar sized group of healthy children. They found that children who used feather pillows were actually less likely to suffer from wheezing than those who sleep with synthetic bedding. If this is true, synthetic fiber pillows may be an important newly identified cause of severe childhood asthma and could account for half of the asthma cases seen in this study."

Although feather pillows are a wonderful nesting place for house dust mites, it may not be advisable to replace them with synthetic fiber pillows. It is possible that problems with synthetic fibers are caused by a low-level release of gasses. Synthetic fibers are generally made of plastics such as polyester derived from petroleum and may tend to release irritating organic compounds over a long period of time. Many asthmatics who come to me have as many problems with their synthetic fiber pillows as with feather pillows. I muscle test them for each pillow and recommend that they use the kind of pillow they do not react to or be treated with NAET for one or both kinds.

Cooked Foods

Allergens can be contained in the steam from cooking foods. I have even noticed that some people cannot stand to be in close proximity to food to which they are allergic. One time I treated a young boy for sugar and suddenly noticed that his mother was about to pass out. "You know," she said, "sometimes even being near foods I might be allergic to I feel symptoms." She was feeling faint as a reaction to the sugar her son was holding.

Research has been done by boiling shrimp and analyzing the steam. The researchers found shrimp allergens in the steam and concluded that inhaling such steam may cause allergic reactions in sensitive individuals.

Smoke and Chemicals

Other inhalants include smoke, smog, pollutants, chalk, perfumes, carpet pad fumes, and formaldehyde which is almost certainly a trigger for asthmatics. Formaldehyde is found in new clothes, clothing labels, rugs, polyurethane foam, perfumes, refinishing materials, plywood, particle board, counter tops, electronic equipment, deodorants, chlorine, and certain foods. Outdoors its primary source is the combustion of gasoline and diesel fuel; indoors it is contained in cigarette smoke, carpets, and furniture. Toxic pollutants can be given off by a number of building products such as wood glue, paint (acrylic, latex, and oil), paint thinner, and turpentine. Household products that emit fumes include chlorine and other laundry detergents, as well as heating and cooking fuels such as diesel, natural gas, propane, and butane. Freon, contained in air-conditioning systems and refrigerators, and hydrocarbons, which are chemical compounds released by the combustion of coal, oil, and gas are problems for some asthmatics.

Smoke includes tobacco smoke and wood smoke. Cigarette smoke is one of the most disagreeable and potentially dangerous indoor pollutants. It is made up of a complex mixture of gasses and particles that contain a variety of chemicals including synthetic compounds added to the cigarette by the tobacco companies. Indoor tobacco smoking substantially increases levels of carbon monoxide, formaldehyde, nitrogen dioxide, acrolein, hydrocarbons, hydrogen cyanide, and many other substances.

Wood burning stoves used in cold, oxygen-poor conditions result in the release of large amounts of carbon monoxide and other inhaled chemicals and particles. Increased use of wood as a heating fuel has raised many concerns about indoor contamination. Wood smoke can be devastating to an asthma sufferer.

Molds

Molds are microscopic fungi made up of clusters of filaments. Unable to produce their own food from sunlight and air, they live on plant, fabric, or animal matter that they decompose for their nourishment. Molds are some of the most widespread living organisms with tens of thousands of different varieties. Bread mold may be the most familiar. Some molds produce penicillin or other antibiotics or are necessary for agriculture. Others produce potent toxins or are major sources of plant disease. Many molds reproduce by releasing spores into the air that settle on organic matter and grow into new mold clusters. These airborne mold spores are far more numerous than pollen grains and can cause allergic symptoms when inhaled.

Molds are found in most indoor and outdoor environments and on food. Their distribution varies from region to region. Unlike pollens, molds do not have a limited season although their growth is encouraged by warmth and high humidity. As a result, they are more prevalent during humid seasons. Outside, molds are present in the air unless there is a cover of snow on the ground. They are most prevalent in shady damp areas, on decaying leaves and other vegetation, and where plant materials have been disturbed. The highest fungal levels are in temperate zones, near oceans, and in areas with the least snow cover.

In North America, grain crops are particularly susceptible to smuts and rusts. Farm workers exposed to these fungi often have many allergic symptoms. Exposure is greatly increased by activities such as thrashing, baling, and combining that release spores. People doing yard work can spread spores by cutting grass or clearing dry brush. Peak levels of the spores of fungi such as Alternaria and Cladosporium are reached on hot, breezy, rain-free days. At night and during rainfall a very different array of fungi is found. They are Ascomycetes, fleshy types called basidiomycetes, and yeast, which require high humidity and splashing water droplets to become airborne.

Some molds are produced in humid areas of the house such as bathrooms and basements, whereas others enter from outside. Houses are never completely free of mold, and exposure is high in areas where plant material has been stored or processed. Molds include mildew and rust, also allergens. Molds also exist in our diet in such foods as blue cheese along with mushrooms, the other member of the fungi group.

Molds are highly irritating to asthmatics. In fact, I have never seen an asthmatic who is not affected by them. Molds can cause a stuffy or runny nose, sinusitis, nasal polyps, eczema, and many other problems. NAET treatment for mold and mold spores can cause dramatic improvement in severe asthmatics as well as in people with chronic health problems such as chronic fatigue and poor digestion. One woman I treated suffered arthritic pain in her back every time she sat on a particular piece of furniture. It turned out she was reacting to mold in the furniture. Chiropractors who find themselves working on the same area over and over would do well to consider that the problem might be caused by an allergy.

Pollens

Pollens, the final group of the inhalants, has a more widespread effect than we previously suspected. For example, I have long surmised that some fruit allergies are really caused by an allergy to the pollen of the fruit tree. Discussed more fully in the case history section, I have successfully treated allergies to fruit by treating for tree pollen. The reverse is not true, however; treating for fruit does not cure allergies to the pollen.

Pollens cannot be avoided but the amounts dispersed vary throughout the year. Tree pollens cause problems in the early spring, grass pollens strike in late spring and early summer, and weed pollens cause flare-ups in late summer. Seasonal patterns vary in different regions of the United States and it is important to know the pattern in your area. For example, ragweed is at its highest level in the east coast and midwest regions from mid-August to late October. In temperate climates such as California, pollens are present year round. Weather and time of day also have an effect on asthma symptoms.

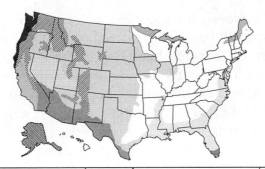

Region	Season	Region	Season
Great Basin		*Great Plains*	
TREES: Juniper, Elm, Poplar, Willow, Sycamore, Box Elder.	February-May	TREES: Mountain Cedar, Poplar, Juniper, Ash, Oak, Elm, Willow, Hackberry, Sycamore, Hickory, Pecan Mulberry, Osage Orange	January-June
WEEDS: Sage, Goosefoot, Amaranth, Ragweed	Mid June-September		
California Lowlands		WEEDS: Sorrel, Dock, Hemp, Goosefoot, Amaranth,Ragweed, Marsh, Elder, Sage.	May-Mid October
TREES: Mulberry, Alder, Ash, Willow, Walnut, Collonwood (Poplar), Elm, Sycamore, Oak, Birch, Olive.	February-May		
		Southeastern Coastal	
WEEDS: Sage, Goosefoot, Amaranth, Ragweed.	Mid May-November	TREES: Red Cedar, Hackberry, Elm, Willow, Poplar, Aspen, Bald Cypress, Bayberry, Wax Turtle, Ash, Birch, Hickory, Pecan, Paper Mulberry, Sycamore, Oak, Walnut, Mulberry.	Mid January-June
Northwestern Coastal			
TREES: Incense Cedar, Ash, Hazelnut, Willow, Alder, Birch, Box Elder, Aspen Poplar, Elm, Maple, Oak, Walnut.	January-June		
		WEEDS: Red (Sheep) Sorrel, Plantain, Nettle, Sage, Goosefoot, Amaranth,Ragweed, Marsh, Elder.	Mid May-October
WEEDS: Plantain, Red Sorrel, Goosefoot, Amaranth, Ragweed	Mid April-October	*Southern Florida*	
Western Mountain		TREES: Oak, Bald Cypress, Elm, Maple, Bayberry, Wax Turtle, Australian Pine, Hickory, Pecan, Mulberry.	January-June
TREES: Mountain Cedar, Elm, Juniper, Alder, Maple, Ash, Oak, Aspen, Poplar, Birch, Walnut.	January-July		
WEEDS: Ragweed, Sage, Goosefoot, Amaranth.	July-November	WEEDS: Ragweed, Marsh Elder Sorrel, Dock, Goosefoot, Amaranth.	April-November
Eastern Agricultural		*Southwestern Desert*	
TREES: Red Cedar, Hazelnut, Elm, Alder, Aspen, Poplar, Box Elder, Maple, Birch, Bayberry, Wax Turtle, Ash, Sweet Gum, Paper Mulberry, Willow, Beech, Sycamore, Oak, Hackberry, Walnut, Mulberry (Red), Hickory.	Mid February-July	TREES: Mountain Cedar, Elm, Arizona Cypress, Ash, Poplar, Mulberry, Olive.	January-June
		WEEDS: Sugar Beet, Ragweed, Gossefoot, Amaranth, Sage.	March- Mid May, July-November
WEEDS: Red (Sheep) Sorrel, Plantain, Nettle, Hemp, Sage, Goosefoot, Amaranth,Ragweed, Marsh, Elder.	Mid May-October	*Alaska*	
		TREES:	May-August
		Hawaii	
Northern Woodland		TREES:	January-Mid July
TREES: Hazelnut, Aspen, Poplar, Alder, Birch, Willow.	April-Mid July	WEEDS:	April-September

Figure 5–2 Pollen chart to identify the pollen seasons in your area.
(For more information on pollen, contact the Asthma and Allergy Foundation of America.)

Ragweed, for example, releases pollen in the early morning. It has been estimated that up to seventy-five percent of seasonal hay fever in the eastern United States is caused by ragweed. There are seventeen different species, and each plant produces up to one billion pollen grains that can be carried five hundred miles by wind.

Pollen is produced by weeds, shrubs, grasses, flowers, and trees. When treating an asthmatic, I always consider all these possibilities. I remember treating one little boy who wheezed whenever he went out to play. We treated for flowers, weeds, and shrubs with some improvement but treating him for grasses made all the difference. We recheck periodically because new kinds of pollens can show up and cause problems.

ENVIRONMENTAL ALLERGENS

In this section I discuss allergens found in the environment. They are classified into two categories: indoor allergens and outdoor allergens.

Indoor Allergens

Indoor pollution is a serious problem with at least five hundred harmful chemicals reported in many buildings. This pollution can come from fumes from room dividers, telephone cables, paint, and carpeting. The worst offender is formaldehyde discussed earlier in the inhalant section. Some sensitive individuals react as soon as they walk into a department store because of the formaldehyde found in new clothing.

Volatile organic compounds (VOCs) are found in many household products including dry-cleaned clothing, paint solvents, cleaning products, wood preservatives, aerosol sprays, air fresheners, stored fuels, hobby supplies, disinfectants, repellents, and automotive products.

Some chemicals appear to penetrate nasal membranes and cause congestion, runny nose, tearing eyes, and, in asthmatics, wheezing and coughing.

Asbestos is a major health hazard that was used from 1945 to 1975 in ceiling materials, synthetic tiles, acoustical wall coatings, stove guards, and as insulation on hot water heaters. It is a dangerous allergen to many and a major trigger for asthmatics.

Indoor chemical sensitivities are becoming more prevalent because there is less ventilation in tight, energy efficient houses and buildings. Media attention has led to increased public awareness of this problem in recent years. Poor indoor air quality in buildings has been associated with a variety of syndromes or groups of symptoms loosely known as building related illness or **sick building syndrome**. These terms are applied when one or more occupants in a building develop certain recognized symptoms that are apparently related to some indoor pollutant. Many of these illnesses involve hypersensitivity of the lungs and respiratory system. In one illness, called hypersensitivity pneumonitis, organic dust can create complex immune system reactions and symptoms including mucus membrane irritation, coughing, chest tightness, headache, and fatigue. People with these illnesses are diagnosed as having multiple chemical sensitivities (MCSs) or environmental illness (EI).

Chemical sensitivities can be triggered through the use of, or exposure to, cosmetics, perfumes, hair spray, hair products, chlorine and other cleaning products, and detergents. A common offender is dichlorobenzene, found in moth balls, insect spray, disinfectants, and solvents. Cooking on a gas stove can also be hazardous to your health. A study of over one thousand British women found that those who cooked with gas were more likely to suffer wheezing, breathlessness, and hay fever—and two and a half times more likely to suffer asthma attacks—during the previous year than women who did not cook with gas.

Your car can be filled with pollutants from plastics and carpets to leather preservatives. I remember a woman who had improved in her treatment until she bought a new car. She spent a lot of time in her car because of her job, and she started to cough and wheeze. When she found a small bottle of leather preservative that had been left in the glove compartment, we treated her for it with NAET. Since then, she has been able to drive long distances without any problems.

The house and car are not the only hazardous areas. More than half a million Americans suffer from asthma caused by breathing some kind of irritant at work. One article reported that five to fifteen percent of all asthma cases are caused by on-the-job irritants. These irritants can cause problems ranging from shortness of breath, wheezing, and lung inflammation to life-threatening attacks. According to an anonymous author, the most common asthma-inducing agents on the job are isocyanates, chemicals used in the manufacture of foam for chairs and car seats and in spray paint and glue. Other common workplace irritants known to cause asthma are latex, molds, animal dander, grain dust, and wood dust. A recent report of a 12-member panel of the American College of Chest Physicians estimates that five percent of workers exposed to isocyanates will develop asthma.

Outdoor Allergens

In combination with drug therapy, food allergies, and other allergies discussed in this book, environmental allergies resulting from outdoor pollutants, chemicals, and toxins are compromising our immune systems and causing severe health problems, especially among asthmatics. The pollutants may not be the direct cause of disease but allergic reactions to pollutants can cause the immune system to link antibody complexes to these substances. An immune system faced with an overabundance of these compromising substances might simply not be capable either of dealing effectively with major diseases such as cancer or with **free radicals** that damage the body's tissue.

Since the Clean Air Act went into effect in the fall of 1995, Methyl-Tertiary-Butyl Ether (MTBE) has been added to gasoline to reduce the amount of carbon monoxide emissions. Unfortunately, this fuel additive is responsible for increased bronchial and lung problems as well as skin rashes and symptoms of disorientation. Most of the public is unaware that some scientists fear MTBE produces elevated levels of formaldehyde. The EPA contends that MTBE is not harmful to the environment or to health but increasing evidence suggests it can exacerbate or cause asthma.

The propellants used in metered dose inhalants for asthmatics contain **chlorofluorocarbons (CFCs)**, chemical agents that when released into the air become part of the chemical brew that can damage the Earth's ozone layer. These CFCs are also found in air-conditioning, hair sprays, cleaning solvents, and other products that rely on propellants.

Other atmospheric environmental pollutants include car exhaust, gas and diesel fuel exhaust, acid nitricum and Acid Sulfurosum (sulfurous acid from coal-fired plants and gasoline exhaust), and asbestos dust generated from automotive brakes in sufficient quantities to be measurable. Fumes, exhaust gases, and pesticides contain ethylene oxide, car exhaust contains cadmium sulfuricum and chromium oxydatum, a by-product of burning jet fuels, and paint (latex, oil, acrylic) contains plumbum metallicum. Fertilizers sometimes contain Calcium cyanamide (calcium nitrate) that is also found in foods, and Potassium nitrate (K-saltpeter); superphosphate; and Thomasmeal, a pre-emergent bud inhibitor.

Radon is a naturally occurring environmental toxin, the by-product of uranium 238. It is formed in soil and rock and can accumulate in enclosed places. Risks to individuals are evaluated according to the intensity of the radiation and the length of exposure to the toxin. Radon absorption occurs through inhalation and drinking ground water. Levels are highest during the warm months of the year and are higher in lower parts of an enclosed space. There is an increased incidence of lung cancer among miners working in a high radon environment and among members of residential households with excessive levels of radon.

Many people are also sensitive to naturally occurring radiation. For example, I used to get a bad headache every time I was in the sun, even if I wore a hat or other head covering. Since I have been treated for a sensitivity to radiation with NAET, I have no problem in the sun. Natural radiation levels fluctuate and are highest during changes in weather. Some people feel sick whenever it starts to rain or the weather changes in some way. Asthmatics especially tend to be worse during a change of weather but treating for radiation with NAET can change this situation.

Carbon dioxide may also cause an allergic reaction in some individuals, leading to a buildup of the gas in the bodily fluids. This allergy is especially apparent when people climb to higher altitudes and takeoff or land in airplanes but it can also be provoked by drinking carbonated water. I have seen people suffer both asthma symptoms and migraines as a result of this allergy. In order to attain normalcy of the respiratory gases, people have to breathe more forcefully. This can lead to dyspnea (labored respirations) associated with the inability to breathe enough to satisfy the demand for air. The allergic reaction to carbon dioxide is referred to as "air hunger," an experience that most asthmatics find very frightening. Since many asthmatics are also allergic to adrenaline, this fear makes the symptoms even worse as adrenaline levels rise.

Outdoor pollution can result from natural causes (the eruption of volcanoes, dust storms, forest fires) or from man-made causes (vehicle exhaust, fossil fuel combustion, or petroleum refining). General air pollution and smog affects us all. Many people have burning eyes or a little congestion but asthmatics experience difficulty breathing. There is substantial scientific evidence linking specific air pollutants to an increase in illnesses and a decrease in pulmonary function, especially in children. Sulfur dioxide can cause bronchial spasms, hives, GI disorders, inflammation of the walls of the blood vessels (vasculitis), and related disorders. Temporary or perhaps permanent bronchial hypersensitivity has been connected to inhaling ozone, and long-term exposure to nitrogen dioxide has been associated with the increased occurrence of respiratory illness. As mentioned earlier, the greatest exposure to airborne pollution occurs inside homes, offices, and other nonindustrial buildings.

Common symptoms associated with environmental allergens include respiratory problems, chronic dizziness, headaches, burning eyes, aching throat, and loss of energy. These symptoms are often mistaken for viral infections such as colds and the flu.

ATMOSPHERIC CONDITIONS

Atmospheric changes can have dramatic effects on asthmatics, especially when the temperature falls and the humidity increases. Even jumping into cold water, eating something cold, or inhaling cold air can provoke an attack.

One asthmatic patient who often traveled to New York told me that as soon as she hit the cold winter weather, she would start coughing. Once we treated her for cold the weather no longer bothered her and she could spend part of the year there without getting sick.

INJECTANTS

This last category deals with allergens that enter the body by injection or puncturing of the skin.

Insects

Stinging insects include the bee, yellow jacket, wasp, and two types of hornets: yellow and white-faced. All of these can cause allergic reactions. There are four basic levels of reaction: (1) a small local reaction; (2) a large local reaction; (3) urticaria, or hives that is not life threatening; and (4) a life-threatening reaction such as swollen throat tissues that block breathing, an asthma attack, or dizziness and fainting. When the throat closes off, a venom amino therapy injection containing actual venom may be necessary. Such injections are successful eighty to one hundred percent of the time.

The best ways to deal with stinging insects are to avoid them and take precautions: wear shoes when walking through grass; do not stand around trash receptacles; limit the use of perfumes; and do not wear bright-colored clothing in areas around insects.

We have had wonderful results treating insect allergies with NAET. Once patients have been treated they should no longer react to being stung by that insect.

One young girl was brought in by her mother because she had apparently been stung by a bee. She had a rash, her arm was swollen, and she was in a great deal of pain. We found that she had been stung by a wasp and we treated for the allergy. Before she left the office, all symptoms of the sting, including the rash, had completely disappeared. I have witnessed similar results with bites from mosquitoes, bees, spiders, and ticks.

One woman patient who was bitten by a tick brought the creature with her when she came to be treated for a reaction to the bite. By the time she left the office, all reactions to the bite were gone.

6 | METABOLIC CAUSES OF ASTHMA

FOOD ALLERGIES

Food allergies are the most obvious of all recognized allergies. At sometime we all have felt a number of varied symptoms from eating foods we could not tolerate or to which we were allergic. Asthmatics can experience this at every meal. They usually cough, develop excess mucous, wheeze, or feel their chests tighten. NAET is the only successful, permanent answer to ending these food allergies and potential triggers for asthmatics.

Walk into an elementary school, sit in a classroom, and observe the number of children coughing. My daughter, who is in the first grade, came home the other day and said "Mom, so many kids in my class are coughing, they are all allergic to some foods." I said "absolutely!" It is a result of their immune systems being unable to fight off the bacteria and viruses they are inhaling, ingesting, and contacting. Food allergies are key allergens to treat for the asthmatic.

Sugars and Carbohydrates

I was grateful when Dr. Barry Sears' book *Enter the Zone* appeared with its intelligent discussion of sugars and carbohydrates. I have felt for a long time that people eat far too much sugar, particularly those who are sugar intolerant or allergic. Here is what Sears had to say about carbohydrates:

> Unfortunately, many people don't really know what a carbohydrate is. Most people will say carbohydrates are sweets and pasta. Ask them what a vegetable or fruit is, and they'll probably reply that it's a vegetable or fruit—as if that were a food type all its own, a food type that they can eat in unlimited amounts without gaining weight.
>
> Well, this may come as a surprise, but all the above—sweets and pasta, vegetables and fruits—are carbohydrates. Carbohydrates are merely different forms of simple sugars linked together in polymers something like edible plastic.
>
> Of course, we all need a certain amount of carbohydrates in our diet. The body requires a continual intake of carbohydrates to feed the brain which uses glucose (a form of sugar) as its primary energy source. In fact, the brain is a virtual glucose hog, gobbling more than two-thirds of the circulating carbohydrates in the bloodstream while you are at rest. To feed this glucose hog, the body continually takes carbohydrates and converts them to glucose.
>
> It's actually a bit more complicated than that. Any carbohydrates not immediately used by the body will be stored in the form of glycogen (a long string of glucose molecules linked together). The body has two storage sites for glycogen: the liver and the muscles. The glycogen stored in the muscles is inaccessible to the brain. Only the glycogen stored in the liver can

be broken down and sent back to the bloodstream to maintain adequate blood sugar levels for proper brain function.

The liver's capacity to store carbohydrates in the form of glycogen is very limited and can be easily depleted within ten to twelve hours. So the liver's glycogen reserves must be maintained on a continual basis. That's why we eat carbohydrates.

Now what happens when you eat too much carbohydrate? Here is Dr. Sears' answer:

> Whether it is being stored in the liver or the muscles, the total storage capacity of the body for carbohydrate is really quite limited. If you're an average person, you can store about three hundred to four hundred grams of carbohydrate in your muscles, but you can't get at that carbohydrate. In the liver, where carbohydrates are accessible for glucose conversion, you can store only about sixty to ninety grams. This is equivalent to about two cups of cooked pasta or three typical candy bars, and it represents your total reserve capacity to keep the brain working properly.

> Once the glycogen levels are filled in both the liver and the muscles, excess carbohydrate has just one fate: to be converted into fat and stored in the adipose, that is fatty tissue. In a nutshell, even though carbohydrates themselves are fat-free, excess carbohydrates end up as excess fat.

Finally, he talks about insulin:

> Any meal or snack high in carbohydrates will generate a rapid rise of glucose. To adjust for this rapid rise, the pancreas secretes the hormone insulin into the bloodstream. Insulin then lowers the levels of blood glucose.

All well and good. The problem is that insulin is essentially a storage hormone, evolved to put aside excess carbohydrate calories in the form of fat in case of future famine. So the insulin that's stimulated by excess carbohydrates aggressively promotes the accumulation of body fat.

In other words, when we eat too much carbohydrate, we are essentially sending a hormonal message, via insulin, to the body (actually to the adipose cells). The message: "store fat."

Hold on, it gets even worse. Not only do increased insulin levels tell the body to store carbohydrates as fat, they also tell it not to release any stored fat. This makes it impossible for you to use your own stored body fat for energy. So the excess carbohydrates in your diet not only make you fat, they make sure you stay fat. It's a double whammy and it can be lethal.

To put it another way, too much carbohydrate means too much insulin."

People generally eat too many carbohydrates. This causes stress on the hormonal system and throws the body out of balance. For an asthmatic or anyone with allergies or an immune system under stress, sugar can produce excessive amounts of mucus and lead to severe asthmatic symptoms. Sugar allergies are a common cause of a buildup of mucus in the bronchi, the lungs, the throat, and the sinuses. Carbohydrates and sugars consist of fructose (found in fruit), lactose (found in dairy products), glucose, and maltose (found in grains, pasta, breads, cereals, and vegetables).

According to researchers at the University of Sydney's Department of Medicine, sugar and fat may be contributing factors to the development of asthma among children with allergies. In their study they recorded the dietary habits of 213 children with common allergies and measured the children's ability to breathe normally while exercising. The children, whose air passages were hypersensitive to exercise (102), ate twenty-three percent more refined sugar and twenty-five percent more high-fat foods than the other children. The children who did not eat excessive amounts of sugar or fat did not show signs of airway hypersensitivity. Based on these findings, the researchers suggest that a healthy diet can prevent the development of asthma symptoms.

Although this data is exciting, it is still a preliminary finding. Nevertheless, in my practice I have often seen children's immune systems destroyed by excessive amounts of carbohydrates and sugar. These children burn themselves out more quickly, their energy fades during a particular time of the day, they lack prolonged focus and attention, and they constantly crave carbohydrates and sugar. Some children come in to my office with a chronic cough. I remove sugar from their diets and much of the coughing stops right away. Treating with NAET for an allergy to sugar diminishes both the craving and the cough.

Sugar is also one of the primary foods that is linked to infectants, especially bacteria and fungi. Eating excessive amounts of sugar can create an allergic reaction that brings to the surface a linked infectant. This starts a cycle of ear, sinus, or bronchial infections. In children, this can result in repeated school absences.

It is also important to clear and desensitize allergies to sugar. We recommend that protein, with its rich supply of amino acids, be eaten with carbohydrates to balance it, but many people are allergic to amino acids as well. People who are allergic to one or all of the amino acids do not absorb or digest them properly and cannot utilize them. This results in a craving for sugar because the body is not able to absorb sugar without the necessary amino acids. Fifty percent of our protein is converted to sugars, another reason that an allergy to amino acids may increase sugar craving. Because the brain requires a constant supply of glucose, it is important to check for, and clear allergies to, amino acids and proteins as well as to sugars.

When large amounts of sugars are eaten, B vitamins and minerals, especially potassium, are depleted. People who have allergies to B vitamins do not get enough because the body is unable to absorb and use them. For these people, it is important to clear the B vitamin allergy with NAET before the sugar allergy is cleared. Otherwise, their already low levels of B vitamins may be further depleted. B vitamin deficiency can cause depression, mental fatigue, low energy, and exhaustion.

Sugar is also responsible for bloating in many people and is strongly linked to fungal infections. I have found that people who are allergic to B vitamins and sugar are especially likely to have fungal infections.

The craving for carbohydrates and sugars is always a result of B vitamin problems. When people tell me they crave complex carbohydrates, I always look for B vitamin allergies and sugar allergies. When people crave sugars I look for the amino acid allergies as well as the B vitamin allergies.

Fats

Fats must be well digested in order for the body to utilize the fatty acids necessary for the health of the nervous system. Fatty acids help to control neurotransmitters and assist in the manufacture and secretion of vital hormones in the thyroid, adrenal, and pituitary glands. They also act as antioxidants and inhibit the secretion of acid in the stomach. Clearing sensitivities to fats can be very beneficial to asthmatics.

Dairy Products

An allergy to dairy products such as milk, yogurt, and cheese is one of the most common and widely recognized form of food allergies. I have found that dairy product sensitivities often can be cleared by clearing sensitivities to calcium and lactose. Sometimes, the dairy product itself has to be treated. With a combination of NAET treatment and enzyme therapy, dairy intolerance or allergy can be eliminated.

One of the most common complaints of dairy product allergy is the production of excess mucus. All of us have had this kind of experience at some time or other: the need to clear our throats after eating a certain food. I remember one woman who constantly had mucus in her throat, especially after she ate dairy products. After we treated her with NAET, she no longer had the problem with any food, including dairy foods. She was surprised because, being in the health field, she believed that dairy products were always mucus producers. Before working with this method I had the same idea and was equally surprised by our results.

Every food is unique and has its own electromagnetic energy field. A person might have a reaction to yogurt, for example, but not to milk. There are many ingredients in the food that may be causing the problem such as **phenolics**, (discussed later in this chapter), sugars, calcium, and B vitamins. For this reason it is necessary to test each member of a food group separately to ensure that eating the particular food will not cause symptoms.

Eggs

Eggs and chicken are the first foods we treat for in our practice. My daughter has always had mucus in her throat: in fact, she had to clear her throat almost immediately after she was born. This became more apparent as she grew older, and by age three she began to comment about it. She also craved eggs. When I treated her for eggs using NAET, her craving disappeared and she no longer needed to clear her throat after eating them. Now if she has mucus after eating a food, she know she needs to be checked and treated. She has turned into a detective to discover her own allergens.

Soy Products

The soybean is an excellent source of protein but it is also frequently an allergen. Many mothers tell me they take their children off milk early and put them on rice and soy milks. The mothers mean well but this practice can result in children with chronic upper respiratory infections caused by allergies to soy.

Soy is now used to make milk, cheese, nuts, flour, and vegetarian "meat," with new products coming out all the time. Lecithin is a soy product often used in candy to prevent drying and to help emulsify the fats. Clearing lecithin often clears a chocolate sensitivity. Soy is also used in many other foods. Soy flour is used in hard candies, fudge, nut candies, and caramels. Some bakeries use soy milk instead of cow's milk in recipes. Soy products are used in custards and coffee substitutes as well as other household products such as varnish, paints, enamels, printing ink, massage creams, celluloid, paper finishes, cloth, nitroglycerin, some dog food, adhesives, soap, fertilizer, automobile parts, textiles, and lubricating oil (for a complete list refer to Part VI). Ford Motor Company uses soybeans to make plastics for window frames, steering wheels, and other automotive parts. They even use soy to make a rubber substitute and an upholstery fabric. As soy becomes more common in the environment, it is important that sensitive people be treated for it.

Grains

Corn is a major grain allergen. Dr. Nambudripad believes it is the most common allergy today. Many foods contain corn in the form of cornstarch and corn syrup. Most prepared foods contain cornstarch such as Chinese food, baking powder, and toothpaste. Additionally, it is the binding product in most pills and vitamins including aspirin, Tylenol®, and other kinds of drugs. Corn syrup is a common sweetener found in many soft drinks. Corn is found in food mixes, canned foods, and foods cooked in corn oil and corn silk is used in many makeup products.

In Chapter 9, I describe how successful we have been clearing wheat allergy by treating for maltose and the B vitamins. Foods that contain wheat are so numerous that I have listed them in Part VI.

Barley, oats, and rye can also be allergens. We have had success treating them by treating for gluten.

Fruits

Any fruit can be a potential allergen. I have seen people allergic to all types including apples, bananas, grapes, pears, and melons. The more acid fruits such as pineapples, strawberries, and kiwi, and the more sugary fruits such as papaya and mangos also cause allergic reactions in some individuals. Many children drink a lot of apple juice that can be mucus forming. Both apple juice and bananas can be particular problems for asthmatics. The chemicals that are sprayed on fruit can also be a problem and serious triggers for asthmatics.

Treating for Vitamin C and sugars often clears these fruit allergies as well as treatment for phenolics, salicylates, and acid, all common ingredients in fruits.

Peanuts

Peanuts are a widely used food and a common food allergen. The incidence of peanut allergy has increased in the last decade, perhaps because of the increased use of peanut products and of peanut butter as a source of protein. Research indicates that many lactating mothers use peanut butter to supplement their protein intake while breast feeding. Because peanut allergen is secreted in breast milk, this can create a sensitivity in an at-risk child.

Reactions from peanuts include mucus formation, asthma attacks, and anaphylactic shock. I have treated adults and children successfully for all of these reactions. Other nuts that can cause problems are cashews, pecans, and walnuts.

Nightshades

Eggplants, potatoes, tomatoes, and peppers are all members of the nightshade family. Any of them can be serious allergens and can provoke immediate asthma reactions. I have seen the nightshades act as irritants for arthritics or others with joint pain. Sometimes what is diagnosed as arthritis is actually an allergy to one of these foods. Studies have indicated that an allergy to eggplant is linked to a certain grass and other allergies such as ragweed, birch, or animal dander.

Vegetables

Most vegetables are potential allergens. Onions are known to be a common trigger for asthmatics. Peppers are sometimes a problem as well as yams, cucumbers, and carrots. I have seen people begin wheezing immediately after eating a carrot. Sometimes treating for Vitamin A will clear a sensitivity to carrots without having to clear the carrots themselves. Before being treated for Vitamin A, I used to get a headache and nausea whenever I ate carrots but not anymore.

Dried beans can also be a problem, especially garbanzo, kidney, and pinto beans.

Fish, Seafood, and Meat

Fish and seafood can cause severe asthmatic reactions. One of the first cases I treated with NAET involved a woman whose throat closed off when she ate prawns.

After the treatment I was still skeptical and I called Dr. Nambudripad. I asked her, "Do you really think this treatment will work, because this woman could die?" She assured me there should be no problem if I treated the woman and made sure she stayed away from seafood for twenty-five hours. After the treatment, the woman's daughter called me up to express her concern that her mother might get seriously ill or die if she tried to eat shellfish or prawns again. Although I said that I was confident, I added that the patient should not be too far from an emergency room when she tried it, just in case. The woman has been eating prawns and shellfish for years now without any problems.

Turkey, chicken, and pheasant are common allergens although I have found chicken to be the most common. A turkey sensitivity is sometimes a reaction to the **neurotransmitter** serotonin which occurs naturally in turkey. Serotonin allergy can produce feelings of depression, tiredness, and mental fogginess.

Chocolate, Caffeine, and Coffee

Chocolate and caffeine are common allergens. Children should be checked for a chocolate allergy because they tend to eat it so often. A craving for chocolate usually indicates an allergy to it. In addition to obvious sources like coffee and tea, caffeine is also a hidden ingredient in some soft drinks and over-the-counter medications such as Excedrin® and other aspirin-based products. Both the allergy to caffeine and the allergy to chocolate that tends to result in heavy mucus production and congestion can be treated with NAET.

I had one patient who ate excessive amounts of chocolate her whole life and noticed that she coughed after eating it. Once, as we were treating her for something else, she ate some chocolate and began to cough deeply and wheeze. When I treated her for the chocolate, the coughing stopped immediately. Her craving disappeared and she never had a cough from eating chocolate again.

Salt and Spices

Salt has been found to be an asthma trigger. A recent study suggests a correlation between levels of salt intake and asthma symptoms, especially among men. High salt intake is also correlated with deaths from asthma in men and children. Other studies show increased bronchial activity in men with high salt intake but not in women.

Most asthmatics have allergies to spices. Garlic is a common allergen although it is regarded by many to be a healthy food. I have seen asthmatics who begin wheezing after eating excessive amounts of garlic. It can also cause indigestion, bloating, and headaches. Vanilla and artificial sweeteners are also allergens to some people.

Combinations of Food Groups

Even after they have been cleared for the foods they are eating, many asthmatics cough and wheeze after eating a meal which suggests they are possibly allergic to combinations of foods. To eliminate these episodes, I have them describe several typical meals then treat them with NAET for the combinations. I also recommend they set aside a portion of each meal so they can treat themselves if they notice symptoms after eating.

Fluoride

Fluoride, another asthma trigger, is found naturally in certain foods and added to the water supply in many areas. Recent studies show an increase of certain chronic health problems with exposure to fluoride. Although much has been written about the benefits of fluoride, people should educate themselves about the possible dangers as well.

Food Additives

Many food additives cause problems for asthmatics and others who are sensitive to food. These include sulfites, MSG, hydrolyzed vegetable protein, sodium nitrate, and sodium nitrite. The sulfites in particular are potentially deadly for asthmatics. I have seen several cases of children who had serious reactions after eating in fast food restaurants. Most food additives are listed on prepared foods. Small amounts do not need to be mentioned, however, so sensitive people eat them without being aware. Preservatives such as butylated hydroxyanisole (BHA) and butylated hydroxytoluene (BHT) used in packaging may cause reactions in sensitive people who eat the food contained in that packaging.

MSG has been used for many years as a flavor enhancer for a variety of foods prepared at home and in restaurants. Manufactured by a fermentation process using starch, beet sugar, and cane sugar or molasses, it is the sodium salt of glutamic acid, an amino acid, that is found naturally in our bodies. Glutamic acid makes up a large part of the proteins found in foods such as cheese, meat, peas, mushrooms, and milk.

The FDA has studied many of the reportedly adverse effects of MSG and unfortunately still considers it a safe ingredient. I disagree. I treat many people who are allergic to MSG and find that it causes particular problems for asthmatics.

Any packaged food with MSG must list this ingredient on the label. Other food ingredients that contain glutamate include hydrolyzed vegetable proteins, autolyzed yeast, extract flavorings, natural flavorings, and potassium glutamate. Hydrolyzed vegetable protein contains five to twenty percent glutamate and is used in place of MSG as a flavor enhancer in many foods such as canned tuna, dried soup mixes, canned vegetables, and processed meats. People who are allergic to MSG can be allergic to other glutamate products as well. Be aware that MSG and the other glutamates do not have to be listed as ingredients if they are a component of an ingredient that is listed such as hydrolyzed vegetable protein. This can have serious consequences for people who are allergic and have no way of knowing they are eating these additives.

It is important to check labels. You can look for MSG in dips, soup mixes, stews, gravies, sauces, prepared meats, poultry, fish, and vegetables. Some restaurants that claim they do not use MSG use commercial sauces or spice mixes without realizing they contain MSG or one of the glutamates. Because it is difficult to avoid them completely, it is best to treat for them if a person is allergic. I have had excellent results in treating for sensitivities to MSG, hydrolyzed vegetable proteins and other glutamates, and food additives. If an individual is not allergic to them, the body will eliminate them quickly and easily.

Gums, such as Acacia, karaya, xanthan, and tragacanth gums are other kinds of additives that can cause problems. They are found in many foods including yogurt, candy bars, cottage cheese, soft drinks, soy sauce, barbecue sauce, macaroni and cheese, and ready-made foods.

Other additives include acidum Sorbicum (sorbic acid found in canned meats), acidum Benzoicum (a food preservative), Diphenyl (a preservative for oranges), and Hexamethylenetetramine (a preservative in canned fruit). Sodium pyrophosphoricum gives the red color to meat, especially processed meats. Sodium o-phenylphenolate, Sodium Sulfurosum, sorbic acid, Urethanum (used in wine manufacturing), and Carbamide (inhibits potato sprouting) can all produce reactions.

Another major additive group is the salicylates. Salicylates are food preservatives that are used, among other places, in the manufacture of aspirin. Many asthmatics have problems with salicylate foods although they appear to build up in the system before provoking a reaction.

Salicylate is both a food additive and an ingredient that appears naturally in many foods. Salicylate food may be tolerated on a four-day rotation diet but not if eaten every day. Most sensitive individuals do not react every time the food is eaten unless it is consumed in excessive amounts. Salicylates are found in a variety of fruits, including apples, apricots, blackberries, boysenberries, cantaloupe, cherries, cranberries, currents, dates, guava, grapes, loganberries, orange pineapple, plum, dark red raspberries, frozen strawberries, gooseberries, and currants. They are also found in vegetables such as chicory, chili peppers, endive, mushrooms, sweet and green peppers, radishes, tomato paste, tomato sauce, zucchini, almonds, peanuts, water chestnuts, bay leaves, basil, caraway, champagne, chili flakes, chili powder, ginger root, mint, nutmeg, cloves, green olives, white pepper, peppermint, port, tea bags, herbal teas, vanilla flavoring, and wine vinegar. A variety of crackers, some cereals, cake mixes, muffins, biscuits, cakes, coffee, pastries, tobacco, mayonnaise, ketchup, Jell-O® and gelatin, candies, gum, and corned beef contain them as well.

Food coloring is another important category of additives. I discuss some case histories involving food coloring in a later section. Many candies, jelly beans for example, contain large amounts of coloring. Even foods sold in natural food stores may contain artificial coloring, so beware! Reactions to food coloring can be serious, from severe constriction of air passageways to coughing, runny nose, and fever.

Pesticides are also food additives and are particularly serious because they are everywhere. Even banned pesticides such as DDT still exist in residues in the soil and in people's bodies. I have worked with people who register a sensitivity to DDT. I remember treating one man who was HIV positive and suffered from severe fatigue and a depressed immune system. One of the breakthroughs in our treatment occurred when I treated him for pesticides to which he was highly allergic. He told me that he grew up on a farm and helped his father spray the plants and trees with pesticides. (A list of different pesticides appears in Part VI.)

We should eat foods that are free of pesticides but they are so pervasive in the environment that they are very difficult to avoid. For this reason, we should treat for sensitivities to them.

Alcohol

Alcoholic beverages such as beer, wine, and liquor cause difficulties for many people and alcohol is the root of the problem. I treat first for B vitamins and sugars, then for alcohol. Our clinic has successfully treated several alcoholics for their addiction to alcohol, and with the help of other therapies, have successfully recovered. Often the craving for alcohol is a craving for sugar and the B vitamins that have been depleted by alcohol consumption. It is a vicious circle because alcohol depletes many B vitamins and minerals.

Alcohol is not just a problem for those who drink alcoholic beverages. It is produced in the body by anyone who consumes large amounts of fruits and sugars. Alcohol was a difficult allergy for me to clear. Although I did not drink it often, I ate lots of fruit, and I was showing signs of becoming addicted. After I was treated for alcohol and sugars, the craving diminished. I also noticed that when I did drink alcohol I no longer had headaches, depression, or the other symptoms I used to experience.

Alcohol tends to aggravate or sustain yeast and other fungal infections. Therefore, it is important to eliminate alcohol cravings when treating for fungi, especially with asthmatics, who tend to have a problem with excessive fungi.

Wines contain other ingredients that can be problematic as well: sulfites, which I have already discussed, and histamines, which I will talk about later in this chapter. Alcoholic beverages made from grains are problematic for anyone allergic to them. Because beer and wine are both made with yeast, they cause problems for anyone with fungal allergies. Other ingredients in beer may also cause difficulties.

Water

Surprisingly enough, some people react to their drinking water. One woman told me she thought she was allergic to the bottled spring water she used. Every time she drank it, she coughed. When I tested her, I found she was indeed allergic. When she stopped drinking it, her cough went away and her mucus production diminished significantly. Some people seem to be allergic to their tap water, others to their bottled water. The reaction may be to something in the water such as fluoride or other minerals, or to the plastic in which the water is bottled.

Phenolics

Phenolics are derivatives of benzene used to give flavor and color to foods and to help preserve them. They also occur naturally in some foods. Once phenolics enter the bloodstream, they are broken down in the liver and excreted into the intestines in bile or eliminated in the urine. Cow's milk naturally contains high levels of phenolics and often provokes a reaction. There are said to be fourteen different phenolics in milk, and people treated for cow's milk, which might normally desensitize them to milk, may continue to react to phenolics until treated for them. Tomatoes and soybean products are also high in phenolics.

Some of the phenolics that asthmatics react to most often are cinnamic acid, coumarin, dopamine, gallic acid, uric acid, rutin, fennel, phenylisothiocyanate, malvin, indole, and histamine.

Cinnamic acid is found most often in fruits, tomatoes, cheese, lettuce, bananas, and such juices as apple, grape, orange, pineapple, and tomato. Coumarin is found in approximately thirty different foods, the most common of which are wheat, rice, barley, corn, soy, cheese, beef, and eggs. Coumarin has been used commercially as a flavor for tobacco, butter, and medicines. Because of the coumarin, it is important to check both for wheat and all the phenolics in an individual with an allergy to wheat.

Dopamine is a neurotransmitter involved with inhibition, coordination, and integration of fine muscular movement such as picking up small objects. It is also involved with memory and emotions. Dopamine has been shown to play a role in Parkinson's disease and has been linked with high copper levels in schizophrenics. There are high levels of dopamine in pineapples, bananas, plantains, and avocados.

In addition to coumarin, gallic acid, found in seventy percent of all foods including food coloring agents, is unquestionably one of the most important phenolics. It can act as an asthmatic trigger, cause chronic nasal congestion, sinusitis, and chronic fatigue and lead to hyperactivity in children.

The amino acid tryptophan is broken down by bacteria to form indole and skatole. When indole is detectable in feces, it indicates bowel toxicity and fermentation of food by putrefactive bacteria. Indole is found in all complete proteins. When ingested, it penetrates the bowel and moves into the liver where it is converted to alcohol and excreted in the urine. Excessive production of indole can be carcinogenic. It is found in oranges, flowers, green vegetables, perfumes, and, in high levels, dairy products. When I find high levels of indole in laboratory tests and a person suffers from bloating and constipation, I suspect poor protein digestion. Based on indole levels and other markers, I recommend enzymes to help digest protein. Chronic bowel problems are fairly common among asthmatics, and they should be treated for indole, skatole, and other by-products of bowel elimination.

Malvin, found in more than thirty foods, is the natural red and blue pigment in fruits and vegetables such as strawberries, tomatoes, and concord grapes. It is also found in oranges, eggs, chickens, milk, soy foods, and dairy products. Like gallic acid and coumarin, it is a common cause of reactions.

Phenylisothiocyanate is found in twenty foods such as chickens, eggs, beets, soybeans, cheese, lamb, peanuts, and legumes. This phenolic can stimulate the sympathetic nervous system and may be a cause of migraines.

Rutin, a bioflavonoid containing glucose and quercetin is found in about fifty foods including eggs and rice, and in plants such as buckwheat, hydrangea, pansies, ragweed, and goldenrod. A rutin deficiency or an allergy to rutin causes a susceptibility to bruising. This is such a common allergen that it is one of the first we deal with when we begin treatment (it is included in the Vitamin C mix).

Uric acid is present in the urine of all carnivorous animals and in cat saliva. The end product of the nitrogenous metabolism of protein, it appears in the urine when the plasma concentration is slightly higher than normal. A high concentration of uric acid in the urine is an indication of poor protein metabolism or excess protein consumption. It may also be an indication of stones or calculi in the kidneys or bladder and may be linked to gout, hepatitis, and leukemia. We look at this level in the twenty-four hour urinalysis we conduct to monitor assimilation of various proteins. Certain foods can produce high uric acid levels including caffeine, beans, nicotine, meat, spinach, and mushrooms.

I have had excellent results treating asthmatics for phenolics. Not only does it help reduce asthma symptoms but also helps desensitize people to many foods that contain phenolics.

ACID- AND ALKALINE-FORMING FOODS

Acid foods are sour and contain the element hydrogen. The sour taste of oranges and lemons, for example, is due to the acid they contain. Alkalies, or bases, have properties opposite to acids, and they neutralize acids. Our body fluids—blood and extracellular fluid—maintain a constant condition of alkalinity or acidity.

Foods can be acid or alkaline, or they can be acid or alkaline forming. The first category refers to how much acid or alkaline the foods contain. The second refers to the condition the foods cause in the body after being metabolized. Protein, for example, is an acid-forming food because acid is the by-product of its metabolism. The same is true of grains. Fruits and most vegetables oxidize when broken down and are considered alkaline-forming foods.

Some common acid- and alkaline-forming foods are:

ACID FORMING	ALKALINE FORMING
eggs	salt
grains	vegetables
meat	fruit
fish	wine
sugar	
nuts	
beans	

Moderate, severe, and childhood asthma sufferers are commonly allergic to acid-forming foods and they tend to become more metabolically acidic (acidotic). This acidity causes sluggishness and increases the rate and depth of respiration that triggers an asthma attack. It also causes gastritis, or reflux, which irritates the mucous membranes of the stomach, duodenum, or esophagus, a condition commonly known as "heartburn." This condition can even be the precursor to an ulcer.

One authority estimates that eighty percent of the millions of asthmatics in the United States suffer from the kind of heartburn known as gastric reflux where stomach acid backs up into the esophagus and causes a burning sensation. He believes that acid in the airways increases the incidence of asthma reactions and suggests testing for acid levels by using a probe in the throat and stomach to measure acid levels for twenty-four hours. If high acid levels are found, treatment with prescription drugs or surgery is recommended.

I use much less invasive techniques because I believe the reaction is due to an allergy to the acids. Sugars, the major allergens for asthmatics, are high in acid. Acid in the airways provokes an intense allergic reaction in that tissue. An allergy can be detected with my normal muscle response testing procedure and treatment with NAET and enzymes. I have found antacid enzymes taken at night are very helpful.

Sometimes acid stomach irritation will mimic a hiatal hernia. This condition is especially prevalent among older asthmatics. There are chiropractic manipulation techniques I teach patients that help them manage this condition (refer to Hiatal Hernia Manipulation in Part VI).

POOR DIGESTION

The by-products of poor digestion can cause allergic reactions. Any undigested food—whether protein, carbohydrate, fat, or fiber—is absorbed into the bloodstream and regarded by the immune system as an allergen. In diagnosing and treating for allergens in our clinic, digestion is a key factor. We make sure that digestion is optimal because after clearing many allergies, we do not want people to walk out and develop more of them. I stress good digestion and talk about it with everyone who comes to see me. I make sure they chew their food well and recommend predigestive enzymes to help predigest their food. In my own experience, I found that using enzymes helped me reduce the reaction to foods to which I was allergic. Until all the foods are cleared with NAET, this can be a lifesaver for asthmatics and prevent them from developing new allergies.

VITAMIN AND MINERAL DEFICIENCIES

Vitamins are important supplements for asthmatics but many people are allergic to the vitamins they need to take. People tend to be deficient in the vitamins they are allergic to because their bodies are unable to absorb and use them. The vitamin allergies I have found most common in asthmatics are to Vitamin C, all the B vitamins, Vitamin A, and Vitamin F (fatty acids).

Vitamin C

We all know that Vitamin C has a wide range of applications in the treatment and prevention of many diseases. Studies have shown it to be important to the health of the immune system and many books have been written about its benefits and the effects of Vitamin C deficiency. It is necessary for healthy skin, connective tissue, and gums. It is the most widely taken vitamin supplement.

As a chiropractor, I know that Vitamin C is vital to combating disease and healing muscle damage. It can also prevent the loss of other vitamins in the body such as A, E, and some of the B vitamins. Vitamin C has been shown to help protect the bronchial airways and lungs from the effects of environmental toxins such as cold temperatures, pollens, smog, fumes, and chemicals. It is also said to protect against viral and bacterial infections, such as colds and the flu, and to protect against radiation. Vitamin C is the primary **antioxidant** vitamin, preventing oxidation from damaging tissue and it is the most abundant antioxidant nutrient found in the lungs' inner lining. Vitamin C also helps deal with some of the adverse effects of smoking by combating the oxidants such as nitrogen oxide that may be a cause of asthma in some people. The lungs of asthma sufferers are weakened from exposure to pollutants, contaminants, and oxidants that cause coughing, wheezing, and chest tightness. The more Vitamin C they take, the better they can combat these symptoms.

Seven studies conducted since 1973 have shown that breathing in asthma sufferers improves with Vitamin C supplements. Other studies have shown a thirty-five percent lower concentration of Vitamin C in the blood serum of asthmatics than in nonsufferers and a fifty percent lower concentration of Vitamin C in asthmatics' white blood cells.

Clearly, the proper absorption and use of Vitamin C is essential for asthmatics and they need to be tested for an allergy to it. As suggested earlier, an allergy to C may be causing many of the symptoms the person is trying to treat by taking the vitamin in the first place. For example, chronic sore throats may be caused by an allergy to Vitamin C and taking the vitamin only makes the symptoms worse. After treatment for the allergy, the sore throat will disappear and Vitamin C can be taken freely without the recurrence of symptoms.

People spend large amounts of money on vitamins recommended by health food stores, doctors, and other practitioners that may not be doing them any good. If people are allergic to a vitamin they will not be able to absorb and utilize it, no matter how much they take. Once an allergy to Vitamin C has been treated, people begin to absorb it from their food. They also are able to better utilize the nutrients from their food without having to take excessive supplements.

Food sources for Vitamin C are tomatoes, citrus fruits, broccoli, strawberries, peppers, leafy greens, and potatoes. I do both laboratory testing and muscle response testing to determine the best dosage for each individual. For those who are not allergic, Vitamin C is harmless. It may increase toxicity, however, in those who are allergic and are not treated for the allergy.

B Vitamins

The B vitamin complex also presents problems to sensitive people. The complex is made up of at least eleven types of vitamins essential for the proper nourishment and functioning of our bodies. Almost everyone, however, is deficient in one or more B vitamins because it is difficult to get enough through normal diet, especially when there is a high consumption of processed foods. Excessive sugar intake can also deplete B vitamins. By reducing the body's reserve of B vitamins, sugar actually decreases the energy available. High levels of caffeine deplete Vitamin B, especially the natural relaxant inositol, as do alcohol, stress, illness, and physical activity. We need a fresh supply of B complex vitamins every day because the body does not store them. Any excess is washed out through the kidneys or through perspiration.

The B vitamins include:

- B_1, thiamin

- B_2, riboflavin

- B_3, niacin or niacinamide

- B_5, pantothenic acid

- B_6, pyridoxine or pyridoxal-5-phosphate

- B_{12}, cobalamin or cyanocobalamin

- folic acid or folicin

- biotin

- inositol

- choline

- para-aminobenzoic acid (PABA)

These eleven vitamins are synergistic which means they work as a team to perform all their vital individual functions properly, and are more potent taken together than separately. Therefore, many nutritionists recommend taking a B vitamin complex rather than single vitamins. For proper metabolism of the B vitamins the body must also maintain adequate levels of other nutrients such as iron and coenzymes. Thiamin, riboflavin, and niacin all bind to enzymes to help them do their job. None of these vitamins could function as effectively without their coenzymes. When treating for B vitamin allergies, it is important to check all the vitamins, related nutrients, and coenzymes for sensitivity.

The primary function of B vitamins is to convert carbohydrates, fats, and proteins into energy the body can use. They are vital to the proper functioning of the nervous system, production of red blood cells, maintenance of muscle tone In the GI tract, and the health of skin, hair, eyes, mouth, and liver. A high potency vitamin B complex helps in recovering from debilitating illness, alcoholism, or excessive use of medication by reducing the effects of stress and supporting the adrenal glands. Vitamin B supplementation is recommended for heavy coffee drinkers, women who take birth control pills, and people with high carbohydrate diets.

B₁, Thiamin   B$_1$, or thiamine, aids in the digestion of carbohydrates, stabilizes the appetite, promotes growth and good muscle tone, inhibits pain, and assists in the normal functioning of the nervous system, muscles, and heart. Thiamin helps the body release energy from carbohydrates during metabolism. People who expend more energy and have high caloric intake need more thiamin than those who eat fewer calories. It can be depleted by excessive consumption of alcoholic beverages. A person deficient in B_1 might experience a loss of appetite and weight, feelings of weakness and fatigue, paralysis, nervousness, irritability, insomnia, unfamiliar aches and pains, depression, heart difficulties, and constipation or gastrointestinal problems. A thiamin deficiency can also cause the disease beriberi that results in weakness, nervous tingling of the body, and poor coordination.

Grain products including bread, cereals, pasta, and rice are good sources of thiamin. Others are meat (especially pork, poultry, and fish), fruits, vegetables, and sunflower seeds. Pasta, most instant and ready-to-eat cereals, and most breads made from refined flour are enriched with vitamins to replace the nutrients lost in processing, including thiamin.

B_2, Riboflavin   Vitamin B_2, or riboflavin, is necessary for the metabolism of carbohydrates, fats, and protein. B_2 also promotes general health by maintaining cell respiration, aiding in the formation of antibodies and red blood cells, ensuring good vision, relieving eye fatigue, and maintaining healthy nails and hair. The body's need for riboflavin may increase during periods of healing and pregnancy and in conditions such as asthma. A person deficient in B_2 might experience sluggishness, itching, and burning or bloodshot eyes, sores or cracks in and around the mouth and lips, purplish or inflamed tongue and mouth, dermatitis, oily skin, slowed growth, trembling, digestive problems, and respiratory problems.

Breads, cereals and other grain products, milk and milk products, meat, poultry, and fish are all good sources of riboflavin. Pasta and most breads made from refined flours are enriched with riboflavin because riboflavin is another of the nutrients lost in processing. To retain riboflavin during storage and cooking, food should be stored in containers through which light cannot pass, vegetables should be cooked in minimal amounts of water, and meat should be roasted or broiled.

B₃, *Niacin*   Vitamin B$_3$, niacin or niacinamide, helps to improve circulation and reduce the blood's cholesterol level. B$_3$ also assists in maintaining nervous system tissue, respiration, and fat synthesis. It aids in metabolizing protein, sugar and fat, helps to reduce high blood pressure, increases energy through the proper use of food, produces acid, metabolizes sex hormones, activates histamines, prevents pellagra (a disease characterized by diarrhea and dermatitis), and maintains healthy skin, tongue, and digestion. The body requires more niacin in periods of stress, acute illness, and low tryptophan intake.

B$_3$ is a good example of how a vitamin can be as effective as a drug in combating disease. Niacin, much less expensive than prescription medication, is successfully used to lower levels of harmful cholesterol **low-density lipoprotein (LDL)** and raise levels of good cholesterol **high-density lipoprotein (HDL)**.

A person deficient in B$_3$ might experience gastrointestinal disturbance, loss of appetite, indigestion, bad breath, canker sores, skin disorders or rashes, muscular weakness, fatigue, insomnia, vague aches and pains, headaches, nervousness, memory loss, irritability, or depression. It can also result in respiratory problems including asthma, chronic bronchitis, or pellagra.

Niacin is formed in the body from tryptophan, an essential amino acid found in meat, poultry, fish, and eggs. If a diet includes these foods, an individual will have less need for niacin from other sources. Good sources are meat, poultry, fish (especially tuna), bread, cereals and other grain products such as wheat bran, vegetables such as mushrooms or asparagus, and peanuts. Pasta and breads made from refined flours are usually fortified with niacin. Loss of niacin from foods due to preparation and storage is slight but vegetables should be cooked in a minimal amount of water, and meat should be roasted or broiled to retain the nutrient.

B₅, Pantothenic Acid B_5, pantothenic acid, participates in the release of energy from carbohydrates, fats, and proteins, aids in the utilization of vitamins, and improves the body's resistance to stress. It helps build cells, aids in the development of the nervous system and the immune system, maintains healthy skin, supports the adrenal glands in the production of cortisone in times of stress, fights infection by building antibodies, detoxifies the body, stimulates growth, and utilizes Vitamin D.

B_5 deficiencies can trigger asthmatic attacks, cause muscle cramping, painful and burning feet, skin abnormalities, retarded growth, dizzy spells, weakness, depression, decreased resistance to infection, restlessness, digestive disturbances, stomach stress, and vomiting.

B₆, Pyridoxine B_6, pyridoxine or pyridoxal-5-phosphate, is necessary for the synthesis and breakdown of DNA, RNA, and amino acids, the building blocks of protein, and is required by the central nervous system for normal functioning of the brain. B_6 also aids in the metabolism of fat and carbohydrates, the formation of antibodies, and the removal of excess fluid and discomfort during menstrual periods. It aids hemoglobin in its function, promotes healthy skin, reduces muscle spasms, leg cramps, and stiffness of hands, helps prevent nausea, and promotes the balance of sodium and phosphorus in the body.

Conditions that respond to B_6 therapy include carpal tunnel syndrome, joint pain, homocystinuria, sensitivity to bright light, sensitivity to MSG, burning or tingling in the extremities, the inability to recall dreams, and imbalances of the liver. Because Vitamin B_6 is used by the body to break down protein, the more protein one eats, the more Vitamin B$_6$ one needs. Deficiencies can produce skin eruptions of dermatitis, loss of muscular control or muscle weakness, arm and leg cramps, fatigue, nervousness, irritability, insomnia, slow learning, water retention, anemia, mouth disorders, and hair loss.

Good sources of B$_6$ are meat, poultry, fish, fruits, vegetables, and grain products. Most ready-to-eat and instant cereals are fortified with B$_6$. To retain B$_6$ during cooking, serve fruits raw, cook foods in minimal amounts of water for the shortest time possible, and roast or broil meat and poultry.

B$_{12}$, Cobalamin B$_{12}$, cobalamin or cynocobalamin, is required for the formation and regeneration of red blood cells to help prevent anemia. B$_{12}$ is also necessary for building genetic material, metabolizing carbohydrates, fat, and protein, increasing energy, and maintaining a healthy nervous system and muscles. It is important for promotion of DNA synthesis in childhood growth, cell longevity, memory improvement, maintenance of the appetite and digestive system, and strengthening of the immune system. It aids in the absorption of iron and calcium and helps prevent inflammation. It also assists in folate metabolism and in the synthesis of DNA and is essential to produce insulation for nerve fibers. B$_{12}$ aids in the conversion of fat to lean muscle tissue. For this reason many athletes, such as weight lifters take B$_{12}$ as a safe, competitive, and legal alternative to steroid hormones. A B$_{12}$ folate complex can be used as a tonic to assist in the conversion of iron to hemoglobin, to help normalize hormonal production, and to improve short-term memory in the elderly. B$_{12}$ is even considered an antiaging nutrient and an agent for increasing sperm count.

There is some controversy today about the best way to get enough B$_{12}$ in our diets. Some claim that B$_{12}$ is only acquired naturally by eating meat, eggs, and milk products, but vegetarians and vegans claim they have found numerous nonanimal sources of this vital nutrient including edible seaweed such as hijiki and wakame, certain mushrooms, sourdough bread, tofu, tempeh, miso, barley malt syrup, parsley, beer, cider, wine, and margarine. Some nutritionists disagree, saying that the only source of B_{12} available to vegetarians is fortified nutritional yeast, fortified breakfast cereals, soy milk, and other soy products.

Supplements that contain spirulina or nori can interfere with B_{12} absorption. Some experts also advise against taking multivitamin products because these preparations may contain products that interfere with the breakdown of B_{12}. By preventing the absorption of B_{12}, they help to create the deficiency they are supposed to correct.

B_{12} can be produced by bacterial activity in the body's own small intestines, mouth, teeth, gums, nasal passages, and around the tonsils, tongue and upper bronchial tree. Because B_{12} is often found in soil, freshly picked raw, unwashed vegetables, especially root vegetables, may have B_{12} on their surfaces. To retain the B_{12} in meat or fish, they should be roasted or broiled.

A person deficient in B_{12} could experience pernicious (life-threatening) anemia, degeneration of the spinal cord and nerves, poor appetite, stunted growth in children, nervousness, depression, lack of balance, neuritis, or brain damage. Symptoms of anemia include a pale yellow, sallow complexion, a shiny or red, sore tongue, weakness and fatigue progressing to paralysis, numbness or tingling in hands and feet, gradual deterioration of motor coordination, moodiness, poor memory and confusion, delirium, delusion, hallucinations, and psychotic states. Paralysis and possible death may occur with the deterioration of myelin sheaths and the failure of DNA production.

A B_{12} deficiency, especially among the elderly, may occur even though the person's diet contains enough B_{12} because other substances needed for B_{12} absorption are lacking. For example, the stomach manufactures an "intrinsic factor" that must bond with B_{12} before the body can absorb it. Other substances needed for absorption include iron, folic acid, and a factor manufactured in the stomach that can be blocked by intestinal parasites. Microorganisms in the stomach can compete for the B_{12} and toxins can block absorption. Enzyme deficiencies, liver or kidney disease, and atrophic gastritis can interfere with the utilization of B_{12}.

B_{12} can be further depleted by disease, **hypothyroidism**, and an allergy to lactose. Consumption of foods such as meat and animal products, refined sugars, carbohydrates, drugs, chemicals, caffeine, alcoholic beverages, tobacco, mega doses of Vitamin C, egg albumen, egg yoke, and allergies to any of those can all use up the body's storage of B_{12}.

Sufficient levels of B_{12} are considered especially crucial for women during pregnancy and lactation. The most nutrient-dense source of B_{12} is organ meat such as the heart, liver, and kidney. Clams, oysters, beef, pork, eggs, and milk are also good sources of B_{12}.

Folic Acid Folic acid (folate or folicin) helps the body form red blood cells and aids in the formation of genetic material within every body cell. Folic acid also works with Vitamin B_{12} in synthesizing DNA and RNA, essential for the growth and reproduction of all body cells. It is useful in amino acid conversion, breakdown and assimilation of protein, stimulation of appetite, the maintenance of a healthy intestinal tract, and nucleonic acid formation. Folic acid may reverse certain anemias, reduce the risk of cervical dysplasia, and lower the likelihood of heart attack. It becomes even more essential during times of growth and cell reproduction, especially during pregnancy, when folic acid seems to be in short supply. It protects the body against neural tube defects in unborn babies and other midline birth anomalies.

Folic acid deficiency during pregnancy can cause the disease spina bifida in the child which can be permanently crippling. Recently it was discovered that folic acid reduces the risk of premature birth. Deficiency can result in megaloblastic anemia in which red blood cells fail to divide properly and become large and abnormal, causing a shortage of red blood cells. Other symptoms of folic acid deficiency are GI disorders, prematurely gray hair, pale tongue, and Vitamin B_{12} deficiency.

Good sources of folic acid include fruits and vegetables, especially citrus fruits, tomatoes, foliage, cooked spinach, lettuce, broccoli, grain products, and organ meats. To retain folic acid, fruits and vegetables should be served raw, if possible, or steamed or simmered in a minimal amount of water. Store vegetables in the refrigerator.

Biotin   Biotin helps to strengthen the immune system, aids in the utilization of protein, folic acid, pantothenic acid, and Vitamin B_{12}, aids in cell growth, fatty acid production, and synthesis, helps in the formation of DNA and RNA, and helps produce healthy hair.

Anyone allergic to this B vitamin is not properly absorbing it or the other B vitamins. An allergy to biotin produces a deficiency in all the B vitamins. A biotin deficiency leads to drowsiness, extreme exhaustion, depression, loss of appetite, muscle pain, and gray skin color.

Inositol   Inositol, found in every cell of the body, is necessary for the growth of muscle cells and the formation of lecithin. It aids in the breakdown of fats, helps reduce blood cholesterol, and helps prevent thinning hair. Inositol is also an antioxidant free radical scavenger and is known as "nature's tranquilizer" for the calming effect it often has. A deficiency may result in hair loss, eczema, constipation, migraines, and high-blood cholesterol.

Choline   Choline is very important in controlling fat and cholesterol buildup in the body, preventing fat from accumulating in the liver, and facilitating the movement of fats in the cells and throughout the bloodstream. It also helps regulate the kidneys, liver, gallbladder, and is important to the health of myelin sheaths that cover the nerve fibers, and to nerve transmission. Choline is known to help improve memory, support brain chemistry, and is an essential component of acetylcholine, an important neurotransmitter.

A deficiency may result in cirrhosis and fatty degeneration of the liver, hardening of the arteries, heart problems, high blood pressure, and hemorrhaging kidneys. Choline should be taken with the other B vitamins for optimal effectiveness.

Para-Aminobenzoic Acid (PABA)   Para-aminobenzoic acid (PABA) is a component of folic acid as well as an antioxidant and membrane stabilizer. It helps to prevent red blood cells from bursting and lysosomal membranes from breaking and releasing tissue-damaging enzymes. PABA helps to produce folic acid and aids in the formation of red blood cells and the assimilation of pantothenic acid. It produces healthy skin and skin pigmentation, helps return gray hair to its natural color, and screens the skin from sun exposure. A PABA deficiency causes extreme fatigue, irritability, depression, nervousness, eczema, constipation, digestive disorders, headaches, and premature gray hair.

Allergies to B vitamins are among the most important to treat with NAET because many foods have high B vitamin content. Eating vitamin-rich food and taking supplements can do more harm than good to B vitamin sensitive people. For asthmatics the most common problems are with Vitamin B_2 (riboflavin), B_5, B_6 (pyridoxine), and B_{12} (cobalamin). Other B vitamins, or all of them, can cause difficulties. With asthmatics and those suffering other chronic problems, I test each of the B vitamins separately.

Eczema is often a precursor to asthma, and I have found that allergies to B vitamins are closely connected to eczema, especially in young children. NAET has been very effective in eradicating eczema and decreasing the likelihood of asthma.

Possible symptoms of B vitamin deficiency are mood swings, behavioral problems, cold sores, herpes, extreme fatigue, severe bloating, malnutrition, chronic sinus congestion, and chronic yeast infection. Chronic yeast infections always involve B vitamin allergies and deficiencies, and treating for B vitamins can sometimes clear the infections before the yeast is treated. I have seen miraculous results with all kinds of symptoms from clearing only one of the B vitamins. These are so important that I sometimes have patients treat themselves at home for several days or a few times in one day, using the acupressure points shown in the Self-Treatment Section of Chapter 5 (p. 66) and some chiropractic reflex points.

Vitamin E

Vitamin E is a fat soluble antioxidant that protects cells from free radical damage and neutralizes the damaging effects of ozone. Because asthmatics tend to worsen after ozone exposure, this can be a key nutrient for them.

Vitamin A

Vitamin A comes in two forms: betacarotene, found in a wide variety of fruits and vegetables; and Vitamin A itself, found in liver, eggs, cod liver oil, butter, and dairy products. Recent research suggests that betacarotene, known to be a precursor to Vitamin A, boosts the immune system and prevent arteries from clogging. Betacarotene and Vitamin A are both fat soluble vitamins. Vitamin A is important for good eyesight, healthy skin, a healthy intestinal tract, and as protection against pollutants. It is important in strengthening the immune system and protecting against infection. High doses of Vitamin A can help fight viral infections and are effective in combatting illnesses and treating wounds.

Excessive consumption of alcohol and the liver damage that results depletes Vitamin A. When the liver is impaired, the body is not able to metabolize Vitamin A and several other nutrients. Smoking also depletes Vitamin A in the respiratory tract. When treating a patient for smoking, it is important to treat for Vitamin A allergy and deficiency as well.

Because Vitamin A is retained in the body, it is important not to take excessively high doses that can build up to a toxic level. An allergy check should always be done before taking supplements.

I have treated many people, especially children, for Vitamin A. This allergy is significant in children who have chronic coughs, chronic infections involving the respiratory system, and asthma. Treating their Vitamin A allergy with NAET and giving them liquid Vitamin A with betacarotene has been helpful.

Food sources of Vitamin A include eggs, butter, fish, oils, and milk. Betacarotene is found in deep green vegetables such as spinach, broccoli, sweet potatoes, carrots, squash (especially winter squash), grapefruit, mangos, and apricots. These foods also contain large amounts of Vitamin C and other antioxidants. People with hypothyroidism have trouble converting betacarotene to Vitamin A and require regular intake of Vitamin A through food or supplements.

Vitamin F (Fatty Acids)

Essential fatty acids help build cell membranes, support the nervous system, and boost the immune system to help ward off disease. Fat also helps slow the release of sugar into the bloodstream and is especially important for those who are hypoglycemic or diabetic. Fat is needed for absorption of Vitamins A, D, K, and betacarotene.

Of all the fats we consume only two are essential. They are the omega-6 fatty acid (linolenic) and the omega-3 fatty acid (alpha linolenic). Eating junk food, including fat-free health store junk food, depletes the body's store of essential fatty acids. Fried foods, margarine, and vegetable shortening cause oils to become rancid and should be avoided.

Omega-6 can be found in all vegetable oils and most grains and beans. Omega-3 is found in flax seed, flax oil, fresh walnuts, walnut oil, pumpkin seeds, soy, and canola oils. It is important to buy oils that are not refined or rancid and to avoid buying oils sold in light glass bottles in supermarkets (look for the dark green bottles instead).

Because good fat metabolism is a key to proper use of essential fatty acids, I use enzyme therapy to ensure absorption of the good fatty acids from the regular diet. This works well in combination with NAET treatment for any allergy to fatty acids or the foods containing them.

Minerals

Minerals that may cause sensitivities include silver, gold, copper, vanadium, potassium, sulfur, copper, chromium, and magnesium. A deficiency of magnesium, the most important mineral for asthmatics, increases the amount of histamine released from cells, causing constriction of the bronchioles and triggering the onset of asthma. Magnesium is a specific smooth muscle relaxant and works magically to eliminate severe acute asthma attacks. It is also a natural laxative and therefore helpful for people with chronic constipation. Large doses are safe with many asthma medications.

A study from Great Britain tested over 2,500 adults with a chemical that can cause constricted airways in asthmatics. They found that people with low magnesium diets were twice as likely to have the reaction as those with high magnesium diets. Another study from France found that asthmatics have lower levels of magnesium in the tissues of their airways than people who do not have asthma. This study spurred further research into the anti-inflammatory properties of magnesium.

This study also prompted me to test asthmatics for allergies to magnesium and to foods high in magnesium such as seafood, whole grains, dark green vegetables, molasses, nuts, and bone meal. As it turns out, many asthmatics are allergic to magnesium and respond well to treatment for it. One asthmatic man with chronic sinus infections and respiratory problems came to see me. After treating for the first few basic allergens, I tested him for minerals and found an allergy to magnesium. When I treated him for this allergy and gave him supplements of 1,000 to 1,500 milligrams per day, he had far fewer asthma symptoms with infrequent reactions. He has not used an inhaler or any other medication for over two years. For infants and children, I supplement their diets with a liquid magnesium that is tolerated at about one teaspoon for twenty pounds of body weight. As with other supplements, I test the individual to find out how much supplement is needed.

Antioxidants

Antioxidants are known as free radical scavengers because they remove dangerous free radical particles from the tissues, strengthen the immune system, build up tissues, and regenerate the body. They are particularly important for anyone with a chronic illness. The basic antioxidants are Vitamins C and E, the B vitamins, fatty acids, and beta-carotene. New antioxidants are being discovered all the time including zinc, copper, selenium, N-acetylcystine (NAC), glutamine, and choline. I test and treat for each one of these because they are so important. Once people are cleared of sensitivities to antioxidants, they should be able to derive them easily from eating a good diet because antioxidants are plentiful in many foods.

One antioxidant worth discussing in greater detail is NAC, an amino acid and building block for glutathione, one of the most powerful free radical scavengers in the body. Glutathione helps the liver detoxify medications and is particularly helpful for asthmatics on large amounts of medication. The immune systems of many asthma patients have been compromised by large doses of chemicals such as cortisone and prednisone. They need help in detoxifying their immune system and building up their energy and stamina.

Selenium, a trace mineral, is another building block of glutathione and is important for detoxification. Selenium also helps Vitamin E prevent free radical damage.

Ginkgo is a traditional herb in Chinese medicine that can also be helpful to asthmatics.

ENZYME DEFICIENCIES

Through muscle testing, the palpation exam, and urinalysis I use for enzyme evaluation, I have found that many asthmatics are extremely deficient in amylase (refer to Chapter 13 for a more in-depth discussion). Because amylase is an important anti-inflammatory, people who are deficient cannot fight properly against environmental pollutants and allergens that cause irritation to the lungs and respiratory system. In combination with other enzymes, amylase is important in digesting carbohydrates. I have found that this deficiency is often linked to an allergy to amylase and to the enzyme amylopsin. Treating the allergies and then supplementing with the enzymes can be very helpful.

Protease is another enzyme that is critical in the treatment of asthma. It is important for digesting protein and as a natural antibiotic, anti-infectant, and anti-inflammatory agent. It can help fight pathogens, repair tissue damage, regenerate tissue, remove tissue debris, and break down foreign bodies that might be identified as allergens or pathogens by the immune system.

Much of the vulnerability to infections that asthmatics suffer is because of a deficiency of protease. I always test for it and then supplement with it in high doses once the allergy is cleared. Since those who are allergic to protease may experience upper gastrointestinal problems or pre-ulcerous gastritis, treating this allergy often resolves such problems.

Cortisone, a synthetic version of cortisol, is commonly used as an anti-inflammatory for asthmatics as well as for other chronic conditions such as Multiple Sclerosis (MS) and rheumatoid arthritis. People who are allergic to their own cortisol also may be allergic to cortisone, causing serious reactions. A study done on seventy-six patients treated with cortisone showed that cortisone therapy tended to cause an inability to digest carbohydrates that may have resulted from a deficiency of amylase. Cortisone can also causes a worsening of gastroduodenal ulcers, bleeding, and even perforation of the intestinal lining. Women over fifty tend to have reflux and gastritis and cortisone therapy can worsen these conditions.

Gastric problems can be helped with several enzymes including papain from papaya, lipase, and protease. Because people who have problems digesting proteins may be sensitive to protease, it can be helpful to treat for cortisone, protease, and food allergens.

Cortisone therapy also lessens the resistance of patients to infection that results in fever, malaise, chronic bronchitis, and sinusitis in asthmatics. Many asthmatics who have been on prednisone and cortical steroids or hydrocortisone therapy for some time are deficient in protease, a natural anti-inflammatory. Supplementing with protease helps them fight infections and deal with inflammation naturally. The enzyme inhibits inflammation without suppressing amino acids, as steroids do, and improves blood circulation and nutrition of the tissue.

Many people with chronic health problems such as fatigue, asthma, and rheumatoid arthritis do extremely well with enzyme therapy. The most noticeable results are with asthmatics who have problems with chronic infections. They generally come in with recurring bronchitis, always on antibiotics, never looking well, and never having enough energy. After enzyme therapy they are able to fight infections without using antibiotics and have far fewer asthma episodes than with steroid therapy. They are happier, feel and look better, and do not age as quickly.

One asthmatic patient of mine was traveling with a friend who showed signs of infection. The patient treated herself for her saliva with NAET using the acupressure points she had learned and increased her protease and antioxidant intake. She was able to resist the infection without using antibiotics which she had been unable to do before.

METABOLIC IMBALANCES

One of the primary causes of metabolic imbalance is the toxicity resulting from the body's inability to rid itself of metabolic waste products. This condition is worsened by incomplete oxidation in the tissues, poor nutrition, and the resulting chronic disease. The liver, the organ primarily responsible for the elimination of toxins, is severely stressed by prolonged treatment with cortisone, prednisone, antibiotics, inhalers, and other medications. Other organs responsible for detoxification include the skin, intestines, kidneys, and lungs.

Good blood and lymphatic circulation is also important for detoxification. The blood supplies oxygen and nutrients to the cells and cleanses, transports, and disposes of metabolic waste through excretion by means of the intestines, kidneys, lungs, and skin. In the lymphatic system, macrophages, the body's first line of defense against infection, travel around, eating up foreign substances and breaking them down into smaller, nontoxic components. Well-functioning macrophages are essential to the effective elimination of pathogens, metabolic waste, and toxins.

In a healthy immune system, the antibodies and lymphocytes are present in the blood and lymph and immediately recognize foreign cells such as bacteria, viruses, fungi, and toxic waste. They bind with these substances to form immune complexes that can be degraded and eaten up by the macrophages. When a small number of immune complexes are present, the macrophages can easily consume them before they do harm. But when an overabundance of immune complexes are present or the macrophages are inhibited by medications and metabolic waste, these complexes affix themselves to body tissue. This calls the secondary backup immune defenses into play that cause autoimmune inflammation and, ultimately, chronic degenerative disorders such as asthma, rheumatoid arthritis, or thyroid disease.

These immune complex diseases do not occur as long as macrophages retain their ability to function properly. Many metabolic toxins and addictive substances such as cocaine, morphine, steroids, and cortisone inhibit macrophage activity and thus contribute to immune complex disease. Certain enzyme mixtures are effective in removing and preventing immune complexes and keeping macrophage activity intact. Treatment of chronic degenerative disorders caused by circulating immune complexes with enzymes and NAET can result in improvement in appetite, reduction in depression, and decrease in inflammation.

To correct metabolic imbalances in asthmatics, it is important to facilitate the excretion and elimination of metabolic waste and toxins from the body. Asthmatics are often constipated, experience chronic loose stools, or fluctuate between the two. They may also suffer bloating and malabsorption. These problems are usually caused by sugar and starch intolerance and poor digestion. I use enzymes to treat this condition rather than more invasive therapies such as enemas or colonics.

In addition to facilitating proper intestinal elimination, I also ensure the kidneys are working properly. They can be stimulated by increasing liquid intake, using herbs such as horsetail and goldenrod, and prescribing enzymes for optimal kidney detoxification. The herbs are mild diuretics that stimulate kidney function. Exercise and diet are also important, as is the process of clearing food allergies and avoiding highly toxic food such as alcohol, caffeine, and excess salt.

The skin is an important organ of elimination and skin brushing is one method of helping the skin detoxify. Using a firm, hard vegetable brush, brush your skin vigorously for five minutes before you take a shower in the morning. Foods that can clog or toxify the skin are food allergens found in dairy products and highly fatty foods. Foods that help the skin with elimination are those high in enzymes and Vitamins A and E such as wheat germ oil and betacarotene.

The liver, the principle organ of detoxification, eliminates inhaled and ingested substances, toxic compounds, and drug by-products from the gastrointestinal organs. Allopathic physicians assess liver function with blood tests or a blood panel that evaluates the combination of liver enzymes appearing in the serum when hepatic tissue damage occurs. Many of these blood tests, however, only show abnormalities when there is liver injury or other physiological problems. Unfortunately, they do not detect toxification. To accurately detect dysfunction, we must inspect other areas for evaluation and diagnosis. There are certain laboratories that do assess liver dysfunction through a specialized "challenge test" to the liver. The test assesses an individual's functional capacity or hepatic detoxification ability. One laboratory doing this type of liver function test is Great Smokies Diagnostic Laboratory in North Carolina (refer to Miscellaneous Resources in Part VI).

Many factors contribute to liver toxification such as drug reactions, pesticides, hormones, inhaled toxic substances, food allergies, and genetic disposition. Genetically determined enzyme processes may vary and influence the individual's ability to detoxify. For example, risk for smoking induced cancer and other health problems depend in part on one's genetic detoxification system. Individuals who cannot adequately detoxify the hydrocarbons in cigarette smoke have increased risks for smoking induced cancers. Exposure to fat soluble toxins, pesticides, and alcohol may also increase the risk of liver damage by depleting important antioxidants and increasing oxidant induced damage. Oxygen free radicals play a significant role in the promotion and progression of liver diseases. Metabolites from gut bacteria as well as substances such as sulfites, naturally occurring compounds in foods that are used as food additives, can deter liver detoxification and contribute to liver damage.

By decreasing allergic response and improving digestion and immune function, NAET and enzyme therapy can help spare the liver unnecessary toxification.

In addition, there are many good liver detoxification programs utilizing supplements and nutrients such as the amino acids, Vitamin B_5 (pantothenic acid), certain hepatic coenzymes, glutathione, and sulfates to rid the liver of drugs, food additives, environmental pollutants, and steroid hormones. Recent studies have shown that people with chronic fatigue, fibromyalgia, multiple chemical sensitivities, and asthma suffer metabolic toxicity and imbalance and, therefore, benefit from such programs.

Liver and bowel detoxification programs are begun after the ten basic allergies and the infectant allergies are cleared. They usually last for two to three weeks, sometimes longer if necessary. For intensified detoxification, I complement the program with enzymes and dietary recommendations.

7 LITTLE-KNOWN CAUSES OF ASTHMA

In Chapters 5 and 6, I covered some of the most obvious causes of asthma. In this chapter I provide both practitioners and patients with insights into some of the less obvious causes of asthma. Some of the least researched allergens found in asthmatics are included in this chapter. These allergens were uncovered because of persistent study and research into asthma and asthmatic individuals. Patients suffering from asthma gave me the tools and their suffering gave me the motivation to find answers that would end their struggles. The findings outlined in this chapter are the results of years of clinical research treating patients for often unsuspected causes of asthma. Sometimes the results were dramatic: in a matter of twenty-four hours their lives were profoundly changed. Many of these results surprised me and gave me the drive to further explore potential new areas of allergies.

CONTACTANTS

Latex

One of the most common but largely unrecognized **contactants** is latex. Over the past five years latex has been used more frequently in a variety of professions. More than 100,000 health-care workers such as dentists, doctors, nurses, and laboratory technicians are exposed to latex on the job. People with high exposure to latex and a history of allergies are at risk for an allergic reaction as well as people who have frequent surgical procedures. Dermatitis and rashes may be irritated by latex exposure. Studies in the United States and Great Britain have found that the body produces specific antibodies to high levels of latex. Latex is used in hospitals and medical practices for such items as anesthetic tubing and ventilation bags.

The American College of Allergy, Asthma, and Immunology (ACAAI) has called for the protection of health-care workers and consumers who are said to use over seven million metric tons of latex every year in such items as balloons, condoms, tires, waist bands, rubber toys, bottle nipples, and pacifiers. The ACAAI wants immediate implementation of FDA regulations that would require labeling of latex, banning the "hypoallergenic" label on some latex gloves, and regulating maximum amounts of extractable allergen in latex products. The organization also recommends improved testing for the allergy, the identification of nonallergenic forms of latex, "latex safe" zones in workplaces, and research into the cause of latex allergies.

NAET offers an alternative approach. I have treated many people successfully for serious latex allergies. Many of them were able to continue using latex in their jobs for their protection and the protection of their clients. One patient was a nurse practitioner who had to wear latex all the time which exacerbated her asthma. Since her treatment with NAET, she has been able to wear latex on the job without any problems. Many dentists I see also wear latex gloves all day. Most sensitive people who wear latex for prolonged periods of time will develop an allergy to it. NAET can provide a way to deal with this new and growing problem.

Formaldehyde

Some contactants also identified as inhalants include formaldehyde, hair spray, bug sprays, clothing labels, nail chemicals, and hair chemicals. Formaldehyde is extremely widespread and probably one of the worst triggers for asthmatics. It is found in new fabrics, the dye on clothing tags, pressed wood, Wite•Out®, plastics, finishing materials, leather goods, decaffeinated coffee, ice cream, embalming fluid, plaster, concrete, antiperspirant, antiseptics in mouth washes, germicidal and detergent soap, hair products, aerosol deodorant, tanning agents, and the like.

Although formaldehyde is used in the formation of slow-release nitrogen fertilizer, it can also be responsible for plant disease. Because it kills bacteria, fungi, mold, and yeast it is used to disinfect equipment used in fermentation processes and in the manufacture of antibiotics. It is used in the synthesis of explosives as well as the synthesis of Vitamin A and to improve the activity of Vitamin E preparations. Formaldehyde improves the strength and water-resistance of paper products and is a preservative and accelerator for photographic developing solutions. It is sometimes used in the manufacture of both synthetic and natural fabrics, making them crease-resistant, wrinkle-resistant, crush-proof, water-repellent, dye-fast, flame-resistant, water-resistant, shrink-proof, moth-proof, and elastic.

Chemicals

Many other chemicals act as contact allergens and more are found to be problems every year. The following is a list of contact chemicals used in a wide variety of cleaning, makeup, and fabric products that I have found to be particularly problematic for asthmatics:

- acetone in nail polish remover

- methanol

- benzyl alcohol
- ethylene oxide
- butter yellow
- estradiol benzoate-8
- Congo red
- sulfa-urea
- carbon tetrachloride used for dry cleaning
- trichloroethylene
- chromium oxide
- benzinum crudum
- mangan peroxydatum
- plumbum bromatum
- plumbum sulfuricum
- polyester
- dimethyl terephthalate
- ethylene glycol
- isopropyl glycol found in many cosmetics and deodorant sprays
- paraffinum
- laundry detergent
- hydrazine sulfate
- toluene
- xylene
- asbestos
- tipa white

- benzanthracene

- cyclohexanol

- amyl alcohol

Fabrics and Dyes

It is important to treat asthmatics for fabrics because any fabric, natural or synthetic, can cause a reaction. I have treated people for reactions to cotton, linen, silk, wool, rayon, nylon, acetate, acrylic, polyester, jute, and kapok. One woman always wore linen. Whenever I did NAET treatments, I could never get a strong muscle response in the testing. It turned out she was allergic to linen and wearing it weakened her. Another woman was allergic to virtually every fabric. We had to treat her lying almost naked, making sure that there was no fabric near her hand when we were muscle testing. Leather can also be a problem, particularly for those allergic to animal dander or tannic acid. A tannic acid allergy can also cause a reaction to tea. I have seen miraculous results from treating for fabrics, sometimes within the first twenty-four hours. One person's smelling and tasting abilities are restored. Another's long-term eczema subsides and yet another client feels more focused and energetic. Itching, dry skin, and chronic ailments can all decrease dramatically or disappear. Treating for the dyes in fabrics is also important in desensitizing people to clothing, wallpaper, mattresses, bedding, and towels.

Several years ago I bought my daughter a bed sheet decorated with Disney characters. Every time she slept on it she would get stuffed up and cough. I found that she was allergic to the dyes in the fabric as well as to the polyester fabric itself. Once she was cleared for these allergens she could sleep on the sheet without any problems. Some of the most important fabric dyes to treat are:

- aniline, the blue-black dye used in newsprint

- anthracene, used in the manufacture of most dye products and fixed with formaldehyde

- anthraquinone, a commercial vat dye

- benzene, used in dye manufacturing

- bromine, used in organic dyes

- chromium oxydatum, a dye used in tannin and in the ink on dollar bills.

Wood

Wood resin is another contactant that should be checked if a person has a lot of exposure to it. I have seen people allergic to wood in musical instruments (a violin bow, piano keys, the wood of a harp) as well as the finishing of the wood itself. Dr. Nambudripad tells of treating one asthmatic for an allergy to bamboo (cane) furniture with very positive results.

Daily Contactants

Contactants also include common household products such as cosmetics, soaps, skin creams, detergents, metal polishes, hair dyes, rubber gloves, acrylic nails, nail polish and remover, metals (silver, nickel, and gold) in jewelry or flatware, gasoline products, celluloid, flowers, and bulbs. Many people are also allergic to computers, computer keyboards, telephones, vinyl chairs, plastic or carton containers, and other disposable products. I have seen women allergic to their panty hose, and people allergic to toilet paper and paper towels. Silicone, found in glass doors, breast implants, and the newest organic fabrics causes allergic reactions in some people. Then there are the less obvious occupational allergens which fall into the contactant group. For example, printers are often allergic to a fine lacquer spray used for drying ink to keep it from smudging.

Allergy to an Individual's Energy Field

Literally anything or anyone, no matter how benign or unlikely, can be an allergen. Surprisingly, we can even be allergic to people: our spouses, children, or parents. I found it hard to believe at first that a mother could be allergic to her own child, or vice versa, or that a man could be allergic to his spouse. It does, however, happen. I have treated many siblings, mothers, and fathers for allergies to their loved ones, and each time there have been dramatic changes. It may be easier to understand when we consider that everything and everyone has its own electromagnetic energy field. One cannot underestimate how severe an allergy can be to another person or the symptoms it can cause. I have seen symptoms such as irritability, constant bitterness, anger, fear, and an inability to be affectionate all respond to treatment. Sometimes being a good detective can transform people's lives and relationships.

Miscellaneous Contactants

Other contactants include plant oils found in plants such as poison oak, poison ivy, asparagus fern, and eucalyptus. Synthetic contactants include adhesive tape, cement, paper products, crude oil, plastics, newsprint, and photocopy paper and materials. I remember one asthmatic who started coughing each time she read a magazine in my office. She was allergic to the ink. When she was treated with NAET, she no longer coughed when she read a newspaper or magazine. I have also treated many people who were allergic to the plastic or other materials in their eyeglasses or contact lenses.

HISTAMINE

Histamine, actually a phenolic, is a very important allergen that plays a major role in all allergy reactions. Histamine is a major neurotransmitter in the brain, particularly in the hippocampus, and throughout the nervous system. It can also stimulate the secretion of hydrochloric acid in the stomach. Studies indicate that about twenty percent of schizophrenics have high levels of histamine whereas rheumatoid arthritics and Parkinson's patients have low levels.

All allergic individuals, especially asthmatics, have high levels of IgE antibodies. When an allergen such as dust reacts with an IgE antibody, an allergen-antibody reaction takes place and the individual experiences an allergic reaction. IgE antibodies attach to mast cells and basophiles, causing them to rupture and release histamine. Increased levels of histamine cause the dilation of blood vessels and the contraction of smooth muscle cells. A number of different abnormal symptoms occur, depending on the type of tissue in which the histamine is released. Asthma symptoms are one reaction. An allergy to histamine greatly intensifies reactions to other allergens.

Besides asthma symptoms, a sensitivity to histamine can cause depression, fatigue, hay fever, hyperactivity, hypertension, night sweats, premenstrual syndrome (PMS), sinusitis, stomach pain, and vertigo. Histamine is found in wine, beer, oysters, perch, salmon, scallops, shrimp, trout, tuna fish, cod fish, flounder, halibut, haddock, lobster, black bass, catfish, crab meat, yeast mix, human milk, cow and goat milk, cocoa, mutton, ham, chicken, and turkey.

I always check asthmatics whose allergies are especially active as well as those with severe eczema or skin reaction for a sensitivity to histamine. I have found this treatment to be highly successful and have seen remarkable changes.

GLANDS AND HORMONES

Many positive results have been obtained by treating asthma sufferers for adrenal and thyroid hormones as well as for the glands themselves. If people are allergic or sensitive to their own hormones, they develop a deficiency because they cannot properly absorb them into their tissues. I also have good success increasing energy and restoring good respiratory function by treating for epinephrine, norepinephrine, and adrenaline.

Adrenal Glands

The adrenal glands lie above the kidneys and are composed of the adrenal medulla and the adrenal cortex. The adrenal medulla secretes adrenaline and norepinephrine and the adrenal cortex secretes corticoid steroids, glycol corticoids, and androgens.

When tissue is damaged by trauma, infection, allergy, or by some other means, it becomes inflamed. In some circumstances the inflammation is more damaging than the trauma or infection itself. The body naturally produces cortisol to reduce all aspects of the inflammatory process by blocking the inflammatory response. It is very important that the adrenal glands function normally and are able to secrete cortisol in a natural form, especially in asthmatics. If artificial sources such as cortisone, prednisone, methylprednisone, or dexamethasone are taken for prolonged periods to remedy a shortage of cortisol, they actually shrink the adrenal glands which, in turn, produce less cortisol. These artificial sources of cortisol also suppress the immune system. This suppression causes reduced numbers of **lymphocytes**, T cells, and antibodies that not only increases the incidence of allergies, but also makes a person more susceptible to infections and chronic health problems.

In my practice, every allergic individual is tested and treated for their own adrenal hormones. Asthmatics always report positive improvement in their health after this treatment. They feel more energetic, less sensitive to their surroundings, and less in need of their steroids and other drugs.

Thyroid Gland

The thyroid, a gland located immediately below the larynx in front of the trachea (windpipe), secretes the hormones thyroxine (ninety percent) and triiodothyronine (ten percent), respectively referred to as T_4 and T_3, that increase the individual's metabolic rate. The thyroid stimulates all aspects of carbohydrate metabolism and enhances the metabolism of fats. Both the heart rate and blood volume can be influenced by the thyroid. Because most thyroxine is eventually converted to T_3 in the liver and other tissues of the body, a healthy liver is essential for thyroid production and function. The thyroid also secretes calcitonin, an important hormone for calcium metabolism. When the rate of thyroid hormone production increases, most endocrine gland secretions increase as well including the production of adrenal corticoid. In treating asthma, it is important to note that the thyroid also increases the rate of oxygen utilization, thereby increasing the rate and depth of respiration. The thyroid has many other effects on the body as well.

Unfortunately, many people are allergic to their own thyroid gland or thyroid hormones. Because this problem might or might not show up in a blood test, I use the thyroid basal metabolic rate axillary test to evaluate thyroid function. The test measures the metabolic rate by using a thermometer in the armpit immediately after waking up in the morning and before getting out of bed. The temperature is taken for ten minutes. A temperature of 97.7 or below is indicative of low thyroid function (hypothyroidism). Eighty percent of the women I see are hypothyroid, although most are unaware of it. Symptoms include dry skin, cold hands and feet, tiredness, insomnia, eczema, overweight or underweight, sluggishness, hair loss, and poor memory.

If people are secreting enough T_4 but are allergic to their own hormone, they might not be utilizing it and can be as hypothyroid as those with low thyroid function. This may also be the case if there is a problem converting T_4 to T_3 (liver dysfunction). Those individuals show the same symptoms of hypothyroidism but the condition is not likely to show up in blood tests. I have found the basal body temperature test and muscle testing to be accurate in diagnosing both low thyroid function and an allergy to the thyroid and its hormones.

Lymph Glands

One gland that sometimes affects asthmatics is the lymph gland. The lymphatic system provides an ancillary route for fluids to flow from the interstitial spaces into the blood. The lymph glands also carry proteins and other metabolites too large to be absorbed directly into the blood away from the tissues. This process is essential for survival. The lymphatic system helps drain the lungs from the connective tissues surrounding the terminal bronchioles and the lung. If the lymphatic channels are not working properly, there is a buildup of toxicity in the body and an overload of the lymphatic system. If the lungs are not drained, an asthmatic reaction can be provoked.

Salivary Glands

Another problem area is in the salivary glands, important because they are involved in producing mucus and digestive enzymes. The principal glands of salivation are the parotid glands, the submaxillary glands, the sublingual glands, and the buccal glands. Saliva contains two major types of protein secretion: (1) a serous secretion called ptyalin, an enzyme for digesting starches that is found in amylase; and (2) a mucus secretion called mucin for lubrication. The parotid glands secrete the serous type of protein and the submandibular and sublingual glands secrete both the serous type and the mucus type. The buccal glands secrete only mucus.

Parasympathetic nervous pathways, particularly those from the salivary nuclei, regulate the salivary secretions. Salivation can be stimulated or inhibited by impulses arriving in the salivary nuclei from higher centers of the central nervous system. For example, when a person smells or eats favorite foods, salivation occurs. The reaction is even stronger when the person smells food that he or she dislikes. The appetite area of the brain that partially regulates these effects is located in close proximity to the parasympathetic centers of the anterior hypothalamus. It responds to a great extent to signals from the taste and smell areas of our brains.

Salivation also occurs in response to reflexes originating in the stomach and upper intestines, particularly when a very irritating food is swallowed or when a person is nauseated because of some gastrointestinal abnormality. The saliva, when swallowed, helps remove the irritation in the GI tract by neutralizing the offending substances. Salivation can also be affected by the sympathetic nervous system, for example, during "fight or flight"—although less than by the parasympathetic system—and by the blood supply to the salivary glands because secretion requires proper nutrition of the tissue.

When there is a sensitivity or an allergic reaction to the salivary glands, there is either a marked increase or decrease in salivation. I most often see an increase, with increased mucus secretion, creating a breeding ground for bacteria and other pathogens. The increase in salivation also overstimulates the bronchioles and **respiratory system**, causing irritation and triggering possible asthma attacks. I had one female patient who was bothered by many allergens and suffered from excessive amounts of mucus and chronic infections, coughing, and wheezing. She often needed to use her inhaler. After I treated her for the thyroid, submandibular, and sublingual glands, in that order, her mucus production diminished, her coughing decreased, and her bronchioles and lungs felt freer.

Hormones

Some people are allergic to the female hormones estrogen and progesterone, the male hormone testosterone, and dehydroepiandrosterone (DHEA), an adrenal hormone. I have found reactions to insulin, androgen, and hormones related to the kidneys and their function.

An allergy to progesterone produces symptoms ranging from premenstrual syndrome, breast tenderness, bloating, and depression to irritability prior to the start of a period. People with estrogen sensitivities are more prone to uterine fibroids, ovarian cysts, endometriosis, fibrocystic breasts, painful periods, and migraines at the start and end of periods. Many women are allergic to both hormones. Menopausal symptoms can also be brought on by an allergy to one or both hormones.

Treating for hormone sensitivities can be particularly effective for women who developed asthma later in life. One study found that women who have taken estrogen for ten years or more were twice as likely to develop asthma as women who have never taken the hormone. Another study looked at 90,000 women with past or current estrogen use and found that it doubled the chances of developing asthma. A third study of postmenopausal registered nurses over a ten-year period found that taking estrogen, with or without progesterone, increased the risk of developing asthma. The higher the dose, the higher the risk of asthma. These research findings suggest that women who are considering hormone replacement therapy should check their sensitivity to these hormones to prevent late-onset asthma.

When I find patients allergic to their hormones, thyroid, or adrenal glands, I treat them with NAET and give them several supplements to take for a period of time to support glandular function. For thyroid, I use high-mineral supplements containing potassium and magnesium. If I find a sensitivity to the thyroid, I also treat for iodine, vegetable and animal fat, mercury and amalgam, tyrosine and tryptophan (amino acids), the thyroid-stimulating hormones secreted by the pituitary, the adrenal glands, and adrenal hormones, especially cortisone. For the adrenal glands, I supplement with certain B and C vitamins.

Menstrual Period and Pregnancy

Hormones that increase during the premenstrual and menstrual periods and during pregnancy can trigger asthma attacks in women who are allergic to their own hormones. If the asthma happens premenstrually or in pregnancy the trigger is usually progesterone. Postmenstrually there are higher levels of estrogen.

One patient of mine had PMS with migraines, increased asthma symptoms, and irritability. When I treated her for progesterone, both her headaches and her asthma symptoms decreased immediately. We have noticed that treating women for hormones is often effective in dealing with migraines. In men the cause tends to be coffee, caffeine, or chocolate.

Women react to thyroid hormone levels during different points of the menstrual cycle. Treating for allergies to the thyroid and thyroid hormones is often helpful in balancing and regulating the menstrual cycle. After clearing for progesterone, I recommend natural progesterone oils (taken orally) or creams (used topically) made from yams and soybeans to increase progesterone levels. When people are allergic to progesterone they are usually deficient, and supplementation is often necessary.

Adrenal hormones can also be treated with NAET for sensitivities and enzyme therapy for supplementation. These hormones are important to women both premenopausally and postmenopausally. The enzymes and NAET treatment are completely safe during pregnancy and can benefit both the woman and her child.

ORGANS

Many people, particularly asthmatics, have allergies to their own organs (also thought of as weaknesses in those organs). For example, asthmatics may react to their own bronchi, lungs, sinuses, or to glands such as the thyroid, adrenals, parotid, or lymph. An asthmatic may be sensitive to the large intestines (colon), spleen, kidney, or liver involved in functions of digestion, elimination, and cleansing. The liver is particularly important to treat with NAET in order to support its function of cleansing and detoxifying the body. This, in turn, keeps the body functioning optimally by supplying scavengers to eat up free radicals.

Suzanne, a woman in her fifties and an asthmatic, had been undergoing NAET treatments and enzyme therapy for three months. After a course of treatments, she mentioned that she was doing quite well but noticed she would wheeze during bowel movements. I decided to test and treat her for an allergy to her large intestines (colon). As the treatment was clearing over twenty-five hours, she called to tell me she was doing well. One week later, she came to see me with a very tight chest and laryngitis. She explained the week's scenario. Things had improved dramatically. Two days ago, however, she felt she was getting sick and considered getting antibiotics. She mentioned she felt nauseous and also looked very pale that day. I said, "Before you do this, let's test you for large intestines to see if you held the treatment or if there is a combination with something else." Not to my surprise, I found an emotional combination. I am always suspicious of this when a person has dramatic symptoms such as severe nausea, wheezing, dizziness, tiredness, and the like. I treated her for two emotional incidences in her life, one of which pertained to her father's death from colon cancer. It was no surprise that such an emotional incident showed up with this treatment. She left that day slightly improved. I talked to her husband the next day, and immediately asked how Suzanne was feeling. He said, "Great! No problem!" I encounter this type of scenario regularly in my practice. Often an organ treatment will have a profound effect on an asthmatic. It is very important to make sure all the emotions have been cleared.

I check to see if there is a weakness or a sensitivity to the lung and bronchial tissues of all asthmatics. When these tissues are normal and healthy, air flows easily through the respiratory passageways. When there is a sensitivity to these tissues, the flow is reduced, often in the smaller bronchioles. Here the narrowness and the presence of smooth muscles makes the flow of air difficult.

The bronchial system is exposed to circulating norepinephrine and **epinephrine** hormones released into the blood by sympathetic stimulation of the adrenal medulla. Both of these hormones cause dilation of the bronchial passageways by stimulation of the beta receptors. A sensitivity to the adrenals or an allergy to the adrenal hormones restrict the secretion of these hormones, thereby reducing air flow in the bronchial system.

The sinuses are another area to check. Most asthmatics have sinus congestion or related sinus problems. Treating for the sinuses themselves often helps open the sinus passageways and allows easier breathing.

CHIROPRACTIC MISALIGNMENTS AND MYOFASCITIS

When I first began to practice chiropractic care, I treated a young man who had suffered from asthma his whole life. He complained of chronic stiffness and spasms in his upper back and neck. When I examined him, I found some spinal misalignments at the thoracic level (T1-7) with extreme mild fascitis (inflamed soft tissue). Because the nerves from these particular vertebrae innervate the lungs and heart area, I thought that relaxing the muscles in the area, increasing his flexibility, and aligning the vertebrae might help his respiration. I was right. After a series of treatments, his asthma improved so much that he no longer required any medication or treatment. Over the years I have had positive results with chiropractic care for asthma and other lung-related problems. There are certain points on the spine where tapping with the fingers or certain tools open up the bronchioles and relieve an asthma attack. (refer to the section on Spondylotherapy in Part VI).

In a recent study, children with asthma showed an overall improvement in lung capacity after only fifteen chiropractic adjustments. There is ample research documenting the intimate connection between the spinal column, the nervous system, and the respiratory system. It has also been shown that vertebral subluxation in the neck and upper back produces muscle spasms that cause lymphatic congestion. With the lymph system unable to dispose of bacteria, debris, and other foreign materials, toxins accumulate in the area. In many cases, chiropractic adjustments produce immediate relaxation of the neck and back muscles, thereby increasing lymphatic drainage, improving respiratory function, helping cleanse the body, and improving immunity.

The chiropractic approach to health care is safe and natural and benefits children and adults of all ages. I recommend that all my asthma patients undergo chiropractic care at the same time they are being treated for allergy elimination. I see quicker results with those patients who use both approaches.

EMOTIONS AND STRESS

Is asthma caused or affected by emotions? Absolutely. One female asthmatic I treated was free of symptoms after she divorced her husband. A man's asthma symptoms disappeared when his father died of cancer after a long and painful illness. Another patient stopped having asthma attacks after being treated for sorrow related to an incident with her mother that happened almost thirty years before.

Over the years I have developed a deep respect for our emotions and the power of dramatic events in our lives. Many people suffering from migraines, digestive problems, chronic fatigue, or joint problems should do emotional clearing. Every asthmatic I have treated has needed to clear certain emotional blockages in the path to healing and regeneration. Problems or symptom complexes inevitably involve unresolved emotions.

Fortunately, emotional clearing is possible with NAET. NAET unlocks the energy around traumas and helps to clear it from the body so it will not continue to create energy blockages and health problems. Many emotional blockages are easily cleared or worked through during treatment of the basic allergies but some traumas and repressed emotions need to be confronted, felt, and then released from the body and nervous system. These emotions can be connected to food cravings, eating disorders, and environmental factors, as well as to family members, friends, and loved ones. The emotions can be related to love, intimacy, finances, health, physical or emotional abuse, rape, or molestation. They might be rooted in specific incidents such as death of a loved one or divorce. They can also arise from a recurring pattern of events such as fighting at the dinner table, financial stress, marital difficulties, or repeated abuse. Minor, seemingly petty incidents in childhood can create serious allergies or blockages in the energy pathways that act as triggers for asthmatics. In Chinese medicine, sorrow is related to the lungs. It is no surprise, therefore, that sorrow is a common emotion found among asthmatics or that asthmatics respond dramatically to treatments for it.

To treat emotional blocks with NAET, we first use muscle or reflex testing to find out how old the patient was when the block first appeared and what other person, if any, was involved: a family member, lover, friend, or business partner. Next we check to see what kind of relationship was involved—intimate, financial, health, business, or spiritual. The last and most important factor is the emotion involved: fear, terror, anger, rage, worry, sorrow, despair, frustration, guilt, abandonment, hopelessness, resentment, disappointment, or joy. Once we have all this information we treat with NAET to clear the obstructions caused by the incidents and emotions identified.

These emotions are often the primary cause of asthma attacks. I have seen children with chronic coughs immediately stop coughing after releasing an emotion related to an incident with their mother or father. I have also worked with my daughter and other children on biting their nails. When they released certain emotions related to their parents, the nail biting stopped.

One little girl had a rough time being weaned. Several months after I treated her for allergies to mother's milk and to emotions about nursing, she weaned herself naturally with no emotional upset and no pressure from her parents. A boy who was having trouble with his writing turned out to be afraid of his teacher. When we treated him for his fear, his problems disappeared. And a man with chronic bloating, indigestion, and fatigue was discovered to have unresolved shame in relation to his parents. Within days of being treated, the symptoms disappeared.

Never underestimate the power of emotions or the seriousness of the illnesses they can produce. Many food allergies are the result of emotional experiences with food. If people eat when they are angry, for example, they may develop an allergy to foods eaten at that time. I always tell my patients, "Please don't eat when you're upset, and please don't argue during a meal." Even positive emotions of elation can create allergies. A meal is a sacred event and should be peaceful, similar to meditation. Leave any discussion of intense issues until after the meal is finished.

People often ask me to have lunch with them but I always take a rain check. To avoid creating allergies through emotional situations or discussions during a meal, I prefer to eat at home in a quiet, soothing surrounding. Many of my meals at home as a youngster were emotionally charged. No wonder I had poor digestion and extensive food allergies for most of my life. Now I insist on eating with serenity and awareness, and I recommend that my patients do the same.

I have begun to experiment with referring patients to therapists who use hypnotic techniques such as **eye movement desensitization and reprocessing (EMDR)** to help reveal and release emotional traumas that have an impact on illnesses such as eating disorders and asthma (refer to Part VI for a full explanation of EMDR). I have recommended this technique to patients who seem to have emotional blockages and need help uncovering or processing them. I find that the EMDR technique is sometimes sufficient to release the energy block. At other times I have to treat with NAET as well.

One woman patient with severe food cravings constantly thought about food, ate constantly, and continually gained weight. After she was treated for many of the basic allergies and some of her main food allergies, her cravings dropped off dramatically, but she was still obsessed with food. Nothing we treated seemed to help. There seemed to be many incidents from the past related to her mother, who had been continually ill when my patient was a child. I decided to refer her to a therapist for EMDR and after the treatment, the food cravings decreased significantly. She lost about thirty pounds almost immediately, her energy picked up, and she reported that she felt freer in her everyday life.

Stress is another important factor in the incidence of asthma. I believe that if people have good health, a strong immune system, an adequately functioning liver, and good digestion, they will not be physically vulnerable to the stresses they encounter every day of their lives. If, however, they have many hidden allergies, poor diges- tion, poor eating habits, poor immune function, high lev- els of immune complexes, and liver toxicity, they will be susceptible to stress that adds just one more strain to an already overburdened system and increases the likeli- hood of illness including asthma. The best way to man- age stress and avoid the physical consequences that often ensue is to strengthen the immune system and overall health.

Stress affects people of all ages, including infants, children, and the elderly. Whether the stress comes from being weaned from the breast, learning to write in school, or going through difficult life changes, everyone needs to strengthen the immune system to help the body resist the effects of stress. This is my goal for each individual and I find that enzyme therapy, allergy elimination, proper diet, exercise, and the maintenance of spiritual and mental good health are all important factors.

8 | TROUBLESHOOTING AND PREVENTIVE MEASURES

Many people with asthma do not know what causes the disease or triggers their attacks. They may be fine for a period of days, weeks, or even months and then suddenly, within hours, they begin to feel a tightness and heaviness in their chest, experience difficulty breathing, and start coughing or wheezing. Sometimes they must go to a hospital emergency room for treatment with steroids. "I know it's probably related to allergies," they tell me, "but I'm not sure which allergies are the worst. What can I do? How can I know why my body is reacting the way it is? How can I eliminate the allergies that are the most severe and causing the most irritation to my lungs?"

DIAGNOSTIC ENZYME EVALUATION

When a person first comes to see me, I do some preliminary work to help find an answer to these questions. One test is a diagnostic enzyme evaluation that includes an abdominal palpation and a twenty-four-hour urinalysis. I ask them to keep a diary of their asthma symptoms, a detailed daily diet, the supplements they take, and so on. With this information I can begin my detective work.

For example, if the urinalysis indicates they are low in calcium, they are probably allergic to calcium. This means they should avoid foods high in calcium until they are treated for it. The same is true for imbalances of sugar, sodium chloride, electrolytes, or minerals. I may find indications of various allergies that are having a major impact or creating inflammation in the body. When I point these out, patients can note in their diaries whether eating dairy products increases mucus or symptoms such as sinus congestion that are precursors of an asthma episode. They can also determine whether their allergies are mainly to food, environmental toxins, or both.

Clearing the basic allergies with NAET often eliminates many other allergies as well, significantly reducing the asthmatic's need for medication. At this point it becomes easier to spot additional allergens that are causing trouble. One woman who came to see me had asthma her entire life. There were times when she was fine, times when she had attacks, and times when her attacks were life threatening and she ended up in the hospital. "Why does this happen?" she wanted to know. "What is the real cause of my asthma? I know it's allergy related, but what allergies are the cause? Is it environmental? I'm a gardener and I'm outside all the time. Is it the flowers, the food, my house, mold, smoke? Sometimes these things bother me and sometimes they seem to be OK. I'm confused."

I began by doing my routine evaluation. On the abdominal diagnostic exam I found inflammation around the liver and gallbladder area. This usually means there is toxicity resulting from the burden of too many allergens on the immune system. She suffered from sinusitis and chronic sinus congestion, and I noticed indications of Candida and other fungi as well as an inability to digest or absorb sugars. She also had a very weak adrenal function. The adrenal gland is intimately involved with inflammation, metabolism of sugars, and the regulation of energy levels in the body. I also noted that she was slightly constipated. After doing the urinalysis and reviewing her diet, we came up with an understanding of her situation. She was sugar intolerant, and her consumption of large amounts of sugar was weakening and compromising her immune system. I recommended a diet with far fewer carbohydrates than the diet she was accustomed to following (refer to the diet section of Part VI).

I gave her enzymes to digest sugars, relieve nasal congestion, support the liver, and decrease toxicity. Through muscle testing I found that she had many of the basic allergies, including several food allergies. Her most severe allergies, however, were to environmental substances such as pollen, dust, mold, smuts, rust, grains, grain dust, rugs, paints, smoke, perfumes, and other inhalants. Her urinalysis showed a sluggish kidney that usually indicates a congested lymph system resulting from an overwhelmed immune system. There was also a reduced sediment level of sugars, confirming that her absorption and digestion of sugars was poor.

KEEPING A DIARY

After embarking on a low sugar diet, she kept a diary to record what she ate, what she was feeling each day, and what allergic symptoms she was experiencing. We treated for the basic allergies and then for the environmental allergies that were not eliminated when the basic allergies cleared. After this initial clearing, her symptoms were greatly reduced and she became much more aware of her sensitivities. She realized there were certain foods that caused congestion and coughing, certain environmental factors that caused wheezing and tightness, and

certain fungi and contactants that created sinus congestion. Through self-diagnosis muscle testing, she was able
to ascertain what particular infectants were the most important to treat and clear. We progressed well with the
treatments and managed to clear her essential allergies.
Today she is doing extremely well and rarely has an
asthma episode.

It is always important that both the patient and I act
as detectives. From long experience working with asthma
patients I can usually determine which allergies are the
most serious for a particular patient. I must know what
they are digesting and not digesting, absorbing and not
absorbing, and what they are deficient in so I can make
adjustments. And they must become more aware of what
they are bombarded with everyday and which substances
provoke reactions.

Most patients, even children, become excellent detectives. They say, "I know that it was the food additive I
ate that triggered the asthma," or "I know it was pollen,
or chocolate, or perfume, or something in my room."
They get to know their own bodies and I listen to what
they tell me.

SUGAR AND CARBOHYDRATES

Since most asthmatics are sugar intolerant, I usually recommend a reduction in their intake of sugars and carbohydrates. For those who are not, I make dietary
recommendations specific to their needs. Dairy products
are highly mucus forming, as are foods such as apple
juice, bananas, and chocolate and I immediately suggest
avoiding them until they are cleared. Later, I sometimes
add them back to the diet slowly. Both pesticides and hormones cause problems for asthmatics and I recommend
organically grown fruits, vegetables, and grains and organically raised, hormone-free meats as much as possible.

Pesticides, nitrates, food additives, and hormones often can be found in red meat, chicken, and other poultry and should be avoided whenever possible. It is important for asthmatics to learn the foods to which they are sensitive and to avoid them or treat for them.

One patient who came to see me from out of town had improved so much over a year of treatments that she could do without her medication for months at a time. Then, when out at a restaurant, she inadvertently ate a dish containing foods we had not treated her for and she had such a severe reaction that she had to use her inhaler. Asthmatics should know what they are eating, where it comes from, how it is cooked, and with what it is cooked. Otherwise, cooking at home from scratch is probably the safest approach until most allergens are cleared.

SUPPLEMENTS

For dietary supplementation I recommend enzymes with some vitamins and minerals. Of course, I always check to make sure people are not allergic to a supplement before I give it to them. Different brands of supplements have different fillers in them, and people need to be checked for each one before taking it. When people first come to see me, they bring all their supplements and I check them for each one. After I clear any allergies to vitamins and minerals, I supplement with these nutrients, in combination with enzymes that enhance their absorption, in order to make up for deficiencies that may have resulted from the allergies.

For example, an allergy to calcium usually indicates a deficiency of calcium, revealed in the urinalysis and abdominal palpation. After we treat for the allergy, I recommend a calcium supplement with enzymes to help the body absorb calcium from foods. Before they take it, I test to see how much supplementation they need and if they are allergic to a specific brand.

An asthmatic named Patti came to me after working with another practitioner who recommended about twenty different vitamins and supplements. Patti noticed that after taking these supplements she had to go back on her asthma medication. When she came to me, she had been on the medication for some time. I immediately tested her for the supplements and found she was allergic to all but one of them. When she stopped taking them she was able to discontinue her medication almost immediately, and she was free of symptoms for some time. This improvement occurred without even the most basic allergy treatments.

When patients are taking allergy medications, I work with their physicians whenever possible. I do not prescribe or take people off medications. I do prescribe enzymes, nutritional supplements, and cleansers and I help people manage their allergies to prevent attacks. Doctor and patient need to decide how much, if any, medication is needed.

MANAGING ALLERGIES

An allergy management plan defines the goals for getting asthma under control. These goals include normal function of the airways and the ability to participate in physical or social activities without respiratory difficulty. They should also include sleeping through the night, no hospitalization, no emergency room visits or unscheduled visits to the physician, and no fear about what to do when breathing problems occur. The plan should incorporate a list of medications and why they are needed. Once a physician has approved of the plan, it should be kept in a place where it can be referred to often. Management plans may change as asthmatics grow older, or according to changes in the environment, seasons, and so on. As allergies are eliminated and controlled, the management plan changes. In formulating and adapting this plan, it is helpful for the NAET practitioner to work in conjunction with a physician who specializes in asthma.

There are several questions that all asthmatics should be able to answer:

1. Do you have an asthma or allergy management plan?

2. Is it written down and do you understand it?

3. Do you know how to recognize and respond to an asthma episode?

4. Do you know how to recognize and respond to an asthma emergency?

5. Do you know what to do when recovering from an asthma or allergy episode?

6. When you are feeling better, should you continue taking medications?

7. Do you know how to keep an asthma episode from recurring?

Asthma sufferers must educate themselves about allergy medications and the different kinds of asthma symptoms. These symptoms can be divided into noisy and quiet types. The noisy symptoms—wheezing, shortness of breath, tightness, coughing—are easily recognized. The quiet symptom, compensatory breathing, is often not recognized as a precursor to the noisy symptoms. Often the body's compensation for breathing problems is so effective that the person does not realize the problem is a precursor to an asthma attack.

Some people delay treating the quiet symptom and hope it will go away. But immediate treatment can often prevent the onset of more serious symptoms. For this reason, it is important that asthmatics become attuned to changes in their breathing. The peak flow meter is an inexpensive, handheld tool that measures the maximum speed with which air is forced out of the lungs. It can be invaluable for an asthmatic because a reduced peak flow rate, which occurs when the bronchial tubes are blocked, indicates a worsening condition. This instrument is particularly helpful with children who are not yet able to identify mild asthma symptoms. A stethoscope is also helpful for all asthmatics, particularly for children, who can be taught to recognize abnormal breathing sounds by a physician or nurse. Recognition of symptoms makes possible early treatment with enzymes and may help the patient avoid the use of medications.

Acupressure provides another approach to early treatment. The diagram of acupressure points appearing in Chapter 5 shows points that can be stimulated for self-treatment. The lung points are particularly helpful. There is also an area of the spine at the cervical level (C7) that can be percussed or tapped. This stimulation helps relieve asthma symptoms immediately.

Asthma and Allergy Medications

Some asthmatics believe that taking a lot of medications will help cure them. But asthmatics should understand that medications only treat the symptoms and do not cure asthma. In any case, it is important to be aware of what each medication does. There are many types of drugs for asthma, including bronchodilators, cortical steroids, sedating and nonsedating antihistamines, decongestants, generic medications, prescription cough medicines, over-the-counter cough medicines, Tylenol, and aspirin. These can be delivered through inhalation, topical application, capsules, or sprinkling on food. Each asthmatic or parent of asthmatic children should know how long each medication takes to work and the dosages appropriate for them or their children. They should know which are fast acting and which are long lasting, how often they should be used, and the best method of delivery. Delivery systems for asthma medication include metered dose inhalers, spacers, holding chambers, and nebulizers.

An inhaler, a canister that injects a medicated mist into a patient's airways, must be used properly and as instructed by a physician. A spacer is a hollow device added to an inhaler to extend the space between the metered dose inhaled and the mouth of the patient. It coordinates the release of the medication and the timing of the slow aspiration to make sure the proper dose is received. This increases the efficacy of the medication and makes sure it is deposited where it belongs. A nebulizer, commonly called a breathing machine, is designed to aerosolize medication into a fine mist of tiny particles and deliver those particles to the lungs. The efficiency of medication delivery is greatly improved with a nebulizer.

Asthmatics and parents of asthmatic children also should know the purpose of each medication, how often it can be safely used in a twenty-four hour period, and what alternatives are available. For example, if they notice the quiet symptom, can they use enzymes and acupressure instead? This information should be written down in the management plan. Asthmatics should also be checked to make sure they are not allergic to their medications, and, if they are, treated with NAET for those medications right away. I have found that most asthmatics are allergic to their inhaler, cough medicine, or some other medications they have been taking.

In many cases, allergy proofing or otherwise altering their environment, changing their diet to eliminate food allergens, and eating only hormone-free, pesticide-free meat is enough to allow an asthmatic to discontinue medications even before much allergy work is done. The more people take responsibility for their own health and do what is needed, the fewer medications they need.

To help asthmatics take more responsibility for their condition, I have put together a list of questions they can ask their physicians about the medications they are taking:

1. What is the name of the medication and what is it supposed to do?

2. How long after I begin taking the medication will it have an effect?

3. When should I take it?

4. For how long should I take it?

5. How often should I take it?

6. What happens if the medication does not work?

7. Are there any foods, drinks, or other medications I should avoid while taking this medication?

8. Are there any side effects? If so, what should I do if they occur, and is there information available about them?

Asthma sufferers should try to manage their condition as much as possible with alternative therapies to avoid further stressing their immune systems with drug residues. They should have a good plan for avoiding episodes and maintaining a nonallergenic environment. As they go through NAET treatment there will be less need for medications or alternative therapies for threatened attacks. It is important to consult with a physician and adjust medications as needs begin to change.

The Adolescent and Asthma

Taking responsibility and doing what is needed for an asthmatic condition can be particularly difficult for an adolescent. Having an adolescent son, I know that it is sometimes hard to communicate effectively with them, but it is essential that they realize they have a potentially life-threatening condition that must be monitored. Because most adolescents feel a need to assert their independence from their parents and are particularly sensitive to the influence of their peers, they may resist or ignore the suggestions of their parents or their physician.

Adolescent asthmatics should participate in their own health care. They should be educated about their condition, how to treat it, and how to manage it to prevent symptoms from occurring. They need to know about nutrition, digestion, and the importance of eating good food to stay healthy. NAET can be particularly helpful for adolescents because it reduces the number of allergens to be avoided and makes the management of asthma relatively carefree instead of overwhelming.

Adolescence, like other periods of life, has its stresses, peer pressures, competition, and temptations to indulge in drugs, alcohol, and tobacco. The recent increase in teen smoking is a serious problem and teenage asthmatics have to understand how damaging smoking or being around smoke can be for them. It has been reported that more than ninety percent of new tobacco users are children and each day an estimated 3,000 youths, ranging in age from ten to sixteen, begin to smoke for the first time. Studies have shown that three-fourths of youths who use cigarettes continue to do so because they find it hard to quit. They may even end up as lifetime users. President Clinton signed a bill in August of 1996 that was designed to prevent the sale of tobacco to underage users.

The tobacco and chemicals in cigarettes such as tar, nicotine, carbon monoxide, formaldehyde, aluminum, sulfur, and lead have all been shown to cause health problems and to irritate and inflame the airways of people with asthma. Exposure to these toxins, either by smoking or by being around secondhand smoke, can trigger severe asthma attacks.

REMOVING ALLERGENS FROM THE ENVIRONMENT

Keeping indoor humidity below fifty percent can reduce dust mites and mold.

Air-Conditioning and Fans

Central air-conditioning is the most effective way of controlling humidity although some people react to the cooler air. Air-conditioning vent openings are prime locations for the buildup of molds. Window fans draw pollens and molds into the house and swamp coolers increase humidity.

Air Filters

Air cleaning devices that filter the air in the home to remove airborne allergens are invaluable for asthmatics. Several filtering devices are available and some can be used in conjunction with forced air cooling and heating systems. One type of filter uses standard disposable fiberglass filters that are changed monthly. Permanent air filters with baffles should be cleaned periodically. A third alternative, an electric filter that uses an electrostatic precipitator, requires frequent cleaning and produces irritating ozone if not well maintained. The most effective filter is a **high efficiency particulate air (HEPA) filter**. HEPA filtration systems require no maintenance and their efficacy only increases with use. An air cleaner that uses a true HEPA filter is the most efficient and reliable method of cleaning the air. The HEPA filter in my office, for example, removes smoke or perfume from the air within seconds.

Among the many things to consider when picking out an air filter is the amount of air the unit can circulate and clean. There are various advantages and disadvantages to the mechanical and electrical methods of air filtering. A mechanical filtration system becomes more efficient with use and does not produce ozone. It can only be used in homes that have forced air heating and cooling systems, however. They also require frequent cleaning, can become coated with tars from tobacco smoke, and lose static charge capability. An ion generator, which has a very low electrical operating cost, does not require filter replacement for basic models. The disadvantages are that they produce ozone, create an ion imbalance in room air, and cause cleaning problems when air particles stick to walls and furniture.

Few air cleaners are listed by the FDA as medical devices. The agency has not established performance standards. One kind of purifier, the HEPA filter, is used in the operating room where human life, health, and safety are most at risk.

Vacuum Cleaners

Vacuum cleaners are another important piece of equipment for asthmatics. It is important to know if your vacuum really eliminates dirt and dust from your home or merely recycles tiny particles back into the air. These particles can linger in the air for up to an hour where they continue to provoke allergic and asthma reactions.

Since many varieties of vacuums are available, I suggest that people do some research. There are vacuum cleaners with HEPA filters that can trap particles as small as .3 microns. Considering that a hair is between 75 and 100 microns thick and a dust mite is approximately 5 microns, .3 microns is tiny indeed; in fact, it is smaller than many of the particles that are breathed into the lungs. These vacuums can be extremely expensive, however. Vacuums that use a water filter are less expensive and have been found useful by many asthmatics. Allergy control filters can also be added to some canister vacuums. The Allergy and Asthma Network, Mothers of Asthmatics, Inc., will provide the results of studies done on the performance of various vacuum cleaner models (refer to Miscellaneous Resources in Part VI).

Heat Sources

For asthmatics, electric and hot water radiant heaters are the best heating alternatives. Forced air can disperse dust and mold, and even if there is a central filter, ducts can accumulate large amounts of dust and mold. If forced air is used, the ducts should be cleaned once a year and bedroom air vents should be closed to keep allergens from other parts of the home out of the asthmatic's bedroom. Fireplaces and wood-burning stoves are not recommended sources of heat because they can emit toxic particles and gasses that cause respiratory problems. Kerosene heaters produce sulfur dioxide and carbon monoxide in the home, both of which are asthmatic triggers.

SLEEPING ENVIRONMENT

It is particularly important to clear the sleeping environment of allergens because symptoms tend to worsen at night and cause the asthmatic to wake up with an asthma attack. Several factors have been implicated in this characteristic pattern. Irritation from food or acid reflux can be a cause of asthma at night, as can allergens such as house dust and molds that are more active at night. Allergens inhaled earlier in the day may cause delayed reactions when the body is less active and certain chemical mediators and hormones in the body known to affect asthma tend to rise or fall during the night. For example, histamine levels go up at night whereas adrenaline and steroid levels fall. This fluctuation can trigger an allergic response or attack. Everyone's lungs, even nonasthma sufferers, tend to constrict slightly in the evening hours. When the sun comes up the body relaxes and the airways open up.

Allergens in the bedroom can be reduced by removing mold, down comforters, feather pillows, and the foam and kapok in mattresses and cushions. We treat with NAET for allergens in the bedroom air by leaving an open jar of water in the bedroom for twenty-four hours and then treating for the water. The bedroom must be avoided for twenty-five hours after the treatment. This technique treats for various gasses that are given off in the bedroom by furniture, fabrics, carpets, and other items that might be difficult to identify individually. We also check for and treat allergies to materials used in bedding such as wool, acrylic, nylon, polyester, and cotton.

I had one young boy who constantly snored and woke up each morning with congestion. We treated him for foods and many environmental allergens but nothing helped with the snoring. His mother mentioned that he might be allergic to his polyester blanket. Sure enough; when we treated him for polyester he stopped snoring and no longer had congestion. It was an incredible over-night change.

I talked to a man who is very allergic to electricity. He had severe problems with asthma until he worked with several doctors and realized that the electricity sur-rounding his bed was the cause of his problem. The electricity included clocks, lights, and other electrical devices. When we treated for electricity, his asthma completely disappeared.

Animals in the bedroom may have left urine, saliva, and hair. Wallpaper, paint, books that collect dust, fabrics, wood floors, and rugs all can cause problems. One asth-matic told me she was bothered by the natural floral scent in a potpourri near her bed. When she removed the pot-pourri, her wheezing and chest tightness subsided.

A skilled NAET practitioner knows many of the bed-room allergens that should be treated. In the meantime, asthmatics and allergy sufferers should check the bed for possible allergens. Fabrics, detergents, and chlorine bleaches are possible irritants. Asthmatics should find a detergent that is not irritating to them and stick to it. Clothes should be rinsed twice to thoroughly eliminate any detergent residues.

Painting and remodeling a house can be toxic for anyone, particularly for an asthmatic. All the materials used and the gasses they emit are possible asthmatic triggers. I test and treat people for latex, oil, and acrylic paints as well as for glues, hardwoods, and hardwood finishes. Until these treatments can be done, asthmatics should avoid exposure to these products.

Dust Mites

Since dust mites are one of the most common allergens that trigger asthmatics, it is important to get rid of accumulations of dust. Treating for dust with NAET is usually effective but until that is done, many steps can be taken to clean the indoor environment. There should be smooth, uncluttered surfaces in the bedroom, with few small objects such as books, knickknacks, CDs, tapes, or stuffed animals. All of these should be put in drawers if possible. Bedrooms should not be used as libraries or studies. Bedding should be washed weekly in hot water—135 degrees Fahrenheit—to kill dust mites. Cool water just gives them a bath. Pillows can be encased in nonallergic and nonpermeable dust-proof covers if the person sleeping on them is not allergic to the material. Otherwise, the cover will do more harm than good. Avoid feather comforters and pillows, and remove carpeting if possible. Carpeting is a major hiding place for dust mites.

There are chemicals that can be used to prevent dust mites but many people are allergic to them as well. Air-conditioning can prevent the heat and high humidity that stimulate mite growth. Special filters can be added to help trap airborne allergens. When using a humidifier in winter, avoid high humidity. Because mites cannot live in humidity below fifty percent, the ideal relative humidity is forty to fifty percent. Avoid wall pennants, macrame hangings, and other dust catchers. Stuffed toys should be machine washable. Keep all clothing in a closet with the door closed. When vacuuming or dusting, be sure to use a face mask.

Mold

After dust mites, the next major asthma trigger is mold. To prevent or eliminate molds, humidity should be kept as low as possible (never over fifty percent). It may be useful to use a gauge to measure the humidity. Keeping the windows closed and using an air conditioner and dehumidifier is helpful. A dehumidifier must be emptied regularly or attached to a drain and the air intake on air conditioners should be sprayed with a mold-killing spray if the air conditioner develops a musty odor. First, check for an allergy to the spray. Special air-conditioning filters can be added to help trap airborne allergens and air purifiers help clear mold spores from the air. Walls should also be cleaned and a mold inhibitor added to any paints before they are applied, if the occupant is not allergic to the product. Mold flourishes in dark, damp places that are poorly ventilated and in areas where water pools. Moisture and warmth accelerates the growth of dormant mold spores on most surfaces. Once areas of mold are identified, they should be washed with a mold-inhibiting solution, and ventilation and drainage should be improved.

Some humidifiers prevent mold growth by a special heating process. Central humidifiers should be checked and cleaned frequently. Window condensation can lead to mold growth on the window frames. Books, leather products, wood paneling, and wallpaper paste all support mold growth and should be avoided or treated with appropriate mold-killing solutions. Indoor plants are not a major source but can have mold in the soil with spores that become airborne when the plant is watered or repotted. Since wood bark harbors mold, fireplace wood should not be stored inside.

Avoiding mold in the bedroom is very similar to treating for dust. Carpeting can be a major breeding ground for mold, as can foam rubber pillows and mattresses. Keep cupboards and garbage pails clean, and dry shoes and boots thoroughly before storing. Clothing with perspiration should be washed after use and chemical moisture removers used in closets.

KITCHEN

In the kitchen, exhaust fans can remove water vapor during cooking. Mold grows in refrigerators, particularly around door gaskets, in water pans below self-defrosting refrigerators, and on spoiled foods. Mold can also grow on garbage, so containers should be emptied and cleaned frequently.

BATHROOM

In the bathroom, excess water should be removed from shower doors, tiles, and tubs with a squeegee. Shower curtains, bath tile, shower stalls, tubs, and toilet tanks should all be washed with mold preventive solutions. Do not carpet the bathroom.

LAUNDRY ROOM AND BASEMENT

In the laundry room, vent the dryer outside and dry clothing immediately after washing. In a basement, do not lay carpet and pads on a concrete floor. Use vinyl flooring instead. Dirt floors should be covered with a vapor barrier. Keep the basement free of dust and remove stored items likely to harbor mold. Allergic individuals should not have their bedroom on a basement level.

OUTDOORS

Outdoors, avoid cutting grass or raking leaves, or use a tight-fitting mask while doing so. Avoid exposure to soil, compost, sand boxes, hay, and fertilizers. Correct drainage problems near the house to get rid of any pooled water. Avoid camping or walking in the woods where mold grows around logs or other vegetation. Remove rotted logs from around the house and yard.

OTHER PROBLEM AREAS

Antique shops can harbor a lot of mold as can sleeping bags, greenhouses, summer cottages, hotel rooms, and automobile air conditioners. Farmers, gardeners, bakers, upholsterers, paperhangers, millworkers, florists, food preparers, plumbers, librarians, and people working around moldy materials all have occupational exposure to mold.

Other highly toxic environments include hair and nail salons that are hazardous to anyone with respiratory problems. Many of the nail chemicals are common allergens, especially acetone used in nail polish remover and hair chemicals. Perfumes can also be a trigger for asthmatics and a problem for others with respiratory problems. The scent contained in perfumes, lotions, soap, cosmetics, detergents, and other products can cause migraines, dizziness, rashes, and eczema. Until these allergies are cleared with NAET, it is important to employ an air purifier whenever possible and to use perfume-free products.

DEALING WITH PETS

Approximately ten percent of the American population, including twenty to thirty percent of asthmatics, are allergic to animals. Most have an allergy to cats which is actually an allergy to cat dander and the proteins in their saliva and urine. It is estimated that twenty-eight percent of the homes in the United States have at least one cat, This totals about fifty million cats. Approximately six million Americans are allergic to cats and early exposure can lead to asthma in a child with a predisposition. Keeping an animal outdoors is preferable but that can create a problem because outdoor allergens—pollen and mold—cling to the fur and come off when the animal is touched. Frequent bathing of a cat is important as is appropriate indoor and outdoor ventilation as well as vacuuming with a HEPA filter vacuum cleaner. Cat allergen can linger in carpets, mattresses, and walls for months and even years. To speed up removal, clean heating and air-conditioning ducts thoroughly, clean walls, have carpets and upholstery professionally cleaned, and use HEPA air cleaners throughout the house.

Studies have shown that washing a cat with water removes much of its surface allergen content and reduces the future production of allergens. Place the cat or kitten in the sink and pour lukewarm water over its body. Wash it weekly for three weeks, then at two- or three-week intervals after that. Wear a face mask when brushing a cat, wash hands and change clothes after touching it. This is another reminder that parasites can be picked up when touching an animal. Vacuuming may blow cat allergens into the air. Use only a vacuum with a high-quality filter. Since small animals such as mice and gerbils also bear allergens, wear a mask when you clean their cage or have a nonallergic person do it.

NAET has been quite successful in treating for pet allergies in asthmatics and others. Because it is important to avoid contact with allergens for twenty-five hours after treatment, the patient may have to wear gloves and a mask or stay away from the home to avoid contact with these pervasive allergens.

INFLUENZA

When an asthmatic is exposed to the flu or cold virus, there is a high risk of developing symptoms that can trigger asthma. To prevent the spread of viruses, cover your mouth when sneezing or coughing, wash your hands frequently, dispose of used tissues, and keep your hands away from your face. Viruses spread from person to person through the air from coughs and sneezes, through hand contact with an infected person, or by touching surfaces that have been contaminated and then rubbing the eyes, mouth, or nose.

Although flu vaccines are supposed to reduce the incidence of flu in healthy adults, I recommend that my patients, particularly asthmatics, be tested for an allergy or sensitivity to the vaccine before taking it. Otherwise, it can result in flu symptoms that lead to an asthma attack. I usually manage to get a sample of the vaccine each year and test people for reactions. Treatment for the flu virus with NAET can be as strong a preventive as the vaccine itself for both children and adults.

CHICKEN POX

Chicken pox (varicella) is a relatively harmless childhood illness but it can be troublesome for an asthmatic. Children who have been treated with cortical steroids may be at particular risk because these steroids suppress the immune system that can lead to serious complications, even death. The symptoms of chicken pox include a rash with tiny clear red-based blisters accompanied by a fever. Once a child who is receiving oral or injected cortical steroids is exposed to the virus, a physician should be notified immediately. The child can be treated within forty-eight hours after exposure with an injection of varicella immune globulin, an antibody preparation. I also find it helpful to treat with NAET for the chicken pox virus.

CHLORINE

The effects of chlorine, a common allergen for asthmatics, are particularly noticeable after a shower. There may be difficulty breathing and the feeling of running out of oxygen. Some asthmatics have found that a chlorine-removing filter on the showerhead is helpful in preventing this reaction. NAET treatment is also recommended, however, since a filter cannot possibly eliminate all the chlorine.

CAR ENVIRONMENTS

Many people are allergic to substances in their cars including fuel, exhaust fumes, plastics, hydrocarbons, carpets, and synthetic leathers. An acquaintance had excruciating back pain whenever she sat on the synthetic leather seats in my car. Use an air purifier in the car but there is no way to escape from fuel or exhaust fumes or to effectively avoid contact with interior materials. These allergies should be treated with NAET.

EATING FOODS AND BREAST FEEDING

Food allergies can be serious triggers for asthma. The best way to avoid them is to treat for them with NAET. When we treat pregnant women, we find that the benefit of the allergy treatment is passed on to the child. There are additional ways to prevent the development of food allergies in children. Babies should be breast fed for at least one year, and it is preferable to wait six to eight months before starting a baby on solid food. If the mother does not breast feed, the child should be put on a milk-free formula. We test infants for various allergies including breast milk and treat them with NAET when necessary.

A mother should not eat large amounts of common allergens while breast feeding because the allergens can be passed on to the child. Children should not be introduced to foods such as dairy products, wheat, nuts, and other foods discussed in the food allergy section until they are at least a year old. Foods that have caused problems for the mother in the past should be avoided during breast feeding. When children start eating solid food, they should be introduced to them one at a time to see if they are allergic. Muscle testing can also help to determine this.

A mother of a young boy who knew that her husband had a serious peanut allergy asked me to check her son for the allergy. Both the child and his father showed a reaction to peanuts in the test. The child was treated and never had a reaction to peanuts. The father was treated and stopped having reactions, even though he had suffered severe asthma symptoms, airway constriction, and difficulty breathing after eating peanuts in the past.

MASSAGE AND CHIROPRACTIC CARE

Another preventive measure proven to be effective with asthmatics is massage. Research has indicated that weekly upper-body massage may help asthmatics find relief from symptoms such as chest tightness, wheezing, and fatigue. In one study asthmatics who received weekly fifteen minute upper-body massages reported drops in chest tightness, wheezing, physical pain, and fatigue. Even with the best results, massage does not prevent asthmatics from having to take medication. The results, however, have led people to realize that stress plays a major role in asthma.

Chiropractic care is also essential. I generally adjust the upper backs of all my asthmatic patients because the nerves in the area connect directly to the lungs and bronchi. Manipulation sometimes can stop an asthma attack.

Stress plays a major role in any chronic illness. In an emotional situation, asthmatics often feel an immediate tightness in the chest and have difficulty breathing. However, if the body is free of allergens, in a state of **homeostasis**, and digestion is good, I believe it is strong enough to deal with any emotional situation without experiencing an asthma attack. A balanced chemistry, good digestion, and a strong immune system are necessary for asthmatics to deal with the stresses that are common to the society in which we live.

ALTERNATIVE THERAPIES

Energetic techniques such as qi-gong and breathing exercises are helpful as well as acupuncture, chiropractic care, and spiritual practices that help provide an understanding of the emotions behind disease. Deep abdominal breathing is best. Avoid chest breathing as much as possible. Inhale and exhale completely.

Homeopathy has several remedies for congestion, wheezing, and shortness of breath including adrenalinum (6x), lobelia inflata (3x), belladonna (4x), Ephedra vulgaris (4x), ipecacuanha (6x), Solidago virgaurea (6x), and sambucus nigra (1x), although some people can be allergic to these remedies. Adrenalinum is known for its ability to dilate or expand blood vessels and bronchial passages. Ipecacuanha is used for shortness of breath and constriction in the chest. Belladonna is used for tightness in the chest and labored breathing. Solidago vigaurea helps to eliminate heavy phlegm, coughing, and catarrh.

EXERCISE

Experts talk about exercise-induced asthma but I believe that many of those reactions are caused by allergies to hormones, adrenaline, and outdoor allergens. Once these are cleared, the patient can be allowed to exercise. It is important to use discretion, however, and an asthmatic should never over-exercise when ill or suffering from an infection.

Swimming may not be the best exercise for asthmatics, especially if they are allergic to chlorine. Whatever the exercise chosen, however, it should be something the asthmatic really enjoys doing. Experts usually recommend activities that involve short bursts of energy rather than exercise for an extended period of time.

I have successfully used NAET to treat many people with exercise-induced asthma. After the treatment they have been able to exercise without problems and enjoy bike rides, running, and walking.

III NAMBUDRIPAD ALLERGY ELIMINATION TECHNIQUE (NAET)

9

DEFINING THE NAMBUDRIPAD ALLERGY ELIMINATION TECHNIQUE (NAET)

STEVE'S STORY

Steve came to see me with severe food allergies. His diet was very limited and he was frequently distressed physically. He could not tolerate, digest, or assimilate most foods. I decided to introduce the NAET chapter with his testimonial, not because he is an asthmatic, but because his life was so dramatically changed with NAET. He is now able to eat all foods without any problems and can live a more enjoyable, relaxed, and normal lifestyle. The dramatic changes Steve has experienced epitomize the power of this technique. NAET should have far-reaching effects on the way we view and treat chronic diseases and ailments such as asthma, chronic fatigue, migraines, and so forth.

I am writing to thank you for helping me to get my health back. When I came to see you in January 1994, I had such severe digestive problems that I had to curtail many of the activities I had enjoyed much of my life. These problems were also intruding on my business life, and I was becoming seriously depressed and withdrawn. All of that has improved significantly since our work together.

As children growing up in the fifties, my sister and I felt fortunate that we could eat everything we wanted without the hives and other problems my allergic mother experienced when she was not careful about what she ate. As a teenager I was obese, and when I was 21 I went on an all-protein diet over the summer that reduced my weight from 235 to 165 lbs. (I'm 6'1"). Nobody recognized me that autumn until they heard my voice. I was thrilled by the weight loss, but I felt weak and experienced some unpleasant side effects for a while, such as double vision. Around this time I also noticed that I would get diarrhea after eating dairy products, so I began to avoid them. My weight stabilized at about 180 to 185 pounds, and for many years my health was fine except that I couldn't eat any dairy.

When I was around 40 (I'm 47 now), my weight increased to 210, and I began to notice symptoms such as gas, diarrhea and bloating after some meals, even when I avoided dairy products. Fortunately, a doctor was willing to try a relatively new technology at the time, IgA allergy testing using blood samples. The doctor found that I was allergic to 35 of the 70 foods he tested. He said that mine were among the worst results he had ever encountered, and he urged me to avoid the foods to which I was allergic. He also offered me a reducing diet.

His advice was very helpful in eliminating the symptoms and losing the extra weight. To the extent that I avoided the allergenic foods, I had no gas, diarrhea, or bloating and my weight fell again to about 185 pounds.

As helpful as this was, however, it was actually a way of coping with a serious disability. Each time I went to a restaurant (once a source of pleasure), I had to interrogate the waiter about the ingredients in every dish. I read menus with fear because I could not eat wheat, rye, corn, barley, oats, most spices, most oils, or any of the other 35 foods to which I was allergic. Often, waiters would assure me that all of my food requirements would be met, and then my dinner would appear, covered with black pepper or some other item I could not eat.

Whenever I ate one of the forbidden foods, the symptoms came swiftly. If there was dairy in any form, I would experience cramping, gas, diarrhea and bloating within five minutes, and this would become much worse about two hours later. Other foods had similar though less dramatic effects that were just as predictable.

For me this was more than a minor inconvenience. My work as an attorney required me to travel extensively and to take clients and witnesses to meals. I learned how central the sharing of food is to our social and business life, and I began to feel excluded. When friends would invite me to a dinner party, I would arrive with take-out sushi (which I knew contained none of the forbidden foods). After a time, I noticed fewer dinner invitations, and in a way I was relieved because I would no longer have to explain my restrictions to my hosts.

Travel for work or pleasure became something to avoid. Imagine carrying an extra suitcase full of food to Europe just to feel secure about finding something to eat. In each city, after I checked into a hotel, I would locate a food market to buy canned goods, which I would then eat in my hotel room rather than braving the restaurants. Explaining to a Parisian client that I could only have lunch with him if there was no sauce on my salmon was a task that I would not want to repeat.

When I discussed all of this with my sister, I was not entirely surprised to learn that she had had similar experiences. After eating at a McDonald's once, for example, she had been hospitalized for internal bleeding. Later she discovered that they soak their french fries in milk before cooking them, and the milk had caused her to bleed. We spent many hours on the phone sharing information about which foods caused which symptoms and what foods to avoid.

Around this time, when I was 44, an attorney friend told me of her success in treating allergies with you. Thinking that I had nothing to lose, I came to see you. When you assured me that I would be eating dairy again within a few weeks, I was incredulous. By this time, I considered my body to be as reliable as a laboratory: give me something that had even the smallest amount of dairy in it, and within five minutes the symptoms would begin.

You performed some diagnostic exams, prescribed a number of food enzymes to eat with meals, and did some allergy testing. It was the beginning of a year of treatment that led to my recovery. Today, with a few minor exceptions, I eat whatever foods I choose, in any location, have no symptoms, and again weigh 185 pounds.

The path from being a disabled person who had to refrain from many important activities to being an ordinary person with normal health and a regular diet was a fascinating and surprising one for me and sometimes required faith and patience. Although I am open minded about alternative approaches in any discipline, I am also schooled in Western science. For example, I know that acupuncture and other methods have been used in the East for centuries with success, but I also know that we do not understand how or why they succeed. Still, everything else had failed, and my friend's allergies had improved dramatically, so I decided to give NAET a try, whether I understood it or not.

The first set-back came immediately. The initial treatment for an allergy to chicken and eggs did not work, and I had to be treated a second time. Fortunately the next several treatments went well, and I was soon eating foods I had not eaten in years—without any symptoms. I felt like a child eating certain foods for the first time. It had been so long since I had eaten a strawberry or Wheaties®, for example, that tasting them was an indescribable new experience. At times some symptoms would return, especially after eating at restaurants, where I was experimenting with a broader selection. The reactions were far less severe than before, however, and we would work to identify what foods were causing the reaction and then treat for them.

For me the real test came a couple of months into the treatments, when you told me that I was ready to eat dairy. Given the painful and serious symptoms that I had experienced over the past 20 years, it was no wonder that I felt fear when I faced my bowl of chocolate ice cream. Waiting until the house was empty, I ate the ice cream expecting the worst.

After 5 minutes, when the cramping and bloating would ordinarily begin, nothing happened, much to my surprise and relief. The next test, I knew, would be in two hours, when the diarrhea and gas used to become far worse. Again, nothing happened. I have been eating dairy products now for over a year without incident. Though there are many dairy products I don't like and seldom eat or drink (like milk), I am not afraid of dairy and eat some every day.

It has been several months now since we ended the treatments, and I continue to enjoy a wide variety of foods. On rare occasions, I will have minor symptoms after a meal, but probably no more often than most people in their late 40's. For the most part, I eat what I want without any difficulty. I continue to take food enzymes because I find them helpful for maintaining my health. I have far more energy than I used to, and my friends have told me how much better and healthier I look. I am no longer a disabled person and can again participate fully in life. To me, the treatments were a miracle.

THE STORY BEHIND THE DISCOVERY OF NAET

Dr. Nambudripad originally discovered this technique by accident while caring for her own extensive health problems. When she was an infant, she suffered from eczema, and when she was eight her parents started feeding her white rice with special herbs to treat a chronic skin disease. In 1976 she moved to Los Angeles where she became more health conscious and changed her eating habits. Nevertheless, she continued to suffer from bronchitis, pneumonia, arthritis, insomnia, depression, sinusitis, and migraine headaches. She was tired all the time but unable to sleep. Although she experimented with a wide variety of techniques, medicines, and herbs she only became sicker. As she puts it, "Every inch of my body ached. I lived on aspirin, taking almost thirty a day to keep me going."

At the time she was a student at the Los Angeles College of Chiropractic and her nutritional teacher advised her to go on a juice diet. In two days she had bronchitis, laryngitis, and a fever of 104 degrees. To care for herself, she cooked some soft white rice which she had learned to do as a child when she was sick. We now understand that white rice is probably the least allergic food although it has few nutrients.

After hearing an acupuncturist speak at the chiropractic college, Nambudripad was so impressed that she decided to study acupuncture as well. One of her acupuncture teachers noticed her raspy voice and told her he thought she had food allergies. Tests showed that she was allergic to almost all foods except white rice and broccoli. This acupuncturist suggested that Nambudripad try eating white rice and broccoli for a few days. Within a week her bronchitis had cleared, her headaches had become infrequent, her joints had stopped aching, her insomnia had disappeared, and her concentration and thinking had become clearer and more focused.

When she began eating other foods again, her complaints slowly reappeared. She decided to return to rice and broccoli and ended up remaining on that diet for three and a half years. Once in a while she would try something else, but her symptoms, particularly the arthritis, would come back. She could not eat any salads, fruits, or vegetables other than broccoli. She was allergic to all grains, sugars, fish, eggs, and spices. She was also allergic to environmental factors such as fabrics and radiation. She assumed she would live on white rice and broccoli for the rest of her life.

One day she absent-mindedly ate a few pieces of carrot while waiting for the rice to cook. In a few minutes she felt tired, as if she were about to pass out. Recognizing that she was experiencing an allergic reaction to carrots, she called her husband, who was also an acupuncturist, and asked him to get some acupuncture needles and treat her. While she waited for him, she massaged certain acupuncture points to keep from fainting. He inserted the needles and she slept for forty-five minutes. When she woke up she felt strangely different. She was not feeling sick or tired; in fact, her energy level was high. As she got up from the bed she noticed that some pieces of carrot were still stuck to her hand. In a panic, she dropped them immediately. She wondered if there was a connection between accidentally holding the carrots and waking up feeling so good. Her study of electromagnetic fields and acupuncture meridians suggested a possible connection.

Using the muscle testing technique, she found she was no longer allergic to carrots. She ate them the next day and had no reaction. When she treated herself for other foods, those allergies disappeared as well. She began using the technique on herself and over time developed the system she calls the Nambudripad Allergy Elimination Technique. NAET is now used by more than 600 practitioners throughout the world, all of whom are having excellent results desensitizing people to allergens. To locate a practitioner in your area refer to Part VI.

MY FIRST ENCOUNTER WITH NAET

I first came across the Nambudripad Allergy Elimination Technique through another practitioner. After doing well on enzymes for many years, I noticed that I still had trouble eating certain foods such as grains (wheat and rice) and dairy products. My digestion was not affected but I noticed that I felt fatigue and depression after eating the grains. As a result I was on the lookout for other techniques or products that would help my allergies and those of my patients.

An acupuncturist began working in my clinic who had been treating people with an allergy technique that used vials of different materials to diagnose and treat allergies. I observed her work and talked to her about her success rate. Impressed, I began to refer patients to her who had severe mold, dust, and environmental allergies that I had been unable to treat successfully with enzymes. She had some extraordinary results. Allergies just completely disappeared. I began to send her more and more of my patients.

One patient I referred was a long-time chiropractic patient of mine named Judy who consistently complained of severe nasal congestion, chronic wheezing, and shortness of breath. I suggested that Judy consult with this acupuncturist about diagnosing her specific allergies and then clearing them so she could be symptom free. Judy followed my suggestion and the acupuncturist found her to be allergic to dust, mold, pollen, cats, Vitamin C, some fruits, some vegetables, and all the B vitamins. After several NAET treatments for these allergens, she was completely free of symptoms—no more runny nose, coughing, wheezing, or chronic congestion.

After watching her success with amazement, I went for treatment myself. I was treated first for the basics including egg white, calcium, and sugars. I clearly remember my sugar treatment. Whenever I ate sugar, I would immediately get a reddened cold, runny nose, cold hands, headaches, and depression. After the sugar treatment I stopped craving sugar, then found that I had no reaction when I ate it. I also felt energized after the basic treatments.

Then I was treated for grains—including rice, which I could never eat without feeling fatigued, and wheat, dairy products, fruits, and hormones. After the treatment for hormones, I no longer experienced any premenstrual tension or irritability during my period. These NAET treatments opened many doors in overcoming my allergies and I became increasingly curious.

Eventually, the acupuncturist told me she was moving to Hawaii and suggested that I take the training to learn the technique myself. I followed her advice and signed up for a seminar. I ended up taking five because I could not believe that such a simple technique could have such success. I also continued to get treatments from another doctor and had more extraordinary results. I was no longer allergic to alcohol, sun radiation, dust, or any food. With NAET treatments and enzymes, I no longer had to limit my food intake in any way.

In light of this success, I added NAET to my enzyme and nutritional techniques and have been using it ever since. Over ninety-five percent of my practice is now NAET and enzyme work. Besides the successes with asthma that have been significant, I have had tremendous results with headaches, chronic fatigue, arthritis, hay fever, sinus problems, obesity, female problems, and symptoms ranging from warts to nail biting. I have also treated many people with depression and various kinds of skin and glandular problems. I have devoted this book to asthma because people die from asthma every day. Yet the disease can be prevented. I feel confident that after a period of treatment, I can get all asthmatic patients off medications they have taken for years, even since childhood.

WHAT IS NAET?

NAET is a breakthrough treatment that uses chiropractic, kinesiology, and acupuncture to permanently desensitize people to all kinds of allergies. The technique can be practiced by any health practitioner including doctors, nurses, acupuncturists, chiropractors, dentists and, to some extent, allergy sufferers themselves. Clinical studies with NAET have demonstrated that it is by far the most successful and succinct treatment for the elimination of allergies. The theory of NAET is based on viewing the body as made up of pathways for the flow of electromagnetic energy. It is easier to understand how and why NAET works if one understands the theories that underlie it.

The whole concept of the body as an energy field was not new to me when I learned NAET. As a chiropractic student, I was introduced to a philosophy that regards the body as more than just matter, muscles, and tissues coming together without any real intelligence. Chiropractic acknowledges that the body is a holistic complex and that the universal or innate intelligence or organizing force that pervades the vast galaxies also pervades the simplest cells of the body. The founder of chiropractic, Dr. D. D. Palmer, talked about the concept of electromagnetic energy fields. He said that mind does not control the functions of the body. Instead, there is an innate intelligence that controls the mind and its functions as well as the functions of the body. This innate intelligence has the power to conceive, judge, and reason about matters pertaining to the internal welfare of the body. The healing art of chiropractic has been around for over one hundred years and has been successful at treating the body and appreciating it as more than just matter.

In the chiropractic view, when a bone is out of alignment or the spine is distorted or misaligned, the energy force in the body is cut off. This, in turn, causes serious disease. When the misalignments or imbalances are corrected, the energy can flow again through the nervous system to the brain and homeostasis is restored.

The work of Dr. Devi Nambudripad is similarly based on the idea that the body is a flow of electromagnetic currents. According to her theory, when an allergen enters or contacts the body, there is a clash between the energy field of the allergen and the energy field of the allergy sufferer. The brain identifies the allergen and alerts the immune system which locates the allergen and responds with antibodies and delayed reactive T and B cells. This type of immune reaction causes the release of toxic substances from the T cells. The fighter cells, called macrophages, then invade the area, intent on digesting the antigens. Immune mediators such as histamine are released. These reactions cause blockage in the electromagnetic pathways as well as abnormal tissue response, delayed tissue destruction, and possible autoimmune reaction. These responses can produce any number of symptoms such as constriction of the sinuses, throat, or breathing passageways to keep the invader from entering the body, or vomiting, diarrhea, tearing, and sinus discharge to remove it from the body. The brain makes an all-out effort to protect the body from any substance that it perceives as harmful.

Any time there are energy blockages in the body, health problems result. Some areas of the body are weaker for **genetic** reasons and they will react the most, weakening other areas of the body. Some of the common symptoms that can be produced by such blockages are aches and pains in the body, sore throats, fevers, chills, painful lymph nodes, weakness, extreme fatigue, headaches, sleep disturbances, irritability, confusion, depression, forgetfulness, a burning sensation in the body, frequent urination, crying spells, suicidal behavior, sores in the mouth, indigestion, bloating, and water retention. Virtually any symptom can be the result of a blockage caused by contact with an allergen. After working with NAET for some time, my experience has been that most health problems are ultimately caused by allergens.

If blockages continue or the body is constantly exposed to an allergen, the blockages spread throughout the system and more serious problems occur. When the immune system becomes overloaded and compromised, autoimmune problems develop. Over time, as it is bombarded with allergens, the body becomes more susceptible to chronic health problems, decreased energy levels, migraines, tumors, and mental problems.

Blockages of different meridians produce different symptoms. If there is a blockage of the lung and large intestine meridians, a person suffers severe respiratory distress, asthma, cold, sinus problems, constipation, or diarrhea. If the blockage is in the kidney meridian, the person suffers water retention or frequent urination. A gallbladder block-age produces pain and swelling in the breast, pain in intercostal muscles, abdominal cramps, heavy menstrual bleeding, severe mood swings, aggressive behavior, or anger. Blockages in the heart and small intestine meridians cause heart palpitations, cardiac arrhythmia, insomnia, dry mouth, heavy sensations in the chest, night sweats, fatigue, and insecurity. Blockages in other areas cause a whole array of symptoms. When allergens repeatedly cause blockages of the lung meridian, the person may develop asthma.

HOW DOES NAET WORK?

NAET uses chiropractic techniques to stimulate the areas of the body that are connected to the blockages in the energy system. If a blockage affects a certain organ, the practitioner stimulates areas of the nervous system connected to that organ by autonomic nerve impulses. For example, a wheat allergy might affect the lungs or cause a blockage in the lung meridian, also referred to as the lung channel. To treat for the wheat allergy, the practitioner stimulates areas of the nervous system related to the lungs. By stimulating those areas located along the spine while a person is holding the allergen, the electromagnetic repulsion to that allergen is eliminated and a chemical or enzymatic change occurs neutralizing the immune mediators and interrupting the allergen or antigen-antibody complex reaction. This clears the energy blockage for the area involved and sends a message to the brain stating that wheat has been desensitized. The body no longer identifies wheat as an allergen and energy blockages in response to wheat no longer occur.

The **desensitization** process is not instantaneous, however. It takes two hours for energy to pass through each of the body's twelve energy pathways or meridians. To circulate through all twelve meridians takes twenty-four hours. As a result, a patient should avoid contact with an allergen for twenty-five hours after the treatment to ensure complete desensitization. Otherwise, the effect of the treatment may be lost when the brain identifies the substance as an allergen again.

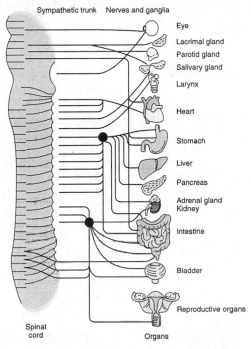

Sympathetic trunk   **Nerves and ganglia**

Eye

Lacrimal gland

Parotid gland

Salivary gland

Larynx

Heart

Stomach

Liver

Pancreas

Adrenal gland
Kidney

Intestine

Bladder

Reproductive organs

Spinal cord

Organs

Figure 9–1 The NAET desensitization process is based on the relationship among the spine, organs, and tissues by way of the autonomic nervous system.

During the twenty-five-hour treatment period, patients are told not to expose themselves to the substance or food for which they are being treated. They must not come within four feet of the substance or eat the food or foods. If they do, they can lose the treatment immediately or in the future, and their symptoms might reappear. People who expose themselves to allergens during the treatment period can experience severe allergic reactions (refer to the NAET Treatment Rules in Part VI).

I remember treating a patient named Karen for a severe sugar allergy. On her way home from my office she accidentally ate a hard sugar candy, immediately passed out, and woke up with an excruciating headache. She learned the hard way how potent these treatments can be. After the twenty-five hour waiting period, however, patients can generally eat foods they have been treated for with no reaction.

ELECTROMAGNETIC PATHWAYS (MERIDIANS)

The concept of twelve primary channels, or meridians, and two governing vessels is important in understanding how NAET works. The treatment with NAET diagnoses and treats blockages in the meridians in relationship to specific allergens. Throughout this chapter the words electromagnetic or energy pathways, channels, and meridians are used interchangeably. They all refer to the same concept. There are fourteen channels in the body, and I will discuss each one separately

> The first channel is the *lung meridian*. It regulates the body's entire energy system and oversees the intake of oxygen. Disharmony in this channel is evidenced as coughing, asthma, allergies, skin problems, bronchitis, and fatigue.

> The second channel is the *large intestine meridian* that regulates the body's waste removal activities. Disharmony here results in a distended abdomen, constipation, and diarrhea.

> The third channel is the *stomach meridian*. It regulates the body's ability to take in food and fluids. Disharmony here leads to mouth sores, nausea, and vomiting.

> The fourth channel is the *spleen meridian*. It regulates the transformation of food into energy and maintains the blood supply. Disharmony results in poor appetite, anemia, menstrual problems, chronic hepatitis, and fatigue.

The fifth channel is the *heart meridian*. This channel rules the head, houses the spirit, and regulates the blood vessels. Disharmony or unbalanced flow here leads to heart palpitations or insomnia.

The sixth channel is the *small intestines meridian* that regulates the organ that draws out energy from food and leaves the remains as waste. Disharmony results in vomiting or abdominal pain.

The seventh channel is the *bladder*. The bladder regulates the receiving and excreting of urine (fluid) waste. Disharmony results in burning sensations when urinating or in incontinence.

The eighth channel is the *kidney meridian* that stores reproductive energy and oversees mainte-nance of bones. Disharmony results in backaches, chronic ear problems, and chronic asthma.

The ninth channel is the *pericardium meridian*. This protects and oversees the heart channel. Disharmony results in stress, sensations of chest tightening, and a variety of breathing problems.

The tenth channel is the *triple burner* that oversees the body's water processing, retaining what is needed and excreting the rest. Disharmony is experi-enced as edema, a stiff neck, or water retention.

The eleventh channel is the *gallbladder*. The gall-bladder regulates the storage and secretion of bile, a fluid that helps transforms food into energy. Dishar-mony is experienced as a bitter taste in one's mouth, nausea, jaundice, and gallstones.

The twelfth channel is the *liver meridian* that regu-lates the entire energy system and oversees the maintenance of blood supplies. Disharmony leads to high blood pressure, dizziness, PMS, muscle spasms, and eye problems.

The thirteenth channel is the *governing vessel* and the fourteenth is the *conception vessel*. They circulate energy through the other twelve channels.

INNER ENERGY

In *The Energy Within: The Science Behind Every Oriental Therapy From Acupuncture to Yoga*, Richard M. Chin, M.D., O.M.D., writes that every person has an inner energy flowing through his or her mind and body that is a reflection of universal energies. When these energies are out of balance or stop flowing, we experience illness or disease. Keeping our energy moving and in balance prevents illness and creates a maximum state of health. He refers to the body as "a matrix of interacting multidimensional energy fields."

This energy, known as *qi* (sometimes spelled *C'hi*) in Chinese, is thought to be the source and the destination of all creation. Qi must keep moving in order to sustain life. In order for energy to move it must have an inherent polarity relationship: it must have somewhere to go.

Eastern practitioners who look at the body from a holistic perspective that considers the energy imbalances of the entire system instead of simply the disease of a particular organ or body part, have discovered a highly organized system of energy channels or pathways. It is another circulatory system, similar to the cardiovascular and nervous systems. Chin describes three types of energy:

Genetic or prenatal energy   The energy level to which people are genetically disposed. It is programmed in the genes like the color of their eyes and hair, their height, and so on.

Core energy A combination of the energy people are born with and the energy that forms their bodies. It is a combination of two prenatal energies.

Acquired energy The energy people acquire during their lifetime by their lifestyles and practices. This is within their control.

Pain or illness results when the flow of energy becomes blocked or unbalanced in some way, because this disharmony then upsets the balance of the body's entire energy system. . . . Although some energetic healing techniques engage the entire system, many only need to work with the body's twelve primary channels and two governing vessels (channels that oversee all others) to create complete balance and health. One method of balancing the body's energy system is acupuncture in which tiny needles are used to stimulate specific points along the twelve primary energy channels and two governing vessels.

Each of the twelve primary energy channels corresponds to one of the twelve primary organs listed above.

ELECTROMAGNETIC FIELDS

The whole universe, from the tiniest atom to the largest galaxy, is controlled by electromagnetic forces. These forces are responsible for the shape of all things and govern their movement, interrelationships, replication, and functions. The electromagnetic forces in the bodies of animals and humans can be seen as lines of force that run near the surface of the body and then pass into deeper structures (the organs).

Acupuncture practitioners employ a variety of techniques to eliminate imbalances or blockages in the natural flow of energy in the body. NAET uses techniques drawn from acupuncture, chiropractic, and kinesiology to locate and remove blockages in electromagnetic pathways that are related to allergens.

Galvanic Skin Response

Several other areas of scientific study give indications of how these energy systems in the body operate and are detected. Studies of **galvanic skin response (GSR)**, for example—the bodily response measured by "lie-detectors"—have provided interesting data. One study found the presence of an organized system of highly electroconductive points on the skin, similar to the system of points used for centuries in traditional Chinese medicine. These points are related to the human autonomic nerve reflexes. Irregularities in the points correlate with clinical medical diagnoses. With a new technique, scientists are now able to use photography to locate and identify those points.

Neurophysicists have known for a long time that when they measure the GSR at different points on the skin, it varies in direct relation to the amount of energy being discharged from the autonomic nervous system. The decreased electrical resistance at certain points on the skin is influenced by autonomic sweat gland activity on the skin's surface, by the concentrations of nerve fibers beneath the skin, and by muscle motor points. This means that any physical disorder that intensifies autonomic activity decreases electrical resistance on those areas of the skin related to the autonomic nervous system.

Ryodoraku: Electrodiagnosis

Skin resistance has been measured in the laboratory by having a person hold one electrode and passing the other over the skin. As early as 1950, one researcher, Y. Nakatani, proposed a system of electrodiagnosis and electrotreatment that was based on correlations he found between differences in skin resistance at certain points and physical illness. His system, called Ryodoraku, is based on the fact that one of the ways internal disease manifests itself is by causing a disturbance in the autonomic nervous system. The disturbance is manifested systematically by increased nerve response at certain points.

Nakatani found that internal disturbances could be detected before they manifested clinically by measuring skin resistance. Nakatani also noticed that anatomical locations of electroconductive points in unhealthy subjects varied with the disease. Subjects with the same disease had most of their points in the same location. All of these electroconductive points were remarkably close in location and about equal to the number of points found in Asian acupuncture charts of the human body. Nakatani used electrical stimulation to normalize highly conductive points.

Kirlian Photography

Another approach to the study of this phenomenon was developed in 1961 by B. K. Kirlian. He devised a method of photographing the electromagnetic discharges emanating from various objects. This Kirlian phenomena and its possible relationship to electroconductive body points triggered much new research on the topic. Researchers wondered if the Kirlian effect was a result of discharges coming from galvanically detectable electroconductive skin points.

Kirlian photography is a good illustration of electromagnetic forces in the body. Perhaps visual and photographic analysis of these points can assist in the detection of diagnosis of diseases that have not yet manifested clinically.

Electromagnetic Points

The interesting thing about traditional Chinese medicine, studies of galvanic skin response, and Kirlian photography is that they all produce evidence of a pattern of electromagnetic points on the skin and all the patterns look more or less the same. We know that these points are related to underlying autonomic nerve activity and that they respond to stimulation by electricity, needles, heat, and pressure.

Researchers who have tested traditional acupuncture meridians to see if they are direct current paths have found that these meridians conduct electricity toward the spinal cord. The researchers concluded that the meridians carry messages to the brain which responds by sending back the electrical current needed to stimulate healing. This concept also helps explain how NAET works. NAET practitioners stimulate the nervous system to send new messages to the brain.

In addition to the acupuncture meridians, many systems identify seven energy centers, called chakras, located in the body along the spine. There are two contradictory views that attempt to explain the body's electromagnetic structure and the chakras. The first is that the biological structures produce the electromagnetic field in the body. In this view, electrochemical activity within nerve plexi is thought to create the energy vortices called chakras. The body is thought to produce an electrical current that is transformed and processed by boosters—the acupuncture points—and carried by power circuits—the acupuncture meridians—throughout the body.

The opposite view is that the electromagnetic energy produces the physical body. In this view, order begins to emerge from random activity in the quantum realm, replicates itself, and becomes a pattern. More precise patterns develop until a physical form emerges from information and energy carried on an electromagnetic wave. The energy pattern of the body, before it becomes physical, is the aura, or what Sheldrake calls the morphogenic field. The role of the chakras—according to this theory—is to process information carried on particular frequencies.

DESCRIPTION OF NAET TREATMENT

When an allergy is suspected, patients are muscle tested while holding a sample of the suspected allergen. When patients are allergic to the substance, a strong muscle weakens in response to a message from the brain. Once the allergy has been identified, patients continue to hold the offending substance while the practitioner checks to see what parts of the body are being blocked in response to the allergy. The practitioner can determine what areas are blocked by palpating or touching reflex areas on the abdomen. A strong indicator muscle weakens in different areas, corresponding to areas of blockage in the body. When the blockages have been identified, patients turn over, still holding the allergen, and the practitioner uses a tool to stimulate areas along the spine that correlate with the areas of blockage.

Stimulation of those areas balances the electromagnetic fields of the body in relation to the allergen and reprograms the nervous system to stop identifying this substance as an allergen. Patients are then retested. If the muscle responses with the allergen(s) are now strong, patients receive acupressure or acupuncture treatments while continuing to hold the former allergen. They are then told to avoid contact with the former allergen for twenty-five hours. At the end of that time they are tested again. If they do not expose themselves to the allergen during the twenty-five-hour period, they usually become desensitized. If they do come in contact with it, their allergy reaction may return over time.

For the first twenty-five hours following a treatment, I recommend that patients do not overstimulate their autonomic nervous systems by taking hot showers, running, watching scary movies, or doing anything that excites the body, either positively or negatively. The first six hours are especially critical because such activities compete with the allergy treatment's stimulation of the autonomic nervous system.

SELF-TREATMENT

The NAET treatment can be self-administered. I teach my patients and their families how to do muscle testing on each other so they can test for certain foods and for saliva when an infection is suspected. Treating for saliva within the first few hours of the symptoms of an infection stops the progression of viruses and bacteria. By using the acupressure points of NAET, the symptoms can be eliminated almost immediately. For example, if a child has a runny nose, coughing, or sore throat, he or she can spit into a thin glass and use it as a sample for muscle testing. If the muscle is weak, it shows that there is something in the saliva that is causing a reaction in the body, usually a virus. Stimulation of the acupressure points while the subject holds the saliva sample stops the allergic reaction, fights the virus so it does not progress, and allows the immune system to effectively get rid of the pathogen.

Any substance can be treated for in an emergency. For example, if one eats a cookie that causes abdominal pain or wheezing and coughing, he or she can hold the cookie in the hand and treat for it using the acupressure points, preferably every half hour to two hours until symptoms subside. If something in the cookie requires a complete NAET treatment, this might prove to be only a temporary solution. It certainly helps in an emergency, however. For more details on Emergency Treatment, refer to Chapter 3. For more information on Self-Treatment, refer to Chapter 5 and to Part VI.

10 NAET TREATMENT PROTOCOL

BASIC ALLERGIES

In my clinic we have a set treatment procedure for allergies, no matter what symptoms or complaints the patient presents. We always test and treat for the basic allergies in the prescribed sequence developed by Dr. Nambudripad after years of research, testing, and experimentation. After years of working with this sequence myself, I recognize how important it is. The complete clearing of each basic allergen in the proper order is crucial for successful results in treating all asthmatics and allergy sufferers.

For example, I remember treating one of my first NAET patients, a young man in his thirties with severe candidiasis and chronic fatigue. Not knowing how critical it was to clear the basic allergies in sequence, I immediately treated him for Candida. When the treatment was completed, he was so fatigued he could not get up off the table. When I called Dr. Nambudripad for help, she explained that we do the basics first to strengthen the immune response. She said he was not ready to treat Candida because his immune system was weak and could not clear such a severe allergen. I treated him again that day for eggs and he was fine. Three months later, after a series of NAET treatments including Candida, he could not remember what it was like to have chronic fatigue.

The basics are vitamins, minerals, and foods that are among the most allergenic and the main ingredients in many foods. When the allergies to these basic allergens are cleared, many other foods are cleared at the same time. These basic nutrients provide support for the immune system and are important coenzymes and cofactors of metabolism. Once they are utilized by the body, health improves dramatically. Before undergoing an NAET treatment, I recommend my patients review ahead of time the list of NAET restrictions so they are prepared to avoid the allergen physically when they leave the clinic. For a list of restrictions, refer to Part VI.

Chickens, Eggs, Feathers, and Tetracycline

The first basic is eggs and chickens. Sometimes it is necessary to treat separately for egg white and egg yolk and for white or dark meat in chickens. Included in this treatment are feathers and tetracycline, an antibiotic commonly given to chickens. When this treatment is done, a patient must stay away from eggs, chicken, feathers, and tetracycline for twenty-five hours.

I always treat for eggs and chickens first, even if people say they never eat them because they are ingredients in many foods and products such as shampoos and conditioners. Twenty-five hours after the treatment I retest patients to ensure they are cleared for each part of the allergen.

Sometimes treatments need to be done in combination. For example, eggs may need to be cleared in combination with another food, an organ, or an environmental condition such as heat or cold. This is important because treating eggs alone may not clear a serious allergy to a combination of eggs and some other substance or condition. On the other hand, clearing eggs may clear other allergies at the same time. Each individual is different. For example, one female asthmatic was tested for the ten basic allergies. When we treated her for eggs and chickens, most of the other allergies went away without being treated. After one treatment she never needed her inhaler again.

Calcium and Dairy Products

The next basic allergy we look at is calcium, an important mineral for the body. Milk, dairy products, and root and green vegetables are high in calcium as are sesame seeds, oats, navy beans, dry beans, almonds, walnuts, peanuts, sunflower seeds, sardines, and salmon. When people, especially women, are allergic to calcium, they are likely to be calcium deficient that causes joint pain, aching, crepitation in joints, osteoporosis, menstrual cramps, tetany, and headache. It also causes leg cramps, hyperactivity, restlessness, and an inability to relax because calcium is important in relaxation and sleep. Many asthmatics with upper respiratory problems respond well to treatment for calcium as well as people with abdominal pain, insomnia, skin problems, nervousness, canker sores, herpes, hyperactivity, obesity, and arthritis. Calcium is an important nutrient for everyone, particularly for asthmatics. To make up for deficiencies it may be necessary to take a calcium supplement after the allergy has been cleared.

One three-year-old boy came to me who had trouble sleeping. His mother thought it was because of his pollen allergies. After we treated him for calcium, he never had trouble sleeping again.

Vitamin C, Fresh Fruits, and Vegetables

The next allergy we treat for is Vitamin C. People wonder how anyone could be allergic to such an essential vitamin, but plenty of people are. In fact, the body can be allergic to virtually anything. Vitamin C is found in fresh fruits and vegetables, rose hips, citrus fruits, black currants, apples, strawberries, guavas, cherries, potatoes, cabbage, broccoli, tomatoes, turnip greens, green bell peppers, green and leafy vegetables, cauliflower, and sweet potatoes. Foods are the best source of Vitamin C, not the high-dosage supplements that many people take. When a Vitamin C allergy is cleared, allergies to many fruits and vegetables are automatically cleared.

Scurvy is caused by a lack of Vitamin C. One of the main symptoms of scurvy is fatigue. One of the main symptoms of Vitamin C allergy is also fatigue. People who have chronic sore throats often start taking Vitamin C immediately when symptoms begin. This is helpful for most people, but if they are allergic to Vitamin C, it may be the allergy itself causing the problem. Sometimes I find that Vitamin C allergies are linked with infectants such as bacteria or viruses. When a person who is allergic takes Vitamin C, it triggers the infectant and starts an infection.

This allergy is particularly important to asthmatics because a Vitamin C allergy also causes chronic bronchitis and respiratory infections common in asthmatics. I always check for and clear this allergy. People who get frequent colds and the flu usually have an allergy to Vitamin C and are therefore deficient in the Vitamin C they need to prevent these problems. If the twenty-four hour urine report shows a deficiency, I put people on supplements.

Vitamin C, especially ascorbic acid, has been shown to be helpful for asthma, but only if the patient is not allergic to it. One woman asthmatic I saw came from another health practitioner who had put her on high doses of ascorbic acid for severe wheezing and restricted breathing. The patient noticed not only that the Vitamin C failed to help, but also that she started experiencing fatigue, joint pain, kidney pain, headaches, and indigestion after taking it.

When I tested her I found her to be allergic to, and deficient in, Vitamin C. I treated her for the Vitamin C allergy and put her on high doses of a Vitamin C complex instead of ascorbic acid. I prefer not to use the ascorbic acid which is perceived as sugar by the body. I use the whole Vitamin C instead.

After the treatment for Vitamin C allergy, the patient needs to avoid all foods that contain it for twenty-five hours. If they don't, their allergy symptoms will return over time. This is crucial for asthmatics who suffer from a chronic and potentially fatal condition and need to clear the allergy to Vitamin C.

B Vitamins

The next, and perhaps most important, allergy we treat is an allergy to the B vitamins. This allergy is vitally important because the B vitamins are found in virtually every food. The only foods I have found that do not contain them are tapioca, Jell-O®, and Cool Whip®, something other than a healthy diet. I am working with others to create a nutritional powder without the B vitamins that will give patients something more substantial to eat during the post-treatment waiting period.

There are eleven different B vitamins, but I include B_{13}, B_{15}, and B_{17} as well in my treatment. The B vitamins were described in detail in Chapter 6. I treat all the B vitamins together, then test them separately to make sure each one has been cleared. Since they are so common in foods, allergies to any of the B vitamins cause serious problems for asthmatics. Most allergies to the B vitamins clear in one session, but some patients take two, three, or even four treatments to clear. Occasionally a patient needs to be cleared on several of the B vitamins separately.

B vitamins are essential for the emotional, physical, and psychological well-being of the body. They contribute to maintaining a healthy nervous system and aid in the digestion of fats and proteins. People allergic to B vitamins suffer severe depression, cloudy thinking, exhaustion, mood swings, and nervousness and can react to virtually any food.

B vitamins are used for the treatment of skin disorders and respiratory problems and help prevent colds and improve memory. Inositol, biotin, and choline prevent hair loss and are essential for healthy hair. Folic acid is needed for the formation of red blood cells and the prevention of anemia. Allergies to the B vitamins must be cleared if good health is to be maintained. Because Vitamin C and the B vitamins are so essential for asthmatics, I usually put the patient on supplements after I have checked and cleared for those allergies. I often include adrenal support as well.

One woman with severe asthma came to see me because her condition had become critical. She was taking large doses of medications, including inhalers and intermittent prednisone, and had become noticeably weaker as a result of her chronic asthmatic episodes. We started treating for the basic allergies. After we had desensitized her to Vitamin C and the B vitamins, I put her on an adrenal supplement that included those vitamins. Overnight her condition improved dramatically and she was able to go for ten to fourteen days without using an inhaler. She even had a fairly good winter for the first time in her life.

Most people who suffer from a chronic health problem have a Vitamin B allergy that needs to be cleared. Clearing it may also clear other allergens such as wheat, carbohydrates, many grains, some vegetables, potatoes, brewer's yeast, meat, and other foods high in B vitamins. Whole grain allergies seem to be the most commonly affected. People who crave carbohydrates usually have a strong B vitamin allergy.

Sugars

The next basic allergy to clear is to sugars. All the B vitamins must be cleared first, however, because they are important cofactors in the metabolism of sugars. Sugars are implicated in many different health problems, especially respiratory problems and asthma. If people are allergic to sugars and intolerant of them as well, eating sugars can cause chronic immune system problems, accumulation of mucus, malabsorption, indigestion, mood swings, weight problems, and a weakened immune response. The sugars we treat are maltose, glucose, dextrose, lactose, fructose, brown sugar, honey, corn sugar, raw sugar, cane sugar, molasses, high-fructose corn syrup, grape sugar, maple sugar, and sometimes gluten which is actually a protein.

Frequently we treat all the sugars at once, although some people are only allergic to one or two of them and should be treated for those separately. During the next twenty-five hours sugars must be avoided. This rules out all foods except meat, fish, or poultry.

Treating for sugar allergies is extremely rewarding. People who have craved sugars all their lives stop craving them. Children who have chronic ear infections, sore throats, or sinus congestion get better. Asthmatics with chronic coughs stop coughing overnight. In fact, sugar allergies seem to be involved in most chronic illness.

Iron and Meats

The next basic allergen to treat is iron. People with an iron allergy do not absorb the mineral from their food and become deficient, causing anemia. Their physicians then put them on iron supplements for long periods of time which doesn't help because they can't absorb iron. Allergic reactions include backaches, headaches, dizziness, menstrual problems, and fatigue. Iron is an essential nutrient that aids in growth, promotes resistance to disease, and prevents fatigue.

Clearing this allergy clears allergies to many foods that contain iron including apricots, peaches, bananas, prunes, raisins, black molasses, brewer's yeast, whole grains, cereals, turnip greens, spinach, beet tops, alfalfa, beets, asparagus, kelp, sunflower seeds, walnuts, sesame seeds, beans, egg yolk, liver, red meat, oysters, and clams. After an iron allergy is cleared, the patient must avoid all contact with iron for twenty-five hours. This involves wearing plastic gloves because iron is used in cars, cooking pots, and metal alloys.

Vitamin A, Betacarotene, Fish, and Shellfish

The next basic allergy treated is to Vitamin A. Vitamin A and betacarotene are important immunostimulants and protective agents crucial for healthy mucus membranes and the prevention of respiratory infections. Many physicians recommend Vitamin A supplements for asthmatics. This is fine as long as they are not allergic to it. A Vitamin A deficiency disturbs white blood cell production in the body and lowers immune function. It is necessary to maintain good vision and prevent night blindness, skin disorders, acne, colds, influenza, and other infections. It helps heal ulcers and wounds and is necessary for the growth of bones and teeth. Vitamin A is an antioxidant and helps protect the cells against free radicals. Betacarotene, found in vegetables and converts to Vitamin A in the liver, is good for the prevention of chronic health problems and is a powerful antioxidant.

When people are allergic to Vitamin A, they do not absorb it properly and become deficient. A deficiency causes skin tags, warts, blemishes, acne, rashes, hair loss, and premature aging. It also causes increased bronchial, lung, and respiratory problems, lowered immunity, infertility, joint pain, vomiting, and GI problems. Vitamin A works in conjunction with other vitamins such as the B complex, Vitamins D and E, calcium, and zinc that are required to mobilize it from the liver where it is stored. Large doses of Vitamin A should only be taken under proper supervision or it can accumulate to toxic levels in the body. Similarly, people who are allergic to Vitamin A and take large amounts are unable to absorb it and accumulate toxic levels in the liver. After clearing the allergy, supplementation may be helpful for a period of time.

Clearing a Vitamin A allergy clears allergies to such foods as papayas, peaches, yellow fruit, asparagus, beets, broccoli, carrots, Swiss chard, kale, turnip greens, watercress, parsley, red peppers, sweet potatoes, squash, yellow squash and other yellow vegetables, pumpkin, corn, spirulina, milk, butter, other dairy products, egg yokes, fish, and fish liver oil.

I saw a four-year-old boy who suffered from chronic respiratory, bronchial, and ear infections. He had been on and off antibiotics for over a year. We tried high doses of Vitamins A and C and took him off dairy products but he continued to get the infections. We noticed that he always had problems after taking Vitamin A and realized it was probably a major allergen for him. When we started the basic allergy treatments, we had to do the Vitamin A treatment three times because his mother forgot and kept giving him the Vitamin A supplement. After the allergy was successfully cleared he was symptom-free for nine months and continues to do well.

Minerals

The next basic allergy we clear is to minerals. Some of the minerals asthmatics are most often allergic to are calcium, chromium, cobalt, copper, selenium, potassium, phosphorus, sodium, sulfur, vanadium, zinc, and magnesium. There has been considerable study of the use of magnesium for asthmatics but I have found it necessary to treat them for the allergy before they take the supplement. Once the allergy is cleared, magnesium can be helpful in reducing asthma episodes.

After the treatment for minerals, the patient needs to avoid contact with metals and should use distilled water for washing and drinking. Calcium is usually cleared in a separate session and sometimes other minerals need to be treated separately as well. I test all asthmatics for allergies to each of the minerals mentioned.

Table Salt and Sodium Chloride

The next treatment is for salt allergies. I use a combination of table salt and sodium chloride when I am treating this allergy. Male asthmatics seem to have more of a problem with salt that can trigger coughing, excess mucus, and even asthma attacks in some people. Salt is hard to avoid because it is an ingredient in so many foods including most canned foods and restaurant dishes.

Clearing a salt allergy clears allergies to other foods such as pineapples, watermelon, celery, lettuce, carrots, beets, artichokes, avocados, Swiss chard, cabbage, cucumbers, tomatoes, asparagus, kelp, coffee, shellfish, and processed foods.

These are the basic allergies I treat in all my patients. For asthmatics there are a few other allergies that are also basic.

Phenolics

The first is to phenolics, naturally occurring compounds that color, flavor, and preserve food. They help in the germination of seeds and protect plants against other invaders. There are certain phenolics that are often problems for asthmatics. When allergies to these phenolics are cleared, many other food allergies clear at the same time. Phenolics also cause problems in combination with other allergens such as chemicals. I have had a lot of success with asthmatics by treating for this allergy.

The problematic phenolics are cinnamic acid, coumarin, dopamine, gallic acid, uric acid, rutin, phenylalanine, phenylisothiocyanate, malvin, indole, and histamine. Although these are the most common allergies, I check for all the phenolics because any of them can be a potential allergen for an asthmatic.

Amino Acids

If an asthma sufferer has symptoms suggesting hypo-glycemia or severe sugar problems, I treat for allergies to amino acids immediately. When people are allergic to amino acids, they do not absorb the protein they need from food. Protein, an essential building block in the body, is important for healing, healthy tissue, stamina, and prevention of fatigue.

The most remarkable aspect of NAET is the sequence developed by Dr. Nambudripad for the treatment of basic allergies. In her genius and her profound understanding of the body and acupuncture, Dr. Nambudripad realized that adherence to this sequence is crucial for success. If it is followed correctly, the results surpass any other treatment method available for allergies. After treating the basics, I go back and test each basic again (using muscle testing) to make sure they are all cleared. I test all the B vitamins, sugars, and minerals separately. If these basic allergies are cleared, a foundation has been laid for a healthy immune system and it is easier to clear other allergies.

I continually research to discover other allergens that should be added to the basic allergy treatment. Every day I have worked on this book, I have learned something new from my patients. They are truly my teachers and have educated me more than anyone else. Not a day goes by that I do not learn something about the mystery of the human body. The complications of the asthmatic and allergic condition and the number and combinations of possible allergens boggle my mind, whereas the incredible accomplishments of this allergy work amaze me. I deeply thank Dr. Devi Nambudripad for her contribution to the field of health and alternative healing and for her genius in discovering and developing this work.

This work has been an incredible gift to my family, my extended family, my patients, and myself. I cannot imagine living without NAET or raising my children without teaching them about NAET. It is an inextricable part of our lives. I believe no one should get sick. With the help of NAET and enzyme therapy, we can live completely free of sickness and physical disorders.

There are conditions other than asthma that I have treated and researched. I will talk about them more fully in later books. These include migraines, menopause, PMS, female problems in general, chronic fatigue, immune suppressive disorders, fibromyalgia, eczema, infertility, and multiple chemical sensitivities (environmental illness).

NAET TREATMENTS: DIFFERENT PROTOCOLS FOR DIFFERENT TYPES OF ASTHMA

After the basic allergens have been treated, I develop a protocol depending on whether the asthma being treated is mild, moderate, or severe, in children or infants, or related to occupation, athletics, or exercise. In the sections that follow I discuss different types of asthma and characteristic protocols for treating them.

MILD ASTHMA

Mild asthmatics are those with mild and infrequent symptoms. They may have attacks two or three times a year, usually triggered by viruses. Their symptoms tend to occur in spring and fall when pollens proliferate. After I clear the basic allergies for people with mild asthma, I start working on the food allergies that did not clear automatically when the basics were cleared.

The significant food allergies I have seen in mild asthmatics include cow's milk, fish, various nuts, seeds, soy and soy products, wheat, and citrus fruits. Others are chocolate, coffee, caffeine, many grains, spices, animal and vegetable fat, dried beans, yeast products, alcohol, baking powder, baking soda, gum mix, vegetable mix, and acid and alkaline foods. Common acid foods are sugars, starches, milk products, dairy products, fruits, vegetables, beans, tomatoes, onions, peppers, and potatoes. Often I treat for the chemical called solanine that is natural to the nightshade family (tomatoes, capsicum, eggplant, tobacco, and potatoes). All of the nightshades contain nicotine and I sometimes treat for it as well.

Treating for mold sometimes clears allergies to foods such as dried fruit, nuts, and cream cheese. Clearing for gluten clears allergies to the grains that contain it (wheat, rye, oats, malt, and barley).

Corn is another common food allergen I check at this point in the treatment. Some commercial adhesives, talcum powder, and starched clothes can all provoke reactions in corn-sensitive patients. Sweat causes some of the corn-laden starch in clothing to be absorbed into the body and can provoke a reaction in asthmatics. Even licking a stamp can cause a reaction in an asthmatic allergic to corn. Clearing an allergy to corn clears allergies to environmental allergens as well.

Next I look at a chemical neurotransmitter called dopamine, a stimulant of the chemical neurotransmitter norepinephrine and found in oranges and grapefruits. It causes problems in some asthmatics, as do salicylates and sulfites, also found in many foods.

Sulfites prevent the browning and discoloration of foods that usually occur at room temperatures and are used to preserve wine, raw potatoes, and fresh vegetables. Ingestion of large amounts of these chemicals can cause problems. By clearing or desensitizing people to sulfites, we can clear many other foods such as avocados, baked products, beet sugar, dried fruits, fresh shrimp, fruit drinks, gelatin, wine, beer, potatoes, starches, vegetables, salads, and cider as well as allergies to cellophane. Sulfites are commonly used in the manufacture of many drugs including asthma aerosols.

Food additives should be checked next. BHA, BHT, sodium benzoine, sodium nitrate, sodium sulfate, tartrazine, and food dyes are common problems. By clearing them we clear allergies to foods that contain the additives.

Treating for oxalic acid can clear foods high in oxalates including chocolate, caffeine, coffee, tomatoes, citrus fruits, spinach, some beans, and mushrooms (refer to Part VI for a more complete list).

After the food allergies have been cleared, most mild asthmatics are significantly improved and can permanently stop taking medication. In many cases, most of the food allergies clear when the basic allergies are treated and do not have to be treated individually. Some mild asthmatics need to be treated for allergies to pollens, trees, dust, grasses, weeds and shrubs as well as for sensitivities to their medications and occasionally fabrics including cotton and some nylons. Smoke, tobacco smoke, perfumes, animal dander, dogs, horses, and molds might also need to be treated but in mild asthmatics, this is usually all the NAET treatments they need.

One mildly asthmatic woman came to see me who suffered from asthma when she was around animals, tobacco smoke, and certain foods. As long as she stayed away from those allergens she was generally free from attacks without taking medications. She was afraid of an emergency, however, and carried an inhaler when traveling. After we treated her for the basic allergies, she no longer needed an inhaler around animals or smoke. It has now been two years, and she no longer travels with an inhaler.

A fourth-grade boy came to me with severe environmental allergies to pollen and trees and mild asthma around cats. Mold seemed to be the worst allergen, causing wheezing, congestion, hyperactivity, attention deficit, and fatigue. He was fine during the spring and summer. We treated him for the basic allergies and then for some food allergies to wheat, yeast, milk, and some fruits. After that, he had no more reactions to pollens or cats, the dark circles under his eyes disappeared, his attention span was normal, and he did well in school.

Occupational Allergens

In all the asthma groups—mild, moderate, and severe—I also treat for occupational allergens that people are frequently exposed to in the workplace. If a person works in a gas station, I treat for gas fumes, chemicals, gas, and diesel exhaust. If a patient is a painter, I treat for paints, chemicals, and other work materials. A person who works in a hair salon is treated for hair dyes and a photographer for photographic chemicals. People in detergent factories are exposed to chemicals that remove stains; artists to adhesives and epoxy resins, and bakers to dyes, flour, and cornstarch. Cannery workers are exposed to bleaches, chrome, fish parts, foods, and oils. Carpenters are exposed to adhesives, exotic wood, plastics, fiberglass, and varnishes, and chemists to antibiotics, formalins, acids, and ammonia. Electricians deal with electricity and isocyanates, florists with mold, and gardeners with dried pots, pollens, fertilizers, and mulch. Garment workers are in contact with cotton, nylon, acrylic, polyester, feathers, formalines, and solvents, metal workers with platinum, chromates, and metal dusts, and printers with cobalt, glue, solvents, zinc, chromates, gum arabic, and pine resin. All of these are potential allergens and potential triggers for asthmatics.

One man I treated sold bread. He was asthmatic and suffered from chronic sinus allergies. When we cleared his wheat allergy, he no longer had problems being around bread. Treatment of occupational allergies such as these keep people from leaving work or going on disability.

MODERATE ASTHMA

Moderate asthmatics develop symptoms more frequently than mild asthmatics. They tend to experience problems every four to six weeks and use asthma medication every day in order to prevent symptoms.

I start by treating them for the basic allergies and follow with a treatment for phenolics. I also include treatments for histamine and prostaglandins, chemicals involved in the body's immune response to allergens. When an allergen or nonspecific irritant contacts the immune cells— mast cells—they begin to leak histamine and prostoglandins into the surrounding tissue. These chemicals cause muscle contractions, swelling, and mucus secretion and an allergy to these chemicals can be serious for an asthmatic.

Next I treat moderate asthmatics for sensitivities to their everyday medications including inhalers and prednisone, if taken. I follow this with a treatment for infectants including viruses, bacteria, fungi, and parasites. Frequently, allergens are linked to infectants in the bodies of asthmatics, creating chronic infections. By treating for the infectants, we stop the cycle of chronic infections and chronic antibiotic use. When clear of infections, the lung tissue heals and the immune system strengthens.

Candida

Yeast infections of Candida in all its many forms are a chronic problem for both moderate and severe asthmatics. Most asthmatics suffer the symptoms of a Candida infection of bloating, fatigue, and possible vaginal infections. Yeast organisms convert sugars to a chemical called pyruvate which is then converted to acetaldehyde and carbon dioxide. Carbon dioxide is the main culprit in bloating and gas and buildup is a problem for asthmatics (refer to the Outdoor Environment Allergens section in Part VI).

When I treat for yeast infections, I also treat for alcohol. Some scientific studies have shown that Candida albicans in the body produces enough ethanol to make the infected individual drunk. Ethanol, one of the phenolics, is sometimes cleared by treating for phenolics.

I find that after I have treated for the basic allergies, phenolics, and some infectants, particularly Candida, many respiratory problems decrease significantly and moderate asthmatics no longer need their medications.

When people are treated for a sensitivity to Candida they must remain on a special diet for ten to fourteen days and curtail their sexual activity (or use a latex barrier) to ensure that Candida is not passed back and forth sexually. Candida can also be spread through toothbrushes, dentures, fabrics, and skin-to-skin contact. If a couple comes to see me and both have Candida, the one showing symptoms is usually the one who is allergic. The person not showing symptoms could still be passing it to his or her mate, so both should be checked. This is not absolutely essential, however, because once the Candida allergy is successfully treated and the yeast removed from the system, symptoms do not reoccur even if Candida is transmitted by another.

It takes as long as two months to completely rid the system of Candida but the ten- to fourteen-day diet is crucial. The pathogenicity—or the ability of an infectant to do harm—is, I believe, a result of an allergy to that infectant. If people are not allergic to Candida, their bodies will be able to deal with it and eliminate it from their system.

I have found that Candida albicans and Candida tropicalis are the most common yeast infectants found in asthmatics. Candida albicans grows rapidly in a medium of sugars, biotin, and organic salts and it prefers an acid **pH**. The higher the biotin level, the more yeast there is. Antibiotics tend to increase the toxicity of yeast and Candida, and the widespread use of tetracycline for teenage acne ends up causing more skin problems by encouraging yeast overgrowth.

Candida adheres to mucosal epithelial surfaces in the respiratory tract and provokes an antibody response in those who are allergic. It has been shown to stimulate histamine release from mast cells, thereby producing a strong allergenic response in asthmatics.

Candida albicans can cause serious problems for asthmatics. Candida overgrowth occurs in the human body when the defenses are locally impaired such as in a disturbance of the gut flora. This disturbance can be caused by parasitic, viral, or bacterial infections. Nutritional deficiencies, allergies, altered glucose metabolism, hypoglycemia, and diabetes can also be factors. Therapies such as antibiotics, cortical steroids, and oral contraceptives are factors in lowering immune defenses. Immunity can be impaired by HIV infections, chemotherapy, radiation, genetic defects, high chemical exposure, high carbohydrate and sugar diets, pregnancy, menses, and thyroid and adrenal deficiencies.

Other symptoms of Candida infection in asthmatics are fatigue, moodiness, depression, anxiety, inability to concentrate, lack of energy, PMS in women, aching muscles and joints, arthritis, fibromyalgia, GI problems such as abdominal bloating, constipation, diarrhea and irritable bowel, skin rashes, vaginal and rectal itching, urticaria, cystitis, and persistent vaginal discharge. A significant number of asthmatics also have other ear, nose, and throat symptoms, recurrent ear infections, throat mucus, postnasal drip, and sinusitis. In males a correlation has been shown between chronic Candida and prostatitis. Both male and female Candida sufferers experience an unusual degree of craving for sweets and carbohydrates.

To clear an allergy to Candida it is necessary to have effectively cleared sensitivities to sugars and B vitamins. Following treatment, patients follow a sugar- and carbohydrate-free diet that includes meat, vegetables, and unsweetened yogurt (refer to the section on Candida diets in Part VI).

When undergoing treatment for Candida, including antifungal medication or dietary changes, many people have what is called a die-off reaction. This can be prevented with NAET treatments for Candida in combination with other allergens. I might treat Candida with certain foods or with DNA or RNA if the person has a genetic tendency toward the sensitivity. I might also treat it in combination with temperature sensitivities—heat or cold—or with certain organs. When all of an individual's Candida combinations are treated and it is completely eliminated, there is no die-off reaction.

One man in his forties came to see me with chronic Candida infections. He experienced fatigue, insomnia, severe bloating, and fogginess. He had suffered for a long time and tried many alternative treatments with only occasional and temporary relief. The woman he was with was also diagnosed with Candida, and they were passing it back and forth. We treated him for the basic allergies and then for Candida and some other fungi we had found. It took several sessions to clear the sensitivity. He went on the special diet for ten to fourteen days and I gave him an enzyme containing probiotic microflora, cellulose, and magnesium, good for detoxification of Candida. After treatments that stretched over a three-month period, he felt better, was able to resume his sexual relationship, and eat the foods that had previously caused difficulties.

Not every moderate asthmatic has Candida but there are certain conditions and symptoms that indicate this problem exists. People who have taken large amounts of antibiotics are at risk. This includes most moderate to severe asthmatics. People with chronic ear infections, athlete's foot, nail infections, skin rashes, oral thrush, colic, recurrent cystitis, jock itch, or loss of libido are likely to have Candida infections as are people who suffer from allergies during infancy and childhood, diabetes, or AIDS. A good indication of a Candida infection is symptoms that start after taking oral contraceptives. Vaginal thrush, pelvic inflammatory disease (PID), and endometriosis all indicate Candida infections and these conditions are treated quite effectively with NAET and enzymes. Recurring nasal polyps can indicate a Candida infection or a respiratory mold allergy.

Treatment with immunosuppressive drugs such as steroids, cortisone, and prednisone for asthma, skin problems, or arthritis can all produce Candida infections. Moderate and severe asthmatics are likely to have taken these medications at one time or another. Another sign of infection is when the symptoms are aggravated after eating foods containing yeast or molds or if the symptoms get worse during wet weather, on humid days, or after exposure to dampness in places such as cellars and attics. Candida infections can cause a craving for sweets, alcohol, and carbohydrates but this can also be caused by allergies to sugars or B vitamins. High sugar diets and multiple pregnancies can bring on Candida infections also.

Infectants: Viruses, Bacteria, and Parasites

Other groups of infectants are parasites, bacteria, and viruses that can cause symptoms ranging from asthma to fatigue. Refer to Part VI for a list of the most common infectants for asthmatics. Some I check for are giardia, Campylobacter, Enteroviruses, and Heliobacter pylori, related to ulcers and a problem for elderly asthmatics. Asthmatics as a group tend to respond well to the parasite and bacteria allergy treatment. Bacterial NAET treatments can turn the corner for a moderate asthmatic. I have found from fifteen to twenty bacterial allergies in most moderate and severe asthmatics. Over the years these bacteria have been controlled by the use of antibiotics. I recommend a good liver detoxification program beginning one month after removing the parasites.

When I finish treating for parasites I move on to food and treat for food allergies in the same way as I do for mild asthmatics. I do detailed and ongoing studies of computerized and muscle response testing on each patient to find and clear all of their food allergies.

Environmental Allergies

After clearing food allergies I move on to environmental allergies and begin treating for pollens, molds, and other outdoor allergens, animal dander, dust, fabrics, wood, chemical irritants, gas, and other indoor irritants. Any of these can be triggers for asthmatics.

There is a process called "outgassing" in which certain products give off gasses or chemicals that can be picked up by contact or inhaled into the body and enter the bloodstream. Perfume, new carpets, and heated plastic, even flowers on a table, all outgas. Many of these can be smelled although chemicals without smell can also be toxic or act as a deadly trigger for asthmatics. Materials in car interiors, formaldehyde, toluene, zylene, hexanes, nitrous oxide, ozone, carbon monoxide, carbon dioxide, alkanes, petrochemicals, and other hydrocarbons can all be health threats to asthmatics and other sensitive people. Photocopy paper outgasses tricholoroethylene (TCE), a solvent used in dry cleaning fluids, carpet shampoos, floor polishes, and furniture glues. Asthmatics should be desensitized to this chemical in particular. Paint fumes also can be a problem, along with cleaning solvents, aerosol sprays, and tobacco and wood smoke.

When I am not aware of which chemical in a room is causing a problem, I have the patient put out a small jar of water and leave it open for twenty-four hours. They close the jar and bring it with them on the next visit. I then treat them for a sensitivity to the water which by now has trapped whatever chemicals are outgassing into the room. I do the same with outdoor allergens. I have the patient put a bowl of water outside the house to collect pollen for forty-eight hours and then treat them for the water. Sometimes I still need to treat for individual allergens such as specific molds and mildew in a patient's bathroom. When I am treating for an inhalant such as tobacco smoke or perfume, I have the patient inhale the substance rather than just touch it during the session.

These environmental allergies are usually the last ones that need to be cleared for moderate asthmatics. Some individuals also need to be treated for certain organs or for cortisol, adrenaline, or other hormones including male or female hormones. At this point in the treatment the moderate asthmatic should be free of symptoms and off all medication.

SEVERE ASTHMA

Severe asthmatics have frequent acute asthma episodes. They wheeze and cough regularly, need daily treatment and medication, and find exercise and sports difficult.

Medications

For severe asthmatics I begin with the basic allergens, starting with eggs, chicken, and feathers. If feathers do not clear I recheck for the allergy and treat again. With severe asthmatics I sometimes treat for sensitivities to their medications even before I treat for the basic allergies, especially if they take medications every day because their bodies may be creating the asthma in order to get the medications. Depending on the individual, I treat the medications all together or one at a time.

I treated one woman for the prednisone she was taking and her need for all other medication disappeared. Another woman in her fifties, a severe asthmatic on frequent but not daily medication, had bouts of severe asthma episodes that were clearly triggered by allergies. She also suffered from severe sinus congestion and sinus infections. When I treated her for the basic allergies, sugar had to be cleared several times because she craved it and had trouble clearing the individual sugars. Once food allergies had been cleared, environmentals such as flowers, pollen, trees, grasses, animals (she had two dogs), perfume (she worked in a large department store), smoke from other workers, and infectants were treated. Within nine to ten months after treatment, when I had finished with the environmentals including mold, she went off her inhalers and medication and has not had an asthma attack in over two years.

Phenolics

After treating for medications and basic allergies I treat for the phenolics, particularly histamine. Caffeine is also a phenolic and I treat for it and others including estrogen as needed. Candida can be considered a phenolic also. I have treated some patients for phenolics and all their food allergies disappeared. They did not need to be treated for anything else. Sometimes I treat phenolics immediately in severe asthmatics.

Amino Acids

Next I treat for sensitivities to amino acids. Because some of the amino acids are considered phenolics they will already have been cleared. The main difficulty with treating for amino acids is that the only food the patient can eat for the next twenty-five hours is lettuce. Everything else has amino acids in it. I am trying to create a nutritional formula without amino acids that will give these patients something more substantial to eat. Although most people can go without much food for twenty-five hours, those who are more seriously ill can undergo treatment for the amino acids separately. This allergy must be cleared so that people can digest and assimilate proteins, necessary to ensure healthy immune function and good tissue repair. In fact, I generally put asthmatics on a low-sugar, low-carbohydrate, high-protein diet as soon as possible.

Parasites and Bacteria

I treat the infectants next in severe asthmatics. Again, I find Candida to be crucial, along with parasites and bacteria. Sensitivities to bacteria are among the most serious problems for severe asthmatics. These bacteria produce large amounts of mucus and chronic infections leading to pneumonia and chronic bronchitis. Much of the problem with bacteria is a result of years of antibiotic treatment and therapy with immunosuppressive drugs such as prednisone and other corticosteroids. Treating asthmatics for bacterial allergies often produces increased stamina and energy levels and a reduction of other allergies.

Vaccines

I also check for reactions to vaccines that people have received as children such as tetanus, DPT, polio, measles, mumps, rubella, or any vaccine taken for travel abroad. I test and treat for each vaccine individually. I find these vaccines can stress and suppress the immune system for years unless allergies to them are cleared.

Once vaccine sensitivities have been cleared I use either muscle response testing or computerized testing to check every food and food group. Some food allergies clear when mold and oxalic acid have cleared but there are still many other foods for which to treat. In pollen season I treat for pollens after—or in special cases before—foods.

Dental Amalgams

Next I treat for dental amalgams. Mercury can severely compromise the immune system and can be a trigger for asthmatics. Many other materials can be used to restore a cavity in a tooth, from plastics to gold and porcelain, although all of those materials must be checked for allergic reactions before they are used. Some dentists can do the testing, or people can be checked and desensitized by a NAET practitioner.

There is quite a bit of controversy about the advisability of removing mercury fillings. At some point it is probably best to remove all mercury from the mouth but there should be careful preparation. People should be treated for, and desensitized to, mercury and other parts of the amalgam fillings before the old filling are removed. During removal, these substances are released into the bloodstream and can cause a strong allergic response that could last for a lifetime. It is also good to take antioxidants when preparing for mercury removal.

Pesticides

Next I treat for pesticides including insecticides, fungicides, herbicides, fumigants, and rodenticides. There are several families of insecticides: organophosphates, chlorinated hydrocarbons, botanicals, and chemical sterilants.

One asthmatic man I treated did extremely well with all the basic allergies and pollens. He had not needed medications for months until he visited his father whose house had just been fumigated by a pest control firm. Because the pesticide residues were lingering in the house, my patient had a severe asthma attack and had to go to the hospital where he was put on steroids. After he was treated for the pesticides, he recovered almost immediately and no longer had any problems at his father's house.

Although DDT was banned as toxic many years ago, it lingers in the soil and we continue to be exposed to it.

Some of the so-called inert ingredients in commercial pesticides are among the most harmful. Carbon tetrachloride and chloroform, for example, are powerful liver and central nervous system toxins. Fruits are sprayed with a pesticide called daminozide, potentially harmful for asthmatics. Even natural repellents such as vinegar and garlic can be toxic to anyone who is allergic to them.

Authorities are reluctant to issue warnings about specific pesticide exposure levels because exact toxic levels are not known. Measuring pesticide levels in one food is not an accurate measure of health hazard, however, because chemical combinations can have a synergistic effect. Pesticides can also leak into water supplies and I always check people for the water they drink, whether it is spring water, filtered water, or tap water.

Just because people are desensitized to pesticides, however, does not mean the chemicals are no longer harmful. Eating them can cause cancer, liver damage, stomach problems, or other symptoms. Washing fruits and vegetables is generally not an effective way to get rid of them. Certain natural products such as grapefruit extract and borax can be used to remove pesticides but people should make sure they are not allergic to those products before using them. By far the best way to avoid pesticides is to eat organically grown food.

Perfumes, Cosmetics, and Toiletries

Following pesticides, I treat for perfumes and cosmetics that can be triggers for asthmatics. Some of the common ingredients that cause trouble are alcohol, aluminum, acetone (found in nail polish remover), ammonium compounds, chloride (a preservative used in some cosmetics to prevent the growth of bacteria), BHA (a synthetic antioxidant), mercury, and colorants, dyes, and color additives that contain coal tar substances. These chemicals can also cause hyperactivity in children. Other potentially allergic products are detergents, soaps, petroleum derivatives, fluorinated hydro-carbons used in aerosols, mineral oils, crude oil, and liquid hydrocarbon, found in hair sprays and a potential problem for both hairdressers and clients. In all, cosmetics and toiletries contain about 8,000 chemicals and chemical compounds, many of which have not been tested by the FDA.

For asthmatics, perfumes and cosmetics derived from petroleum or coal tar can be as bad as cigarette smoke. Even flower oils are chemically extracted with petroleum ether. Unfortunately, it is becoming impossible to walk into a store, wash clothes, or flush a toilet without being assailed by scents and chemicals. Perfumes can linger in the air, on clothing, on furniture, in busses, theaters, restaurants, and workplaces long after the person wearing it has gone. An effective air purifier is helpful in reducing the exposure to tolerable levels.

Fragrances are among the few chemicals in products for human use that are not regulated although they pose an extreme danger to many people. There should be clear labeling with precise information about ingredients and restrictions on chemicals used in scented products.

Clearing patients for cosmetics and perfumes is difficult because they must avoid these ubiquitous products for twenty-five hours after the treatment. During this period they must wear a mask and gloves unless they are in a room that is perfume free. When I do a treatment, I wear a shower cap and gown over my clothes because I spray a little perfume for the patient to inhale. I do the same when treating for smoke allergies.

Fabrics

The next group of allergens I test for in severe asthmatics is fabrics including cotton, rayon, nylon, dacron, polyester, and acrylic. I usually treat for all the other fabrics first and have them wear all cotton. This is crucial for those asthmatics with severe sinus problems, difficulty smelling or tasting, sinus congestion, runny nose, wheezing, and frequent night attacks.

Chemicals

Next I treat for chemicals found in household products, home and work spaces, public places, and cars. We treat for formaldehyde, synthesized from methyl alcohol and found in insulation, particle board, foam rubber, detergents, carpet underlay, new clothes and other textiles, newsprint, household and industrial cleaners, propellants, plywood, resin, glue, concrete, and dyes. It is also found in name tags, correction Wite•Out®, leather goods, decaffeinated coffee, and embalming fluid. Formaldehyde is so prevalent in our environment that patients must wear masks and gloves after the treatment to keep from being exposed. Fingertips are sensitive and should not be exposed within four feet of an allergen if not covered with gloves during the twenty-five hour period.

Carbon Dioxide (CO_2) and Oxygen (O_2)

After treating for chemicals, I treat for carbon dioxide and oxygen. This is especially important for those asthmatics whose symptoms become worse when they climb to the top of a mountain or fly in airplanes because these are times when their bodies produce more carbon dioxide. Candida can also produce a large amount of carbon dioxide that creates bloating. For people allergic to carbon dioxide, this excess can stress the immune system (refer to Chapter 5, Outdoor Environment Allergens).

I next treat for the miscellaneous allergens for which the patient has tested positive. Those might include freon from air-conditioning, radon, plants and ferns, all the various gums, kapok from mattresses, poison oak and poison ivy, rubber, adhesive tape, cement, chalk, all the pesticides, hydrocarbons, paper mix, newsprint, photocopy paper, fabrics, plastics, radiation, benzene, labels, nail chemicals, hair chemicals, and bug spray.

Hormones

I also check for sensitivities to hormones such as adrenaline, estrogen, testosterone, progesterone, thyroid hormones, and cortisol, the natural inflammatory hormone that reacts to allergens in the body. People who are allergic to cortisol may have an asthma attack in response to the inflammation caused by an allergen. The other adrenal hormones such as insulin, glucagon, and DHEA are also important. Women who become more asthmatic during PMS are usually allergic to progesterone. If their symptoms increase after the menstrual cycle, they are probably allergic to estrogen. These sensitivities respond well to treatments with NAET.

I have found that many asthmatics who experience fatigue, temperature change intolerance, weight gain, depression, and test positive for Candida allergy are thyroid deficient or allergic to their own thyroid. A common name for this is autoimmune thyroiditis (**Hashimoto's disease**). These patients do well when treated for the thyroid hormone, iodine, vegetable fat, animal fat, mercury, and some amino acids. Animal fat is particularly important. This thyroid condition is common in those with severe asthma but rarer in those with mild or moderate cases.

Organs, Glands, and Cells

The next group of allergens I test for is organs, glands, and parts of the nervous system. The treatment for these conditions is one of the most successful and helpful for asthmatics by itself or when combined with a treatment for bronchial asthma.

The main function of the lungs is to inhale air containing oxygen and to exhale carbon dioxide from the body. That is why it is important to treat and eliminate any allergies to oxygen and carbon dioxide. The essential exchange of these gasses takes place in the air sacks—alveoli—and I test to see if patients are sensitive to their own lung alveoli. A sensitivity to this area of the body not only causes an autoimmune reaction that destroys cells, but also interferes with the lungs' ability to function optimally.

Before the air reaches the air sacks in the lung, it passes through the windpipe (trachea), then through a series of tubes called the bronchial tubes. I find many asthmatics, particularly severe asthmatics, allergic to their own bronchial tubes. The main bronchial tubes also divide into smaller tubes called bronchioles, and some people are allergic to them as well. In people who are allergic to their own bronchial tubes or bronchioles, the exchange of gases is not normal. Additionally, there are hundreds of thousands of cells in the walls of the bronchial tubes called mast cells. When an allergic reaction occurs, the mast cells secrete toxic chemicals that we call mediators. Mediators cause the walls of the bronchial tubes to swell up. Muscles go into spasm and create an obstruction in the lung. There is the added danger that people might be allergic to the mast cells and the mediators, one of which is histamine. There is also a newly discovered group called leukotrienes to which people can be allergic.

The mediators histamine and prostaglandins cause smooth muscle to contract and cause edema, swelling, and increased mucus secretion. This mucus production is intended as a defense against infectants but is also produced by allergic reactions when there are no infectants present. When this occurs, cells such as eosinophils, lymphocytes, T cells, macrophages, epithelial cells, and neutrophils in the bloodstream move into the bronchial tubes and attach themselves where the walls are inflamed. If the body is allergic to any of those cells, an autoimmune reaction occurs and the immune system attacks the lung tissue. The eosinophils play the biggest role in this reaction.

When a bronchial tube is totally inflamed, fibrin, a kind of scar tissue, is deposited in the bronchial tube to aid in healing. The scarring causes the tube to contract. An allergy to the fibrin intensifies the reaction and causes more fibrin to be deposited.

When these allergic reactions occur, the bronchial tubes do not let air pass in and out of the lungs, resulting in the common symptoms of asthma. Therefore, treating these allergies in asthmatics can be very helpful. Treating the lungs can be helpful to other patients as well. Treating the mast cells and specific cell mediators with NAET, enzymes, and other anti-inflammatory natural products work extremely well for asthmatics. Sometimes the inflammation is aggravated by medications and it is important to check for reactions and allergies to these medications.

The Immune System

The immune system should also be thoroughly checked and treated, if necessary. There are three major parts of the immune system: the thymus gland, the lymph nodes (lymph glands), and the bone marrow. Many times it is necessary to treat all three to boost the immune system. These organs produce two major types of blood cells: B cells and T cells. They are the main warriors that defend the body against invaders of any kind—bacteria, viruses, cancer, and other diseases. The B cells produce antibodies or immunoglobulins, and the T cells secrete chemicals called cytokines. These cells protect the body against any antigen seen as a threat. For example, when someone is exposed to an allergen, the B cells produce antibodies and the T cells produce cytokines designed specifically to fight that allergen. The next time the person encounters this antigen, whether allergen or bacteria, the antibody blocks it and the cytokines neutralize the toxin. During a lifetime, the body makes many different antibodies, most of which protect it from diseases.

IgE Antibodies

To protect itself against invaders, the body produces IgE antibodies. Unfortunately, these antibodies can also be harmful because they can trigger allergic reactions by attaching themselves to mast cells in the skin, nose, intestines, and bronchial tubes. These antibodies are most commonly produced by the body in reaction to parasites, pollen, and dust. Severe asthmatics tend to produce large amounts of IgE antibodies and develop reactions to many foods, environmental allergens, and other allergenic substances. I have had good results treating asthmatics for the IgE antibodies, B-cell antibodies, and the T cells. If people are allergic to these antibodies, their bodies are not producing the proper antibodies or are producing too many. Either situation can be dangerous.

Sympathetic and Parasympathetic Nervous Systems

All NAET treatments utilize the nervous system but there are parts of the nervous system that should be checked in asthmatics to see if a patient is allergic to them. The nervous system controls all our bodily functions. The brain and spinal cord constantly send and transport nerve impulses throughout the body. The nervous system is made up of the sympathetic nervous system and the parasympathetic nervous system. The sympathetic nervous system slows down certain functions, whereas the parasympathetic nervous system stimulates organs and tissues. They act in harmony with each other. For example the sympathetic nervous system opens or dilates the bronchial tubes and the parasympathetic closes or constricts them. If there is an allergic reaction to one or both of these parts of the nervous system, an imbalance can cause too much dilation or constriction. When we treat with NAET, we treat to stop the interference with, and imbalances in, these areas of the nervous system.

Emotions

Another allergen to treat for in cases of severe asthma is emotion. Many reactions in the body are related to core emotions such as anger, fear, sorrow, grief, shame, disappointment, and frustration. Reactions often are related to significant experiences in the person's life. I discover what the core emotion or experience is by using the muscle testing procedure, having the patient feel the emotions or recall the experience, then treating him or her with NAET.

One young girl lost her voice when her singing teacher told her she needed to lower her voice and practice speaking more softly. When we treated the girl for rage toward the teacher, her voice began to return.

Sometimes it is necessary to determine the particular incident that triggered the reaction. I narrow down the times in the patient's life by muscle response testing for particular age ranges such as 0 to 5 years old, 5 to ten years old, and so on. Then I check any relationship involved with the incident—mother, father, sister, brother, child—and the kind of incident—love, financial, business, health experienced. While patients recall the incident and feel the emotions, I treat areas on the spine related to the pathways or organs that are blocked. This treatment is inevitably successful.

Similar to material substances, emotions can be allergens and cause an electromagnetic disturbance in the body. Some emotions can cause an exaggerated response to another allergen or an allergy treatment, always an indication to me that there is an emotional allergy involved. An emotional allergy means that something happened in connection with food, a family member, or friends and an emotional component is stored in the body tied to this allergen. The body is not able to eliminate this allergen unless the emotion connected to it is treated as well. Within minutes after a treatment for an emotional allergy, patients generally feel better, look different, and can eat former food allergens without problems. When treating for emotional allergies to foods, the twenty-five hour restricted diet is not always necessary.

One young boy started kindergarten and began having trouble with his teacher. This manifested as a learning difficulty and some behavior problems. I treated him for an emotional allergy connected to an incident that happened between him and his father that he did not remember. Immediately after the treatment his expression and bodily attitude changed, his learning difficulty went away, and his behavior improved.

Combination Allergies

Some people have combination allergies. Although they are not common, they can occur in severe asthma cases. The combinations can be anything from another food to an organ. After I have treated for an allergen, I always check to see if there is any combination with that allergen to which a person may be allergic. There may even be more than one combination with a given allergen. For example, Vitamin C may be combined with DNA, meaning there is a genetic tendency towards that sensitivity. The same person may also have a Vitamin C allergy in combination with a food, organ, or infectant. Sometimes these allergies are so strong that it takes many acupressure self-treatment sessions to clear them. It often helps to make up a vial of the allergen for people with combination allergies, send it home with them, and have them treat themselves several times a day for a week or two, or until the combination clears. We do not need to know the other part of the combination, nor do they have to avoid it. Clearing for the one allergen while doing the acupressure self-treatment described in Part VI eventually clears the combination.

This self-treatment has proven very effective but only after people have been completely cleared of the original allergen (for example, Vitamin C). Otherwise, the self-treatment could aggravate some symptoms. This does not apply to the saliva self-treatment described in a previous chapter, possibly because it is a treatment for a virus that has only recently contacted the body. The immune system can more quickly and easily attack, fight, and eliminate such a virus, and people experience instant relief.

I recently treated Wendy, a young woman with eczema, severe itching, and lesions on her eyelids and neck. Her symptoms increased around citrus foods. I treated her for ascorbic acid four times and, thinking she was cleared, had her self-treat with ascorbic acid at home. Two days later Wendy reported that she was itching so severely she had drawn blood. She had noticed that the itching intensified when she treated herself. I had her come in immediately, retested her, and found she was still allergic to Vitamin C. We had to treat her again. When she finally cleared Vitamin C, she was able to self-treat. Her symptoms subsided and now she eats citrus fruits with no problems.

Bronchial Asthma

The next step is to treat severe asthma patients for a sensitivity to bronchial asthma. If we can clear this allergy, the body can rid itself of the disease. In mild or moderate asthmatics, this allergy usually clears automatically before we reach this treatment. For severe patients, however, I sometimes need to clear bronchial asthma specifically. This may also be necessary for people who have not been diagnosed with asthma but have a genetic tendency toward the disease and suffer from coughing and chronic bronchitis.

For moderate and severe asthmatics, I have treated many different allergens in combination with bronchial asthma such as DNA, RNA, lungs, bronchus, mucus, and the ten basic allergens. To help clear these combinations, I recommend that people treat themselves over and over until the combinations are cleared. In fact, many patients have found self-treatment to be effective at the onset of an asthma attack. Massaging the acupressure points (refer to Figure 5–1) while holding the bronchial asthma vial can soothe the breathing, coughing, and wheezing and prevent a severe episode. But it must be done immediately and the patient completely cleared of the allergy to bronchial asthma. Otherwise, self-treatment could cause an aggravation of the symptoms.

DNA and RNA

In a recent case, a female patient of mine caught an infection on an airplane, a common place to pick up infectants because of the poor ventilation. (I recommend that people do the saliva treatment right after getting off a plane to prevent infections.) She developed a severe cough and, because she was away, she was unable to get treatments. We treated her after she returned for quite a few bacteria and viruses and some foods, but the cough lingered. When I treated her for a sensitivity to bronchial asthma, her cough almost completely disappeared. We had to treat the asthma in combination with DNA and RNA before the cough went away completely. The patient told me her grandmother had asthma and there was a genetic tendency in her family. I treated some additional combinations of bronchial asthma with lungs, bronchi, histamine, IgE antibody cells, and emotions. There were so many combinations that I had her take the bronchial asthma vial home and treat herself for a while.

By treating for the DNA and RNA I treated for the genetic inherited tendency. I believe that anyone with a chronic illness will develop it again over time unless it is cleared in combination with the DNA to clear the genetic tendency. I do this in cases of arthritis, herpes, and bronchial asthma. Some doctors are using it for cancer as well.

Digestive Metabolic Enzymes

Sometimes it is also necessary to treat severe asthmatics with digestive and metabolic enzymes to support metabolism, nutrient absorption, and the integrity of the immune system. These enzymes can have a profound effect on digestion and on building stamina and immune function. Digestion is key to any chronic health problem. I always test asthmatics before giving them enzymes to ensure they are not sensitive. If people are allergic to enzymes, their digestion is usually poor. For asthmatics, this can mean an accumulation of mucus from foods that trigger attacks. Taking enzyme supplements is not useful to people who are allergic to them and treating for allergies to enzymes can be critical in their therapy.

A patient of mine with chronic stomach pain and heartburn had tried everything without success. I found she was allergic to certain digestive enzymes. After treating for that allergy, she has not had a bout of heartburn in three months. She told me, "You're a miracle worker. Nothing has ever worked for me."

EXERCISE-INDUCED ASTHMA

Exercise-induced asthma is a special kind of asthma which I believe is caused by allergies to things people come into contact with while exercising. Some of the allergens I have found in athletes are cold air, wind, hot air, humidity, and freon. Carbon dioxide, oxygen, and adrenaline allergies can also bring on asthma attacks, as can allergies to the body's own bronchial tubes, adrenals, sinuses, or nasal mucosa. Pollens might be one of the problems for athletes who wheeze when pollen counts are high. Emotions related to stress can also be a problem for athletes. Other possibilities include mold and chemicals in pools and dust in gymnasiums. Food allergies can also play a big part.

Athletes with this condition tend to have more rhinitis than other asthmatics and might not be able to smell or taste. They need treatment for allergens particular to the sinus cavity. I treat for sinus and sinus in combination with foods, environmental allergens, dust, and mold.

ASTHMA IN CHILDREN AND INFANTS

Children and infants are treated somewhat differently than adults. With a few exceptions, children under the age of eight will clear an allergy within six hours after treatment and don't have to avoid the allergens after that.

I always check the basic allergies in children diagnosed with asthma, then immediately go to food unless they have chronic sinusitis, ear infections, or bronchitis. The bronchitis is not as common in children as it is in adults. If children have chronic ear infections I treat for infectants such as bacteria, viruses, and parasites. I have had extraordinary success treating ear infections with a combination of NAET and enzyme therapy including protease as a natural antibiotic enzyme. If treated properly, they almost never develop an ear infection again.

I also treat children for vaccines, food additives such as sulfites, and food coloring. Occasionally I treat bronchial asthma as an allergy. I also sometimes treat for pollens, trees, and grasses. Children tend to have more severe allergies to foods than to environmental allergens that show up in tests and case histories. It usually takes less time for them than for adults to clear the allergies and they are often medication-free within the first few treatments, especially after the treatment for Vitamin C.

When infants are diagnosed with asthma, I treat them for mother's milk or formula first. Sometimes they clear right away. Then I begin treating for the basic allergies and food. I also check for mercury and amalgams because mercury has been known to be passed through breast milk. Vitamin C, sugar, and mold are common allergens for children and infants and are important to treat. I have also found that alternaria, a common seasonal mold, can be a severe allergen for children and infants.

NOCTURNAL ASTHMA

When asthma symptoms occur at night or in the early morning, the condition is called nocturnal asthma. Studies have repeatedly found that ninety percent of asthmatics wake up coughing and wheezing sometime during the night, most commonly from 3:00 to 5:00 A.M. In acupuncture this is the time when the lung meridian is most active or charged. Many patients are not able to return to sleep without asthma treatment. A patient who no longer wakes up needing medication at night will sometimes still wake up at the same time. This indicates that something happens at that time that produces a strong awakening response.

A major consequence of nocturnal asthma is loss of sleep, resulting in a deterioration of daytime performance. Other symptoms associated with lack of sleep include attention deficit and problems with homework for children and ability to work for adults. Other family members are affected as well as the person who is not sleeping.

There are many possible explanations for nighttime asthma and I have had many sleepless nights myself wondering about the possibilities. I intend to experiment with treating people during the night to see if it proves effective.

One possible explanation is that cortisone and epinephrine levels fall during the period when the asthmatic awakens with symptoms. Cortisone combats inflammation, whereas epinephrine causes bronchial constriction. Low levels cause increased inflammation and bronchial inactivity, triggering an aggravation of symptoms. Another possible explanation is that **gastric reflux**—the regurgitation of food or acid from the stomach—is common at that time, especially in elderly people.

A third explanation is that people who are sleeping are exposed to common allergens that can trigger asthma attacks such as fabrics, feathers, dust, and animal dander. A forth possible explanation is related to the position of the body while sleeping. Studies have shown that airway inflammation is more severe when people are lying down than when they are standing up.

Any of these factors could cause coughing or wheezing serious enough to awaken someone. Because the lung's bioenergetic pathway is most active at that time of the night, the organ might be more easily stimulated to react.

WINNING THE WAR AGAINST ASTHMA: THE HEALING JOURNEY

The amount of time it takes to treat a chronic ailment with NAET varies from patient to patient. Every individual is different, and every individual's program is different. In evaluating the program and making recommendations for different people, the practitioner must become familiar with the symptoms, history, immune response, and particular allergens. Everyone's response to NAET is influenced by these factors.

People who identify themselves as severe asthmatics may actually respond quickly, whereas those who think they are moderate may require extra sessions. I base my identification of mild, moderate, and severe on how people respond to treatment after the basics and some of the more obvious other allergies have been cleared. If they do not respond fairly quickly, I start treating by using the sequences described in this chapter.

The healing inevitably takes time. For some asthmatics it takes a couple of months, for others it could take as long as two years. Having worked with many hundreds of patients with a wide variety of problems, I know that with persistent NAET treatment, good digestion, and enzyme therapy, homeostasis will eventually be restored to the body. Asthmatics and people with other chronic problems who pursue this approach will eventually find themselves feeling vastly improved. They should understand, however, that it takes some time.

For example, a fourth-grade boy, John, came to me with hay fever, allergies, asthma, and about twenty warts on each hand and arm. We went through all the basic allergies, some foods, and moved to the pollens and environmentals. He asked me if I could make his warts go away before the school year started. I told him I had very good results with warts and that we would treat the virus that caused them with NAET. We treated for many wart combinations, and he treated himself at home. Nothing happened; not a single wart fell off. At that point, we took a break because it is often a good idea to give the immune system time to catch up with the treatments and to give the body time to detoxify. I talked to his mother about bringing him in for evaluation at the end of the summer but he did not come. One month after school started he walked into my office, and there wasn't one wart on his body. His skin was as smooth as silk, and the dark circles were gone from under his eyes. He told me what had happened. Seven weeks after we ended the treatment he woke up in the morning and found that he could brush off the warts. Within one week all his warts were gone. He had no more problems with mold or pollen and has been around cats and other animals without any reaction. His mother was so impressed that she started treatment for herself.

The lists of allergens I have discussed in this chapter and others are simply examples. Patients should be tested and evaluated by a competent practitioner (refer to Part VI for an NAET practitioner in your area) to find out exactly what their allergies and sensitivities are. Then they should observe responses, test possibilities, and research their own bodies.

12 | STAMINA

Fatigue is often the result of allergy reactions, poor digestion, and a buildup of toxins that slow the body down. Most people react to low energy levels by drinking coffee, eating sugar, smoking cigarettes, or relying on other drugs that give them a boost of energy. These short-term solutions make the real problem worse, cause complications, and aggravate chronic health problems. The maintenance of high levels of energy is achieved by eliminating allergies, improving digestion, absorption, and assimilation, removing toxins from the body, and increasing nutrients. Good energy levels, stamina, and a resistance to aging are all by-products of optimum health and homeostasis.

ENERGY LEVELS

There are many things that hinder the maintenance of healthy energy levels. To determine the cause of low energy, I use an abdominal diagnostic palpation exam, an enzyme evaluation exam that includes the twenty-four hour urinalysis, and muscle response testing. Many factors relating to energy levels show up on these tests.

Digestion

The first indicator is the efficiency of digestion and absorption of nutrients into the body. People can eat the best foods but if they do not digest or absorb them properly, they cannot benefit from them because they are not getting the vitamins and minerals necessary for the metabolic functions of the body and a healthy immune system.

Digestion is the key to high energy levels, and problems with digestion differ from individual to individual. Some people are sugar intolerant, some are fat intolerant, and some are complex carbohydrate intolerant. These intolerances show up in the urinalysis and palpation exams and can be treated with enzymes.

Impaired Thyroid Function

The next indicator is impaired thyroid function that can cause a decrease in energy because the thyroid influences many other metabolic processes, hormonal processes, and tissue function in the body. Impaired adrenal function can have similar effects.

Deficiencies and Allergies

Other possible causes of low energy levels include vitamin and mineral deficiencies resulting from poor absorption, allergies to foods and other allergens, poor liver function, an overgrowth of yeast, bacteria, or parasites in the gastrointestinal system, lack of sleep, insufficient exercise, and mental and emotional illnesses and imbalances. Fatigue can also be caused by other medical problems and serious pathologies. All possibilities should be checked.

In dealing with food and environmental allergies, it is helpful and appropriate to remove the allergenic foods from the diet and the environmental toxins from the patient's surroundings. Because some allergens are extremely difficult to avoid, however, treating with NAET is an important alternative to permanent avoidance. Often, the foods people are allergic to are the ones they like best. Food cravings are frequently connected to food allergies or to a deficiency of some nutrient. If the body is lacking in B vitamins, for example, the individual might crave grains and meat high in B vitamins.

By eliminating the allergies, often the cravings are eliminated as well. Over time, allergic reactions can inhibit good immune system function and impair energy levels and stamina. When the allergy is eradicated, the process of toxicity and immune system damage ends. Feeling tired after eating a particular food is a common experience that signals an allergy to that food. When a food allergy is cleared, a person feels a change of energy either immediately or within ten days.

Good digestion is critical to high energy levels. When undigested food gets into the bloodstream, it creates possible autoimmune reactions, autoaggressive disease, and severe immunosuppressive response that, in turn, causes vulnerability to infection. It also consumes essential metabolic enzymes needed to complete the process of digestion. The extra energy used in this process reduces the amount of energy gained from the food. This is one of the main causes of severe chronic fatigue.

DETOXIFICATION

Toxic buildup in the body is another common cause of fatigue. The toxins come from chemicals in our environment, food and environmental allergens, and by-products of the body's everyday metabolism. Smog and pesticides, food additives, alcohol, drinking water, medications, and drugs can poison our systems. Sometimes these toxic buildups occur because the organs of elimination—skin, colon, lungs, and kidneys—are not working properly. Detoxification requires healthy digestion and elimination and an awareness of what is put into the body. NAET can be a lifesaver for the detoxification process. Effective detoxification can be achieved through a combination of desensitization to environmental allergens, reduction in consumption of foods grown with pesticides, fungicides, and herbicides, and elimination of rancid fats, refined carbohydrates, and chemically prepared fats and margarine. Rancid oils, margarine, and fried foods contain partially hydrogenated oils that can interfere with the production of ATP, a substance in cellular metabolism that helps produce energy at the cellular level. Partially hydrogenated oils can also toxify the liver. Smoking and exposure to secondhand smoke should be avoided and water should be filtered to remove chemicals such as chlorine, fluorine, and other toxins. Finally, stimulants such as caffeine and sugars that lower energy, deplete vitamins and minerals such as potassium and weaken the immune system should be avoided.

The liver is an important organ in maintaining good energy levels and detoxifying the body. Good digestion, allergy elimination, and good nutrition keep the liver working optimally. In addition, the liver should be cleansed at least once or twice a year. I recommend the "Ultra Clear" program developed by Jeffrey Bland, one of the most thoroughly researched products of this type. An effective detoxifier, it tastes good and is simple to use.

A liver detoxification program works particularly well after a person has been treated for the ten basic allergies. When those allergies have been cleared, the person experiences fewer side effects such as detoxification symptoms and the cleansing is quicker and more effective. Liver cleansing is highly recommended for anyone with energy and stamina problems and for those with chronic infections or degenerative diseases.

EXERCISE

Exercise is one of the most important factors in increasing energy levels because it brings more oxygen into the body through increased circulation. Higher oxygen levels help burn off sugars and fats in the body which, in turn, can increase energy levels. Exercise also increases circulation to the brain and stimulates the lymphatic system that removes toxins and aids digestion. Daily exercise can be revitalizing. People should develop their own exercise routines that work for them and not overdo it or overstimulate the body. The point is to stay in balance and thereby maintain good energy levels.

SKELETAL ALIGNMENT

Skeletal alignment is also a factor in maintaining energy levels. As a chiropractor I have had a lot of experience treating people for structural problems by aligning vertebrae and bones that are out of alignment. Misaligned bones affect nerve function and tissue and good muscle tone is essential for optimum energy. When a muscle is inflamed or a vertebra is out of alignment, there is an impeded flow of nerve impulses to the brain and back to the specific muscles, ligaments, and organs as well as poor circulation in that area. This reduces the amount of energy available in the body, no matter how healthy the diet, or how well the liver is cleansed. If there is a structural imbalance or abnormality, the energy does not flow through the body the way it should and it is impossible to exercise well. Correction of problems and proper maintenance through chiropractic care can restore good alignment and a healthy nervous system, basic necessities in achieving good energy levels.

YEAST, BACTERIA, FUNGI, AND PARASITES

Yeast, bacteria, fungi, and parasites in the intestinal system and bloodstream can overload the immune system and prevent it from dealing with other kinds of infections and illnesses. Two of the many symptoms of Candida or candidiasis (yeast infection) are fatigue and insomnia.

Sugar, simple carbohydrates, and alcohol all fuel the growth of this yeast; merely taking acidophilus, a bacteria that aids digestion, without changing the diet does not help with Candida infections. Using enzymes without NAET treatment does not work either. Both are essential and effective.

It is important to understand the importance and seriousness of these infections. Both sexes are capable of succumbing to them, and the infections—viral, bacterial, and fungal—can be passed back and forth sexually.

SLEEP

Sufficient and restful sleep are all important for good energy maintenance. Many people overwork and do not get enough rest. A great deal of repair work occurs during sleep: hormones are manufactured, glands are rejuvenated, and toxins are removed. When people do not get enough sleep, they use more stimulants to compensate for the insufficient rest. They need to understand, however, that the body cannot endure long hours of work and overstimulation forever.

Sleep is essential. When we are deprived of it, aging is accelerated and we burn out. Burnout can happen over a long period of time or in one day. People come into my office and say they used to be able to go, go, go, and thought nothing could happen. They were immune to the physical problems other people had. Overnight, they were suddenly unable to get out of bed and have been unable to function well for years. Or they might say they cannot work anymore and have no appetite.

Not everyone needs eight or nine hours of sleep a night, but people know what rest they need. When people wake up naturally, without an alarm clock, they have had the sleep they need. If they have to use an alarm to wake up, they probably need more sleep.

Some people are now using melatonin to help them sleep. I find that many people are allergic to the melatonin produced in their own bodies. Released during sleep, melatonin is thought to be an antiaging and antioxidant chemical. When treated for melatonin sensitivity, people can use their own melatonin rather than taking it orally. If there is no allergy, the body should be producing enough melatonin and other antioxidants and there should be no need to take an excessive amount. I prefer to have all nutrients, hormones, and other metabolic chemicals absorbed from the food of a good diet and from the body's natural production rather than from using supplements. By taking large amounts of supplements they are allergic to, people may do more harm than good.

MENTAL HEALTH

Mental health is important for all age groups because it is a product of homeostasis and freedom from allergies. When energy levels are low, people are more vulnerable to physical, mental, and emotional problems. When they are tired, it is difficult to relate, hard to function properly, or deal with everyday stresses. I know from experience, that by strengthening digestion, eliminating allergies with NAET, adjusting the diet, exercising, and receiving good chiropractic care, we can not only strengthen the body, but also reduce the impact of mental and emotional stresses. It is easier to have a positive point of view when one feels rested and energized.

When allergies are cleared, digestion and nutrition are improved, the body is detoxified, and the patient gets enough rest stable energy levels are generally easy to maintain. Some people need some forms of supplementation such as enzymes or thyroid or adrenal supplements. They might also use a green drink such as spirulina or blue-green algae that is not toxic to the system. When used in moderation, supplementation of this kind is helpful in conjunction with a good diet and efficient digestion.

Energy levels sometimes improve dramatically; more often they change slowly. After bodies have been abused with coffee, alcohol, and smoking, it takes time to restore adequate energy levels. I prefer to see the energy rebound slowly in order for the body to heal in its own time. I always do a post-treatment abdominal exam and allergy testing and there are usually remarkable changes, especially seen in the urinalysis.

Depression and feelings of anxiety ease as energy levels rise and the body detoxifies itself. With detoxification, stable energy levels can be established and maintained. Each person must pursue health on every level to maintain abundant energy throughout his or her life.

Part

IV ADJUNCTIVE THERAPY

13 ENZYME THERAPY

After many years of working with others, I am delighted to be able to share my own story. At forty-six I am healthier now than I was twenty years ago. I owe this feeling of well-being to Dr. Howard Loomis who changed my life, my health, and my practice as a healer and taught me many mysteries and miracles of the human body. Above all, he taught me about balance, homeostasis, and a healthy immune system.

MY PERSONAL EXPERIENCE WITH ENZYMES

For as long as I could remember, I suffered from digestive problems. I was constipated, bloated, tired, and depressed, especially at the end of a day of eating. No matter what I ate or when, how, or with whom, I would end up feeling as if I was three months pregnant. As a result, I always wore loose clothing with an elastic waist. When I was young, both my father and grandmother had complained of digestive problems. I assumed it was an inherited condition I would have to live with for the rest of my life.

In the seventies I became involved in healing with an emphasis on massage and polarity therapy. I went on to study homeopathy and nutrition with various doctors including Dr. Bernard Jensen at his ranch in Escondido, California. Refusing to believe that my problem and other digestive problems were all inherited, I was determined to find a solution. I studied every book about natural healing available at the time. I tried every vitamin, explored homeopathy, and experimented with diets including fasting. But nothing ever changed my digestive abnormalities. At times I despaired of ever finding the answer I was seeking.

After years of studying nutrition on my own, I decided to get a degree in chiropractic. My twin brother had gone into conventional medicine, but I was drawn to a more natural approach. Unlike medical school, chiropractic college offered a good course in diet and nutrition. I enrolled in 1972.

During my first year there, probably because of the stress of the study, my symptoms worsened. Everything I ate aggravated my digestion and I became severely constipated and bloated. At the chiropractic clinic affiliated with the school, I had X rays, barium studies and various blood tests, and I proceeded to do colonics, fasting, and food rotation. I remember doing a grape fast for almost three months. When I fasted, my symptoms seemed to improve slightly but I would relapse after I began to eat regular foods. I tried different chiropractic treatments, homeopathy, and other new diets. Nothing seemed to help.

After graduating from chiropractic school and practicing for a number of years, I decided to enroll in a three-year post-graduate chiropractic orthopedics training program. This course changed my life, my health, and my professional practice forever. It was here that I was introduced to enzyme therapy by one of my instructors and the work of Dr. Howard Loomis, a chiropractor and biochemist.

At my first seminar with Dr. Loomis I took exhaustive notes that I still read over from time to time. He began the seminar by saying, "The most profound thing we do every day is eat." He went on to explain that the body's ability to maintain homeostasis, crucial for the life of every cell, is based on its ability to digest what it eats. A twenty-four hour urinalysis examines how well the body digests and metabolizes food by looking at what the body discards and keeps. The body strives to resist change and withstand disease by maintaining its internal environment relatively constant. It does this, Loomis said, by keeping the intracellular fluid within certain narrow limits of temperature, volume, pH, and concentrations of various solutes. Laboratory tests can detect deviations from normal homeostasis.

"By definition," Loomis explained, "if blood chemistries are not normal, homeostasis has already been compromised and the body is evidencing exhaustion or an inability to adapt to an excessively strong or persistent stimulus. In order to prevent disease, this process must be identified before deviations in blood chemistry are evidenced."

Loomis told us that studies showed that significant digestion from salivary enzymes alone occur in the stomach before hydrochloric acid and pepsin begin their work. In fact, thirty-five to forty-five percent of starches can be digested before HCl is secreted. The problem is that we do not chew our food long enough to allow this to happen.

Loomis said, "Since the resting pH of the stomach is between 5.0 and 6.0, many nutritional and physiological tests do not consider predigestion in man to be significant. The enzymes in plants will work in a pH environment of 3.0–9.0 and continue digesting until inactivated in the stomach when the pH reaches 3.0. Therefore plant enzymes play a significant role in predigesting food, offering a solution to many acute and chronic digestive disorders, and a means of delivering food past an incompetent digestive system."

After his talk, Dr. Loomis performed an abdominal palpatory diagnostic evaluation and a twenty-four hour urinalysis on some of the doctors in the seminar, including me. The next day I helped him to analyze the urine so I could learn the lab work myself, and he helped me evaluate the test and compare it with the abdominal palpation exam. The purpose was to uncover enzyme and nutritional deficiencies and specific food intolerances. We discovered that I was carbohydrate intolerant, a poor assimilator of sugar, and that I was unable to digest foods containing sugars and other carbohydrates including grains and breads. We also saw that I had moderate bowel toxicity that showed I had some fermentation and putrefaction in the bowel and probably constipation. I was **hypoadrenal** and presented with a slight inflammation of the liver, and I was deficient in calcium, potassium, magnesium, and Vitamin C.

Dr. Loomis recommended I take an enzyme consisting of disaccharidase, cellulase, maltase, sucrase, and lactase to help me digest sugars and carbohydrates. He also recommended I take an enzyme for calcium, minerals, and Vitamin C and a bowel cleanser to help with the bowel toxicity. Two weeks after beginning the enzymes, the bloating and constipation I had experienced my whole life disappeared and they have never returned. It was miraculous!

After this total regeneration of my digestive system, I studied enzymes and enzyme therapy extensively with Dr. Loomis and began to utilize his work in my practice. I performed an abdominal palpation on each patient along with a twenty-four hour urinalysis. I then recommended enzymes and created diets for each individual based on their specific food intolerances. These diets can be found in Part VI of this book.

After careful study, trial, and error, I developed a sugar-intolerant diet for myself. I have found that eighty percent of the people who come to see me are sugar intolerant. Aside from bloating and constipation, sugar intolerance can lead to diabetes, adrenal dysfunction, asthma, hyperactivity, attention deficit, depression, fatigue, poor assimilation of foods, obesity or malnutrition, frequent sore throats, ear infections, and colds. Sugar intolerance can be responsible for **Crohn's disease**, an inability to tolerate lactose (milk sugar) and for **celiac disease**, an inability to tolerate gluten. Furthermore, it can also be responsible for chronic yeast infections and chronic food and environmental allergies. I suffered from many of these problems myself, and the sugar-intolerant diet I developed has changed my life. This diet is low in carbohydrates, grains, fruits, and sweet vegetables and high in protein. I recommend this diet for all sugar-intolerant people.

This regeneration occurred almost thirteen years ago and I continue to be grateful to Dr. Loomis' research and his enzyme formulas. Since I seem to have inherited this sugar intolerance, I will always need supplementation for the predigestion of sugars. Therefore, these enzymes are essential to my health and the health of many of my patients. Indeed, I believe enzymes have saved my life and made me a happier and healthier person. We will hear more and more about enzymes and their miracles in the twenty-first century. This book is only the beginning.

WHAT ARE ENZYMES?

Enzymes are complex proteins in the body that cause chemical changes in other substances in order to provide the labor force and energy necessary to keep us alive. They are energy catalysts that are essential to the successful occurrence of over 150,000 biochemical reactions in our bodies, particularly involving food digestion and the delivery of nutrients to the body. Enzymes help convert food into chemical substances that pass into cell membranes to perform all of our everyday life-sustaining functions. By supporting normal function, enzymes keep our immune system strong enough to fight off disease. Enzymes help to nourish and clean the body, making possible the human body's miraculous capacity for self-healing. They also make available the energy needed for a normal body to burn hundreds of grams of carbohydrate and fat every day. Without enzymes, life could not be sustained.

Enzymes perform so many important functions in the body that they have been called the basis of all metabolic activity. Some of their responsibilities are as follows:

1. Transform foods into muscles, nerves, bones, and glands.

2. Help to store excess nutrients in muscles or the liver for future use.

3. Help to rid carbon dioxide from the lungs.

4. Metabolize iron for utilization by the blood.

5. Aid in blood coagulation.

6. Decompose hydrogen peroxide and liberate healthful oxygen.

7. Attack toxic substances in the body so they can be eliminated, essential for patients with chronic health problems.

8. Help convert dietary phosphorus to bone.

9. Extract minerals from food for use.

10. Convert protein, carbohydrates, fats, vitamins, and nutrients for the body's use.

In other words, enzymes deliver nutrients, break down and carry away toxic waste, digest food, purify the blood, deliver hormones, balance cholesterol and triglyceride levels, feed the brain, build protein into muscle, and feed and fortify the endocrine system. They also contribute to immune system activity. White blood cells are especially enzyme-rich in order to digest foreign invading substances.

While one of the advantages of enzymes is that they can cause a chemical reaction without being destroyed or changed in the process, the number of enzymes we can produce is limited. Every person is born with an enzyme potential or number of enzymes he or she can produce in a lifetime. This number is determined by the DNA code. In addition, each enzyme can only perform a certain amount of work before it becomes exhausted and must be replaced by another. Along with digesting processed food, enzyme supply can be diminished by caffeinated and alcoholic beverages, colds and fevers, pregnancy, stress, strenuous exercise, injuries, and extreme weather conditions. If we do not eat an enzyme-rich diet, we deplete our enzyme potential without replenishing it. This is why supplementation and a good diet are essential. When all enzyme activity stops, the body stops functioning and the person dies. However, humans have the capacity to store external food enzymes to ensure the body's ability to metabolize the needed nutrients. This explains an abundance of new enzyme health products and the recommendations from experts that people supplement their diet with raw foods and manufactured food enzymes.

Enzymes save peoples lives by restoring energy and homeostasis, reversing the aging process, turning a dysfunctional digestive system into a healthy one, and strengthening the immune system. In my fifteen years of working with enzyme therapy, I have witnessed enormous success with a variety of illnesses. The most noticeable and immediate change in each case has always been in the energy level. Patients no longer feel that "crash" after meals, especially after lunch, the most common time.

Enzymes also have been utilized by many industries in various products and processes including laundry detergents, skin care, meat tenderizers, agricultural processes, and waste conversion.

WHAT IS THE FUNCTION OF ENZYMES?

When I began the study of enzymes many years ago, I encountered the phrase "acid-base balance." I did not really understand it until I met Dr. Howard Loomis and learned about the urinalysis and its nutritional evaluation. One of the first evaluations done on urine is the pH level, the degree of a solution's acidity or alkalinity. An alkaline pH is 7.0 or above; an acid pH is below 6.5. To maintain homeostasis, the blood has to have a neutral pH of 7.5. The body keeps it from becoming too alkaline or too acid by buffering it with hydrogen or bicarbonate ions. In doing this, it can rob the digestive system of substances necessary to digest foods or perform other tasks efficiently.

For example, an alkaline urine indicates that the blood does not have adequate quantities of hydrogen and chlorine to aid digestion in the stomach in the form of hydrochloric acid. This condition is called hypochlorhydria, or HCl deficiency, and is characterized by difficulty digesting protein and severe bloating immediately after eating. The opposite is true when the urine is acid: the blood is not capable of supplying enough bicarbonate ions to the pancreatic secretion for proper digestion of starches and fats.

Asthmatics usually have a chronically acid urine that leads to flatulence and bloating two hours after a meal. A twenty-four-hour urinalysis determines how the body compensates to maintain homeostasis. The pH is calculated over the twenty-four hour period because if urine is checked over the course of a day, the pH varies with waking and after meals. The twenty-four hour catch indicates the overall pH for an entire day and gives more accurate information on the compensations the body is presenting. This incredible tool provides information on tendencies toward certain illnesses and imbalances including respiratory problems, diabetes, anxiety, chronic bowel problems, and poor thyroid and adrenal function.

Stanley, a professional pilot, came to see me a few years ago suffering from chronic fatigue and chronic allergies that greatly affected his performance. He loved to fly but was afraid he would fail the physical and lose his job. I did a thorough evaluation and prescribed an enzyme for digestion and carbohydrate absorption. Within two weeks he had so much energy that his coworkers were amazed. He passed his physical easily. In fact, his physician said his health was better than it had ever been. By predigesting foods, enzymes save the body's energy to perform other metabolic functions effectively.

The pH is one aspect of the useful information the urinalysis provides. The urine pH also reflects a person's diet and basic dietary imbalances. For example, an alkaline pH is usually representative of a vegetarian who eats mostly vegetables and fruits and is perhaps deficient in grains, meats, eggs, and proteins. An alkaline urine can also represent more serious problems including insomnia and anxiety. On the other hand, an acid urine usually reflects an excess of protein in the diet and possibly a deficiency of vegetables and fruit. An acid urine causes sluggishness and lethargy. Respiratory acidosis, emphysema, and asthma produce a persistently acid urine by interfering with respiration and causing an accumulation of carbon dioxide in the body (pH below 6.0). Carbon dioxide becomes carbonic acid and the excess acid causes a loss of hydrogen in the urine. The body holds bicarbonate to buffer the acidity, and the loss of hydrogen limits HCl production for proper digestion. If it is possible to discover this aspect of the nutritional makeup early on, a person can be given enzymes that prevent late-onset asthma and other chronic respiratory problems. We treat people both to prevent and to heal existing respiratory problems.

The best way to handle patients with respiratory spasms is to alkalinize them with enzymes. Over the years, we have seen many asthmatics and patients with chronic coughs helped with the use of enzymes that change the pH of the urine. Enzymes soothe an asthmatic's respiratory problems, help with insomnia, increase energy, and create long-lasting excellent digestion.

Bob, age fifty-three, came to see me recently for chronic insomnia. He had been on medication for over nine years. Because of the severe side effects of the medication, he went to see an Asian physician and herbalist in New Mexico who helped him to get off drugs and detoxify his body. Unfortunately, his insomnia slowly returned, and with one to two hours sleep a night, he became weaker and more depressed each day. Palpation showed poor protein and fat utilization and digestion as well as low levels of calcium. A urinalysis revealed a pH of 8.1, metabolic alkalinity, indicating a nervous individual with possible insomnia. We put him on enzyme supplements to lower his pH, raise his calcium, and help digest protein and fats. Within two to three weeks he began to sleep five to six hours a night. Today he sleeps six to seven hours without interruption and is able to function with clarity and peace of mind.

WHY DO WE NEED ENZYMES?

Enzymes enable our bodies to digest the food we eat. They break down the various foods we consume—proteins, fats, carbohydrates, vitamins—into smaller compounds that the body can absorb. They are absolutely essential in maintaining optimal health.

Enzymes are present naturally in raw foods but are destroyed in the cooking process. It is important to eat as much raw food as possible, to subject food to as little heating as possible, and to chew food well because enzyme production begins in the mouth. Because we often fail to follow these guidelines, we do not receive all the enzymes we need to do the job of digestion. Enzyme supplements provide the missing pieces.

Maintaining the body's enzyme levels is critical today when so much of the food in a typical American diet is processed or cooked, as much as eighty-five percent according to recent studies. Enzymes are only found naturally in raw foods such as vegetables and fruits that contain the very enzymes needed to digest them. Food enzymes are extremely heat sensitive, especially at or above temperatures of 118 degrees Fahrenheit. When raw foods are processed or heated in any way (steamed, baked, boiled, stewed, fried, microwaved, canned), they may lose one hundred percent of their enzyme activity and up to eighty-five percent of their vitamin and mineral content. Even the raw food we eat could be enzyme deficient if it was grown in nutrient-lacking soil. In addition, enzyme deterioration begins the moment the food is picked or killed. For all these reasons, supplementing with enzymes is crucial to achieve a more efficient digestive process and better utilization of our food's nutrients.

When digestion is not properly completed, partially digested proteins putrefy, partially digested carbohydrates ferment, and partially digested fats turn rancid. These toxins remain in the body, harming the system. Fermented toxins in the digestive tract can be absorbed into the blood and deposited as waste in the joints and other soft-tissue areas.

The results of enzyme deficiency include digestive disturbance, fatigue, headaches, constipation, gas, heartburn, bloating, colon problems, excess body fat, and problems as serious as cardiovascular or heart disease. Enzyme deficiencies have been linked to premature aging and degenerative diseases as well. Research has also shown that white blood cells are increased to compensate for an enzyme-deficient diet. Making use of the immune system to aid in digestion whenever enzymes are lacking compromises the body's ability to defend itself from disease.

Digestion has first priority on the limited number of internal enzymes available; metabolic enzymes must be satisfied with whatever is left. When food enzymes are introduced from outside the body, the body does not need to manufacture as many digestive enzymes, allocating more of the enzyme potential toward the production of the metabolic enzymes needed for growth, maintenance, and repair. Studies have shown that diets deficient in enzymes cause a thirty percent reduction in animal life span and low enzyme levels are associated with old age and chronic diseases. Cancer research has discovered that certain enzymes are completely lacking in the blood and urine of cancer patients.

When we eat food that is devoid of enzymes, the body must draw on its own internal supply of enzymes, both metabolic and digestive. Eventually we deplete our limited reserves, forcing the immune system to aid in digestion instead of rebuilding the body and fighting illness. The pancreas, salivary glands, stomach, and intestines all might contribute the enzymes needed for digestion, robbing the body of metabolic enzymes needed for muscles, nerves, blood, and other glands.

Enzyme supplements help create more energy, promote faster and easier digestion, and encourage superior nutrient absorption. It is the responsibility of our digestive system to release the nutrients that are trapped in our food by breaking the food down. But our digestive system works best when enzyme supplements assist in setting the nutrients free for the body to absorb and use. Receiving all the nutrients in the food we eat is critical, because these nutrients are needed to build and repair the body's tissue, produce energy, and maintain a strong immune system.

In my practice I see many patients with chronic food intolerances. For example, people can inherit or develop intolerances to proteins, sugars, fibers, complex carbohydrates, or fats. These patients lack the enzymes they need to break down the food that causes them trouble. Through palpation examination and testing (described at the end of this chapter), I am able to ascertain which foods a person cannot tolerate and which enzymes they should take as supplements to restore homeostasis. With the proper enzyme supplements, these patients regain the ability to digest their food properly and thoroughly. Human saliva contains the necessary factors needed to activate plant enzymes in the food we eat but because we fail to chew foods well, we are unable to digest foods. We need to chew each mouthful at least seventy times for complete predigestion!

Protein Intolerance

People who do not digest proteins crave sugars. They tend to experience anxiety, osteoporosis, edema, eye or ear inflammation, endometriosis, or bone spurs. Many of these patients also have an allergy to calcium that further promotes osteoporosis. When one is allergic to particular minerals or vitamins, he or she is usually low in those same minerals or vitamins.

Carla, age fifty, came to see me with a family history of osteoporosis and arthritis. Two years ago she was screened for osteoporosis and the results suggested she might have already developed the disease. She was advised to eat dairy products and take 1,500 mg. of calcium daily. After two years she was tested again and the results were even worse. She also complained of bloating and indigestion. Worried, upset, and afraid, she came to me for a nutritional consultation. An abdominal diagnostic enzyme exam, twenty-four hour urinalysis, and complete allergy test were performed. The results showed that she was deficient in calcium and allergic to calcium and the dairy products she had been eating. After putting her on an enzyme for the digestion of sugars that would help ease the dairy allergy, I treated her with NAET for calcium and dairy and prescribed calcium supplements with her enzymes. In one year her test results were significantly better. I often wonder how many of the millions of women taking calcium supplements to prevent osteoporosis and arthritis are allergic to it.

Sugar Intolerance

People who are sugar intolerant tend to crave protein and suffer from depression, malabsorption, bloating, acute food allergies, hyperactivity, Crohn's disease, asthma, chronic ear infections, and constipation. They usually are very allergic to B vitamins as well.

Starch, Fiber, or Fat Intolerance

People who are starch and fiber intolerant tend to crave fat and suffer from spastic colons, high blood fats, obesity, irritable bowel, ulcerative colitis, and occasionally constipation. People who are fat intolerant tend to crave sugar and suffer from eczema, liver and gallbladder disease, and toxicity.

TYPES OF ENZYMES

There are three main categories of enzymes: metabolic, digestive, and food.

Metabolic Enzymes

Metabolic enzymes are produced internally and are responsible for running the body at the level of the blood, tissues, and organs. They are required for the growth of new cells and the repair and maintenance of all the body's organs and tissues. Metabolic enzymes take protein, fat, and carbohydrates and transform them into the proper balance of working cells and tissues. Metabolic enzymes also remove worn-out material from the cells and keep them clean and healthy.

Digestive Enzymes

Digestive enzymes also are produced internally and deal with the digestion of food and the absorption and delivery of nutrients throughout the body. The most commonly known digestive enzymes are secreted from the pancreas into the stomach and small intestine. Each enzyme is specific to a particular compound which it can break down or synthesize. The three most important enzymes for digestion are protease, amylase, and lipase. They digest protein, carbohydrate, and fat, respectively.

Food Enzymes

Food enzymes, the only ones produced externally, are derived solely from raw fruits, raw vegetables, and supplements. They help the digestive enzymes break down food. Food enzymes must also have the presence of vitamins and minerals, called coenzymes, for proper functioning. Unlike raw enzymes, coenzymes are not completely destroyed by cooking. Because raw food enzymes become useless after heat processing, coenzymes in our diet are not utilized to their full potential.

Enzymes perform best at a certain pH. For example, animal enzymes perform best at a pH of 6.5–9.0. On the other hand, plant enzymes have a broader pH range of 3.0–9.0. I prefer to use plant enzymes because they can survive transport through the acid pH of the stomach (pH 2.0) and can be used in the pancreas and small intestine to further digestion.

Some of the reported benefits of consuming food enzymes are the elimination of:

- heartburn

- bloating

- gas

- constipation or loose bowels

- colon problems

- overweight and underweight problems

- headaches

- food allergies

- hay fever

- fatigue after meals

- stress

- weakened immune system

Some people have claimed that supplemental enzymes cannot survive the strong acids in the stomach. However, manufacturers reply that these enzymes might disintegrate when mixed with acid in a laboratory test tube but not in a living human body. The stomach normally allows salivary, food, and supplementary enzymes to digest food for up to an hour after eating. When they have finished their job of performing predigestion, food and supplementary enzymes that function at a low pH continue digestion of protein, carbohydrate, and fat for a longer time than salivary or pancreatic enzymes. As the stomach acid level increases, the acid enzyme pepsin continues the digestion of protein where the others left off. This information has been elicited after the stomach and upper intestinal contents have been pumped out and examined at various intervals following meals.

Some of the products on the market have a natural enteric coating to protect the enzymes from stomach acids thereby allowing them to pass through the stomach into the small intestines for assimilation. Taking enzymes on an empty stomach minimizes the presence of damaging stomach acids.

The following list contains the names of the main digestive enzymes that are used therapeutically to help restore the body's homeostasis and strengthen the immune system, along with a brief description of each enzyme's function:

Protease breaks down protein into amino acids; acts on pathogens such as bacteria, viruses, and cancer cells; works best in the high acidity of the stomach; also found in pancreatic and intestinal juices.

Amylase breaks down carbohydrates (starches) into simpler sugars such as dextrin and maltose; found in our saliva, pancreas, and intestines; secreted by the salivary glands and the pancreas.

Lipase along with bile from the gallbladder, breaks down fats into glycerol and fatty acids and the oil-soluble Vitamins A, D, E, and F; helpful in losing weight and for cardiovascular conditions.

Cellulase breaks down fiber and cellulose found in fruits, vegetables, grains, seeds, and plant material; increases the nutritional value of fruits and vegetables; foods high in cellulose must be chewed well to allow cellulase to do its work to prevent putrefaction, bloating, and gas.

Pectinase breaks down pectin-rich foods such as citrus fruits, apples, carrots, potatoes, beets, and tomatoes.

Lactase breaks down lactose, the complex sugar in milk products; ideal for lactose-intolerant individuals; production usually decreases with age; NAET treatment for lactose combined with lactase enzyme effectively takes care of lactose intolerance.

Cathepsin breaks down meat from animals.

Antioxidant enzyme protects us from the negative effects of free radicals, highly reactive compounds that can damage almost any cell in the body.

Bromelain   breaks down food protein into smaller peptones by hydrolysis; helps the body to fight cancer, improves circulation, and treats inflammation; after a musculoskeletal injury it can reduce inflammation as well as, or even better than, any anti-inflammatory drug; said to improve the effect of some antibiotics; assists in the absorption of nutrients from foods and supplements; reduces swelling after dental surgery and helps in dysmenorrhea; increases tissue permeability; prevents the narrowing of arteries that contributes to heart attacks.

Papain   breaks down food protein into smaller peptones by hydrolysis; aids the body in digestion.

Glucoamylase   breaks down maltose (the sugar in all grains that may cause cravings for breads and carbohydrates) into two glucose molecules, allowing greater absorption of this energy-giving sugar.

Invertase   helps to assimilate and utilize sucrose, a sugar that contributes to digestive stress if not properly digested.

Some herbs also aid digestion. Aloe vera provides relief from peptic ulcers and helps with constipation, and slippery elm is good for hiatal hernias and acid reflux. Both are common symptoms in asthmatics.

THERAPEUTIC USE

One of the most common complaints I hear from my patients is "I don't have enough energy." Before I discovered enzymes, I had no response. Now I know they can change the situation immediately. For the most part, low energy occurs because people are not digesting their food properly and they cannot benefit from the energy that food provides. Instead of deriving the needed enzymes directly from the food itself, the body has to borrow enzymes from metabolism. Energy is required to accomplish this. In fact, digesting food without an adequate amount of enzymes actually uses more energy than the food provides. Reversing this situation can free up the body's energy for other tasks because the stealing of enzymes from other parts of the body causes certain metabolic dysfunctions as the enzymes are distributed among other organs and tissues. Chronic degenerative diseases, as well as energy depletion, can be the result of metabolic dysfunction.

The regular consumption of enzyme supplements brings numerous positive benefits in terms of ongoing general health, including:

- the prevention of toxic waste buildup in the intestines

- more efficient assimilation of fats and proteins in the body

- more comfortable and efficient absorption of nutrients

- more comfortable digestion of large amounts of carbohydrates

- accelerated digestive process because of catalyzation from enzymes

According to Dr. Edward Howell who researched the effect of enzymes for more than fifty years, it is very likely that every degenerative disease could have its origin in a raw food enzyme deficiency. In response to this research, enzyme advocate William E. Frazier, M.H.P, N.C. remarked, "Not to realize that most, if not all, degenerative diseases are traceable to a common denominator, and that common denominator being the food that we eat for nourishment, is an insult to human intelligence." In my fifteen years of practice with enzyme therapy, I have seen many different illnesses helped by the addition of enzymes.

Digestive Aids

After a large meal, one might notice a sudden feeling of sluggishness and energy loss. The body is faced with an overload of calories and nutrients to break down and deliver to the bloodstream. If the food eaten was cooked, there are no enzymes included to assist in the energy-consuming task of digestion. If an enzyme supplement is taken at the beginning of a meal, the body is armed and prepared to handle the new food entering the digestive system. Without this additional supply of enzymes, it can take the body up to sixty minutes to gather the needed enzymes, sometimes borrowing them from other metabolic processes. When supplemental food enzymes are used, time and energy is conserved, allowing for more complete absorption of nutrients from the food consumed. When enzymes are taken between meals, they are absorbed into the bloodstream and distributed throughout the body instead of being used for digestion.

ENZYMES AND THE IMMUNE SYSTEM

Enzymes play a vital role in building and strengthening a healthy immune system, one of my major goals when working with patients. A strong immune system enables a body to be less vulnerable to viruses, bacteria, parasites, and other toxic invaders. It also helps the body stay healthy during times of stress or when a complete and balanced diet is not followed.

Circulating Immune Complexes (CICs)

According to the theories of Dr. Anthony Cichoke, a well-known enzyme therapist, when digestion is poor and substantial amounts of food remain undigested, these undigested food residues seep into the bloodstream. There they are viewed as antigens and quickly become attached to tiny antibodies and form antigen-antibody complexes known as circulating immune complexes (CICs). These tiny immune complexes float freely in the blood or the lymph until they are eaten by the large macrophages, the "Pac Men" of the body. If these CICs are overlooked by the macrophages, or if chemotherapeutic drugs, steroids, or excessive antibiotics suppress the macrophages, the CICs grow in size and latch themselves onto body tissue. Then the backup immune defense system, T and B cells produced by the bone marrow, start destroying their own tissue cells in an attempt to destroy the CICs. Unfortunately, the body's noble effort backfires and an autoimmune response occurs, creating inflammation, redness, and swelling. Glomerulonephritis, colitis, arthritis, fibromyalgia, migraines, and asthma are examples of autoimmune activity at work. Certain enzymes, especially protease, can break up the CICs. When I put an asthmatic on protease, the immune system is enhanced and there is an immediate decrease in chronic bacterial and viral infections as well as chronic mucus.

Inflammation

Characterized by heat, redness, swelling, and pain, inflammation has a variety of possible causes from a minor cut or sunburn to a major infection such as appendicitis. All inflammatory conditions respond well to enzyme therapy. Inflammation is a sign that many bodily processes are occurring in sequence. The first is the body's fight against the infection, the second is the reparation of the destructive tissue, and the third phase of the inflammation process is the clearing and cleaning up of debris and dead tissue.

Whenever there is an injury, there is an invasion of white blood cells to repair and clean up the area. These white blood cells circulate in the blood and lymph all the time. During the dynamic process of inflammation and repair, blood flows to the area, causes blood clots, and obstructs blood flow that, in turn, causes swelling and oozing. A barrier of fibrin is formed to encircle the area of inflammation.

Supplemental enzymes such as proteolytic enzymes and amylase can help bring more oxygen to the area and reduce swelling by breaking up the fibrous tissue and eating up the dead and infected tissue. This speeds healing and reduces pain. Enzymes remove foreign bodies such as bacteria, viruses, and other microorganisms and help to clean up the area so new nerve tissue and new cells can be formed.

Both acute and chronic inflammation are helped with the use of enzymes. Taking high amounts of amylase with bromelain reduces inflammation. Many acute inflammatory processes such as colitis can become chronic when there are repeated cycles of damage and repair. Enzymes, by restoring digestion, cleansing the area, and preventing the formation of circulating immune complexes and autoaggressive reactions, can be beneficial to sufferers of colitis, Crohn's disease, and irritable bowel syndrome. In conventional medicine, cortisone therapy is often used to treat chronic inflammatory problems such as Crohn's. Cortisone helps stop inflammation but in the long run, makes the situation worse because it blocks the body's natural immune function. Bacteria, parasites, fungi, or other pathogens cause irritation and continue to destroy and invade the body, but the immune system is paralyzed by the cortisone and unable to fight. Even though the inflammation is curtailed, the pathogenic process still prevails and can worsen, causing more irritation and other autoimmune problems. Unlike cortisone, enzymes do not inhibit the immune system. Instead, they promote the healing process by attacking the pathogens and ultimately reducing swelling and inflammation. Enzyme preparations can be used to treat a wide variety of chronic inflammatory conditions including candidiasis, bronchitis, asthma, bacterial infections, kidney infections, ear infections, sinusitis, herpes zoster, and herpes simplex 1 and 2.

Asthma

Antioxidant supplements and enzyme therapy have been used to strengthen the immune system of asthmatics. Dr. Howard Loomis and I have both observed that asthmatic children are sugar intolerant, not surprising given that the annual sugar consumption in the United States is now 150 pounds per capita. In fact, recent studies indicate that eighty percent of the population is sugar intolerant. Sugar intolerance involves all sugars including sugars found in fruits, vegetables, and grains and artificial sugars such as sorbitol, Equal®, NutraSweet®, and mannitol. Asthma is frequently characterized by a B vitamin deficiency, caused by an overabundance of sugar and an allergy to B vitamins.

Linda and Neil, eight-year-old twins with asthma, came to see me a few years ago. A thorough enzyme evaluation indicated they were sugar intolerant. I took them off all refined sugar, limited their intake of grains and fruits, and prescribed large amounts of amylase and protease. Their asthma almost disappeared entirely, and their wheezing and coughing stopped completely.

Overconsumption and underdigestion of protein adds to the excess acidity caused by respiratory distress in asthmatics. Hypothyroid, hypoadrenal, and chronic intestinal toxemia also contributes to asthma. Most asthmatics benefit from an enzyme that contains the four food enzymes plus three disaccharidases—sucrase, lactase, and maltase—and a respiratory formula containing enzymes and herbs that nourish the lungs, help expectorate mucus, and relieve coughing and wheezing.

Arthritis

Osteoarthritis is a degenerative joint disease characterized by pain, heat, and swelling. Rheumatoid arthritis is a systemic disease of unknown origin with similar symptoms.

Rheumatoid arthritis is thought to be related to the invasion of the joints by circulating immune complexes and the autoimmune reactions that occur as a result. By interrupting the immune complexes and causing their elimination from the body, enzymes—particularly protease, bromelain, and lipase—can be extremely beneficial in reducing symptoms and restoring a balanced life.

Enzyme therapy, in conjunction with NAET treatments for allergies, can also benefit those with osteoarthritis. In particular, I focus on allergies to foods that have an acid by-product such as meats, nightshade family vegetables, certain fruits, and sugars. I also treat bacteria as an allergy in working with arthritis and other joint problems. Enzymes that digest proteins and sugars can also be helpful as can lipase (for fats) and protease. Lipase also helps soothe the inflammation.

Jan, a woman in her fifties, came to see me with chronic severe hip pain and stiffness. She had tried everything from anti-inflammatory drugs to homeopathy and acupuncture with no relief. Reluctant to depend on drugs, she decided to see me for nutritional and enzyme evaluation. My examination revealed that she was sugar intolerant, hypothyroid, deficient in the essential minerals potassium, phosphorus, calcium, and magnesium, deficient in Vitamin C, and very acidic (low pH). I immediately gave her a sugar-digesting enzyme and created a diet low in sugar and acid forming foods. I treated her with NAET for calcium, Vitamin C, and acid from the acid-producing foods. Within days of rigorously adhering to the diet and taking the enzymes, she was free of stiffness and pain and looked ten years younger. Needless to say, she was elated.

After one year, she is doing quite well. Because her hip joint had already degenerated, she might have to have it replaced. But in the meantime, she can continue to work and enjoy participating in her children's activities without distraction.

Hypoglycemia

Hypoglycemia (low blood sugar) has a number of causes and eating protein is not always the answer. In fact, the most common cause of hypoglycemia is a problem with protein consumption. Fifty percent of the protein we consume is converted to sugars in the body to provide nourishment and energy. When intolerant of or allergic to protein, the body cannot utilize the amino acids needed to make sugar, and we become hypoglycemic. We must digest and tolerate protein in order to make use of the amino acids. Although elimination of the allergy or intolerance to protein is crucial, enzymes, particularly protease, can also be helpful.

Sugar intolerance or allergy is also important in understanding hypoglycemia. If one cannot digest and absorb the sugars, then hyperglycemia (high blood sugar) and hypoglycemia can develop. When blood sugar levels are too high as a result of overconsumption and poor digestion of sugar, the pancreas secretes too much insulin that brings blood sugar levels crashing. Ultimately, this can exhaust the pancreas and cause diabetes.

Cathy, a twenty-six-year-old aerobics instructor, came to see me for severe hypoglycemia. She had moments of low energy during the day that created difficulties conducting her classes. She turned out to be both protein intolerant and protein deficient. I put her on an enzyme high in protease and treated her for her allergies to sugar and amino acids. Her hypoglycemia disappeared, her day-to-day energy level was restored, and those dark circles under her eyes vanished.

Environmental Toxins

Toxins in our environment, chemotherapy treatment, radiation, and unhealthy lifestyles contribute to the breakdown of the immune system. Enzymes interrupt the damage and inflammation to the immune system that go along with these stresses.

Prevention of Aging

By observing my patients, I have come to believe that enzymes help retard the aging process by breaking up the circulating immune complexes and restoring energy and vitality. People feel more vibrant and have more clarity after working with enzymes. I can see changes almost immediately when my patients begin enzyme therapy. A healthy diet not properly assimilated cannot benefit the body and keep it vital.

Women's Health

Enzymes play a role in many health issues affecting women such as PMS, unpleasant symptoms of menopause, vaginal infections, fibrocystic breasts, endometriosis, menstrual irregularities, and infertility.

The Endocrine System

Enzymes play an important role in maintaining normal, healthy adrenal and thyroid glands by reducing autoimmune reactions and conserving the metabolic enzymes needed for glandular function.

Other Systems

Enzymes help maintain a proper electrolyte balance by regulating the retention of water. Enzymes are excellent for reducing swollen lymph nodes and the fatigue related to lymphatic congestion. Enzymes also prevent the formation of kidney and gallstones by breaking up the oxalic acid that is the most common cause. In this case, NAET can be used as a complimentary therapy to help desensitize a person to oxalic acid and calcium. When a person is allergic to these nutrients, their absorption ability is reduced and there is a crystallization of calcium and oxalates and a formation of stones.

Intestinal Toxemia

Intestinal toxemia causes many symptoms, among which are fatigue, allergies, asthma, arthritis, nervousness, gastrointestinal conditions, impaired nutrition, skin disturbances, low back pain, sciatica, and many more. By restoring proper digestion, enzymes prevent intestinal toxemia and help restore normal intestinal flora.

A diet high in protein causes a predominance of proteolytic putrefactive bacteria in the intestine that produce toxic compounds, some of which are absorbed. If these compounds are incompletely detoxified by the liver, they enter the systemic circulation and cause or aggravate many diseases. The products of the putrefactive flora include indole and skatole from tryptophan, phenol from tyrosine, and hydrogen sulfide from the products of protein breakdown. A widely used measure of intestinal putrefaction is the amount of indican (a form of indole) in the urine. Skatole formed from bacterial action on tryptophan causes bad breath.

Histamine, another toxic decomposition by-product of tryptophan, causes headaches, head congestion, nervous depression, and nausea. Tyramine, a toxin decomposed from tyrosine, can cause high blood pressure.

When I was a young student of nutrition, I studied with Dr. Bernard Jensen. His lectures always included a discussion of intestinal toxemia (bowel toxicity) which he believed was the cause of many chronic health problems. Because the intestines were the hub of the body, he taught, a toxic colon could leak toxins into the bloodstream and cause anything from arthritis to early aging and cancer.

A seventy-year-old friend of mine named John came to see me about five years ago with frequent urination, pain, and burning associated with urination. A complete twenty-four hour urinalysis and abdominal diagnostic exam revealed that his pH was 4.5 and his indican level was 14, the highest I had ever seen. The indican measure usually represents a value that has been there for many years. His bowel toxicity had been poisoning his system for a long time and I suspected he had bladder cancer. Because he had other serious problems beyond my level of expertise, I referred him to another practitioner. He died a year later of bladder cancer. I always wonder had we done the test earlier and corrected his condition with enzymes, would things have turned out differently? Bowel toxicity is usually an inherited condition but it can certainly be reversed with enzymes and dietary changes.

A twenty-four hour urine test is a useful nutritional assessment of chronic enzyme deficiencies and digestive intolerances. It is effective in evaluating intestinal toxemia and excess protein, sugar, or fat in the urine that reflect poor digestion. It analyzes assimilation, calcium and vitamin deficiencies, as well as kidney, adrenal, and thyroid activity. With all these clues to a person's nutritional makeup, we can detect a predisposition to diabetes, heart disease, and osteoporosis. The supplementation of enzymes to a proper level can help prevent these chronic problems in the future.

Parasites

Enzymes help the body rid itself of parasites. With the addition of magnesium and other herbs, parasites can be eliminated as well as prevented.

Herpes and Other Viruses

I have used protease in treating children's illnesses such as runny nose, sore throat, and flu-like symptoms. Early detection and treatment with enzymes eliminates troublesome viruses, including herpes, and prevents recurrence. Because enzymes prevent infections, my family and I take protease every day.

Whenever a child or an adult asthmatic reports any symptoms of infection, I immediately give them high doses of protease every half hour until their symptoms subside. I also recommend NAET treatment with their own saliva every two to five hours (refer to the Self-Treatment section of Chapter 5). This usually eliminates the symptoms and prevents further complications or the progression of the infection.

Skin and Joint Problems

Enzyme therapy controls and treats psoriasis, eczema, joint swelling, and back problems. As a chiropractor, I have seen how enzyme therapy (protease, bromelain, lipase) speeds up recovery when used to treat sprains, strains, misalignments, swelling, and inflammation.

Margo, a woman in her twenties, came to see me for severe psoriasis, a condition she had been plagued with her whole life. After a thorough enzyme evaluation, I found that her pH was very acid (indicating an inability to digest fats and oils), chronic Candida, and another fungus. I recommended an enzyme for digesting fats (high lipase), a liver enzyme, and an acidophilus enzyme with cellulase for Candida, fungi, and intestinal toxemia. After eight months her psoriasis had almost completely disappeared. She has been on enzymes for years now and her condition is hardly noticeable. She would never be without her enzymes. They changed her life.

Chronic Diseases

Autoimmune diseases such as Crohn's disease, colitis, lung disorders, and systemic Candida infections all react to enzyme therapy. Enzymes restore digestion and free up a compromised immune system. Then those living defender cells can do their job fighting organisms and maintaining a clean inner environment, one that is not involved with diseases such as heart disease, malignancies, skin problems, low and high blood sugar, stomach and colon pains, eye trouble, and headaches. Enzymes destroy toxins and free radicals and antigens in the liver and bloodstream.

Research has found that the impaired ability of an enzyme to protect against free radicals may lead to damage to motor neurons in the brain and spinal cord. This research sheds some light on nervous systems disorders such as Parkinson's disease and ALS (Lou Gehrig's disease). Researchers now report early promise in treating a devastating childhood immune deficiency disease with injections of a manufactured form of the missing enzyme that causes the disease. In addition, recent research in Germany has found that MS can be held in check and in some cases improved through the use of enzyme therapy. Children previously treated unsuccessfully for acute lymphoblastic leukemia have achieved complete or partial remission with a newly developed enzyme: one hundred percent of the young patients responded favorably to treatment.

Allergies

Many allergies today are actually related to a lack of certain enzymes needed to digest the substance that causes the allergic reaction. Joint pain and gout often result from undigested proteins, fats, and minerals that form uric crystals that get caught in the joints. Yeast and fungal growth starts with undigested foods in the bloodstream and can be compounded by the white flour and sugar we eat. Extreme fatigue might be a consequence of an inability to digest proteins and fats that cause poor circulation. When blood cells clump together, they cannot carry as much oxygen which leads to slow and muddled thinking. It is also more difficult for white blood cells to travel where they are needed.

Proteolytic and lipolytic enzymes found in some supplements help break down unwanted toxins and irritants partially responsible for allergies and inflammation. The enzymes break the toxic substances into smaller, more manageable components that are then eliminated from the body.

Higher Energy

About half of the body's energy is spent digesting food. Studies find a definite correlation between the amount of enzymes a person has and their energy level. For example, athletes who take enzyme supplements have been able to work out more often with greater intensity and require less recovery time.

Obesity

There is a connection between eating a diet full of cooked, enzyme-deficient food and problems with excessive weight. Raw foods rich in enzymes aid the body in reaching and maintaining its normal weight and firmness. I have had wonderful results with enzyme therapy. Correcting digestive intolerances with enzymes and adjusting the diet based on the specific food intolerances help with either weight reduction or weight gain, whichever is desired.

Doctors throughout the United States have been researching the effects of plant enzymes on various clinical conditions including poor digestion, malabsorption, pancreatic insufficiency, celiac disease, lactose intolerance, arterial obstruction, and thrombotic disease. Results have shown that enzymes are effective for treating a wide range of conditions.

THE VALUE OF ENZYMES AND ANTIOXIDANTS

According to Hippocrates, "Man is not nourished by what he swallows, but by what he digests and uses." With the increasing pollution and depletion of healthy soil, the foods we eat today have only a fraction of the nutrition our ancestors consumed in centuries past. At the same time, we now have an advanced technology that allows us to replenish the nutrients we lose through food processing by producing enzyme supplements to be taken with every meal. Once known only to alternative health professionals, enzyme therapy has achieved such amazing results (measured by patient evaluations as well as by microscopic blood analysis) that the treatment has recently excited even the medical mainstream.

Superoxide Dismutase (SOD)

Superoxide dismutase (**SOD**), a copper/zinc-containing enzyme found in all body cells, is a primary defender against free radicals. SOD eliminates destructive superoxide molecules, a common free radical produced in the body, and soaks up free radical oxygen molecules in the bloodstream. Reactive oxygen molecules, or oxygen radicals, can destroy healthy tissue. Normally, the body makes enough SOD to hold oxygen radicals in check. But when the immune system destroys bacteria or other infectants and invaders, the surge in the number of white blood cells or antibodies triggers a rapid proliferation of oxygen radicals. In many autoimmune diseases, the white blood cells or immune reactors identify certain tissues as foreign and attack them. SOD scavenges the free radicals and interrupts the progress of this autoimmune reaction.

SOD also inhibits fats in the cells from becoming rancid which helps prevent premature aging. It also helps wounds to heal and alleviates symptoms related to radiation sickness. People deficient in this enzyme should use a supplement. The food sources of SOD are green vegetables, yeast, sprouted seeds, and grains.

Coenzyme Q_{10}

Coenzyme Q_{10} is important for the production of energy by all cells in the body because they help activate enzymes. For example, copper, iron, and other minerals and vitamins, including the B complex, are coenzymes. We need to absorb those important vitamins from our foods so that our enzymes and coenzymes can function optimally. Coenzyme Q_{10}, which occurs naturally in the body, has been found useful for heart problems, high blood pressure, diabetes, cancer, obesity, tumors, and Candida. Athletes take CoQ_{10} for increased endurance.

Streptokinase is an enzyme that, according to recent research, helps establish blood flow to the heart. Administered as an injectant into the patients coronary artery, this enzyme acts to dissolve clots and has contributed to an encouraging survival rate among heart attack victims.

Enzymes help the body to build new muscle tissue, nerve cells, skin, and glandular tissue. For example, one enzyme assists in converting dietary phosphorous into bone. Other enzymes aid in digestion, regulate respiration, facilitate better elimination, and stimulate the immune system. There is another enzyme used for burn patients that helps reduce scarring and blood loss. The enzyme acts on dead tissue to expose tissue better able to accept skin grafts.

ABDOMINAL PALPATION AND TWENTY-FOUR HOUR URINALYSIS

The abdominal palpation examination that I learned from Dr. Howard Loomis is based on the recognition of superficial pain or tenderness found in the muscular abdominal wall. When palpated or stretched, these muscles elicit a reflex contraction in the body. This contraction is measured through applied kinesiology or postural deviation, indicated in pelvic leg measurement and leg length discrepancy. These are all reflexes used by chiropractors and health practitioners in many fields to determine and correct areas of imbalance.

Each area of the abdomen, when stretched or palpated, relates to a specific organ or tissue function by means of sensory nerve affiliation. When the palpated area elicits a reflex, a possible inflammation, deficiency, or imbalance is evident. These areas and a brief description of symptoms are discussed below:

The *epigastrum* refers to the stomach, esophagus, and duodenum. A positive reflex in this area indicates gastritis with symptoms that include heartburn and bloating immediately after eating, reflux, and acid indigestion.

The *upper right quadrant* of the abdomen represents the liver and gallbladder. Symptoms include possible gallstones, pain onset several hours after eating a large meal, and poor digestion of fat.

The *upper left quadrant* refers to the jejunum. A positive reflex here can indicate celiac disease, gluten intolerance, or problems arising from poor digestion and absorption of sugars. Symptoms include bloating, diarrhea, chronic fatigue, asthma, and weight loss or gain.

The *lower left quadrant* is related to the colon, particularly the sigmoid colon. Symptoms include irritable bowel, diarrhea, poor digestion of complex carbohydrates and fiber foods, obesity, and the overconsumption of fats, leading to high levels of triglycerides and cholesterol in the blood.

A positive reflex in the *lower right quadrant* represents acute appendicitis or poor protein digestion evidenced by a high urinary indican level. Symptoms include bloating, pain in the ileocecal valve that connects the small intestine to the large intestine, and possibly calcium deficiency with poor digestion of protein. Palpation of this quadrant can elicit a strong reflex and severe pain on even superficial pressure.

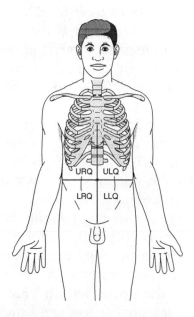

Figure 13–1   Abdominal Diagnostic Palpation Exam developed by Dr. Howard Loomis to determine specific dietary stresses and intolerances. When a trained practitioner palpates the different quadrants, a positive reflex usually is indicative of dietary stress or intolerance.

Abdominal Palpation Reference Chart	
Positive Reflex in:	*Problem:*
epigastrum	excess acidity or alkaline deficiency
upper right quadrant	fat intolerant
upper left quadrant	sugar intolerant
lower right quadrant	protein intolerant
lower left quadrant	fiber intolerant

I use this palpation examination with patients to help me decide on the appropriate enzyme to aid them in the digestion of their food. As discussed earlier in this chapter, good digestion is the key to health. If digestion is poor, undigested food residues are deposited in the blood and lymph, creating an immune reaction that leads to the creation of CICs. These immune complexes inhibit the immune system from working adequately and they inhabit tissue and organs of the body that cause autoimmune reactions including inflammation, swelling, pain, and increased activity of pathogenic organisms in the body. Health declines, the liver overworks, and stress is internal as well as external.

Every one of our patients is put on a digestive enzyme formula to predigest food. I determine the appropriate formula by using the abdominal diagnostic enzyme evaluation. For example, many asthmatics elicit a reflex related to the upper left and lower left quadrants meaning they are unable to digest sugars and fibers. Much of the mucus created in an asthmatic is caused by the improper digestion of sugars and starches. Probably the asthmatic's diet, like the diets of most people, is made up largely of sugars including dairy products (lactose), fruit (fructose), pasta (maltose), breads, crackers, rice (rice sugar), and other grains. With this information, I put the asthmatic on an enzyme that helps digest and utilize sugars and starches and that includes cellulase, sucrase, lactase, disaccharidase, amylase, protease, and lipase. I also put the person on a diet low in sugars and starches since he or she is intolerant to these foods (refer to Part VI for specific diets).

In combination with the abdominal palpation examination, I employ a twenty-four hour urinalysis laboratory exam developed by Dr. Howard Loomis to evaluate inherent food intolerances and dietary excesses, bowel toxicity, and other critical areas such as kidney function and vitamin deficiencies. The kidneys help the body maintain blood homeostasis by filtering the blood and discarding excess waste in the urine. Careful monitoring of the urine reveals what the body is holding and throwing away in its efforts to maintain homeostasis.

For example, the body regulates the pH of the blood by discarding excess acid and base. The inability to do this adequately is revealed in the urine which reflects the many stresses and strains the body experiences. Analysis of the urine can point out sick individuals whose bodies are struggling to cope better than can an analysis of the blood because the body maintains the homeostasis of the blood at all costs. The urine reveals dietary excess in the form of precipitated fat, carbohydrate, and protein that indicates poor digestion of, and/or overreaction to, these foods. The urine shows mineral deficiencies, anxiety, respiratory stress, sugar problems, prediabetic tendencies, gallbladder problems, bowel toxicity, and sluggish or overworked kidneys. With this evaluation and the abdominal palpation, we are able to recommend the appropriate diet and digestive enzymes to better serve an individual's homeostasis and to reinforce or maintain a healthy immune system.

V | CASE STUDIES

14 | NAET AND ENZYME CASE STUDIES

GENETIC

If both parents have allergies, their children will have allergies one hundred percent of the time. I have seen these statistics change after treating mothers with NAET when they are pregnant. I have treated quite a few pregnant mothers for their allergies and then tested their newborn children to find them completely clear of the allergies for which they were treated.

CASE I

Jeanette, pregnant with her second child, came to see me. Both she and her husband were highly allergic and both had severe asthmatic reactions to peanuts, cats, and dogs. Her first child was also highly allergic and constantly sick with colds and respiratory problems. To avoid the problems her first child encountered, we began to treat her during her pregnancy, thereby treating the unborn child at the same time.

Today, she has overcome her allergies to peanuts, cats, and dogs, as well as many others such as wheat, corn, chocolate, and seeds. After the child was born, we found that he was clear of all the allergies for which Jeanette had been treated. The real test came when her son was older. One day he ate peanuts by mistake and had absolutely no allergic reaction. Another day the family was visiting one of their friends (a medical doctor) who had a dog. Jeanette and her son had absolutely no allergic reactions. The father and the medical friend, both of whom had been skeptical up to now, were impressed and amazed given Jeanette and her family's long history of severe asthma symptoms when exposed to dogs. These profound changes have been permanent.

CANDIDA, FUNGI, AND MOLD

CASE II

Leslie, a five-year old who had suffered from severe asthma since birth, came to see me with Jane, her mother. Jane was frustrated, distressed, and frightened about her daughter's health. The day they came to see me, Leslie had been given a variety of medications including antibiotics, steroids, cough syrup, and inhalers. Her mother explained she was not herself because the medications caused severe mood swings, behavioral eccentricities, and tantrums. Then Jane began to detail Leslie's medical history. Every two weeks, sometimes more often, Leslie was sick with colds that developed into wheezing, coughing, and labored breathing. Her constant absences from school caused her mother to miss work frequently.

Using a muscle response testing procedure, I found that Leslie was allergic to eggs, chicken, milk, cheese, calcium, wheat, grains, fruits, certain vegetables, chocolate, sugars, salt, chloride, yeast, food additives, food coloring, modified starch, sulfites, Vitamins A, B, and C, betacarotene, minerals, and toothpaste. Besides foods, the list included fabrics, dyes, down feathers, perfumes, mold, dust, pollen, flowers, grasses, chemicals, animals, fumes, heat, and cold. When I performed an abdominal diagnostic palpation exam, I found she was unable to digest sugars and fats. I immediately put her on an enzyme formula to help digest sugars and fats. I also gave her extra high doses of protease enzymes to help fight bacteria in the body and strengthen her immune system. Then I began to treat her for her many allergies with NAET.

Leslie responded immediately. She didn't get sick as often as before, and her need for drugs diminished. After we treated her for sugars, she stopped having bouts of bronchitis and wheezing. I decided to visit her home and check to see which allergens she was encountering. I was not surprised to find that her bedroom was moldy, and housed an aquarium covered with algae. In fact, I was convinced that her lifelong asthma and wheezing were largely caused by her exposure to mold and mildew. After I treated Leslie with NAET for the specific mold found in her bedroom, her health changed dramatically. She has not missed a day of school in two years now, and she rarely experiences a runny nose or sore throat. Her coughing, wheezing, sleepless nights and, most importantly, her life-threatening breathing problems are gone.

INFECTANTS: BACTERIA, VIRUSES, IMMUNIZATIONS, AND PARASITES

Two years after our last visit, Jane called to tell me Leslie was coughing again. After a series of muscle tests and a thorough investigation of her food intake since her coughing began, I still could not pinpoint the cause of her symptoms. Then Jane mentioned that Leslie had received a DPT vaccination the day before she began to cough and wondered if that might be the cause of her daughter's episode. I told her that vaccinations are a major cause of allergies. When I treated her for the DPT vaccination, Leslie responded almost instantly. Her coughing stopped completely and she is once again a healthy young girl.

CASE III

Jenny, the two-year-old daughter of a family I was seeing for allergy treatments and chiropractic care, experienced severe fevers, runny nose, and wheezing for no apparent reason. Her mother, Jodie, seemed to recall that these symptoms occurred when her daughter was teething. She also commented that Jenny's breath was exceptionally foul when she was teething which seemed unusual for a two-year old.

Concerned that she might have some bacteria in her mouth that were causing an occasional infection of the gums, I did some reflex testing and uncovered three specific bacteria. Then I treated her with NAET for an allergy to these bacteria and recommended that she take some good antibacterial enzymes for about ten days. I also suggested that Jodie treat her daughter at home if necessary for another week to reinforce the treatment. Twenty-four hours later Jenny's fever was gone and she was her normal self again, with sweet breath and tons of energy. Since this treatment she has not experienced any problems with fever or wheezing.

CASE IV

A young woman named Hillary came to me for help with her chronic asthma that had started as a child. She had been in and out of hospitals and on and off medications including antibiotics her whole life. When she coughed and wheezed, which she did often, she would bring up large quantities of colored mucus. I treated her for many allergens including pollen, flowers, dust, and all sorts of foods. I put her on high doses of enzymes for good protein digestion and sugar metabolism as well as high doses of protease to boost her immune system. These treatments improved her energy level, relieved the tightness in her chest, and reduced the frequency of her infections.

However, it was not until I treated her for bacteria, viruses, fungi, and parasites that her asthma totally abated. It took quite a few treatments to clear the fungi, but fewer treatments to clear the bacteria. Now Hillary no longer displays infectious symptoms such as excess or colored mucus and chronic coughing. Her need for her inhaler has decreased, and she is pleased that these improvements have maintained themselves. We are still working on environmental allergens.

CASE V

Michael, a two-year-old child, had chronic coughing and ear infections every other month. His mother commented that she could not remember a day when her son hadn't coughed. His breathing at night was labored and he would scream with pain from ear infections. Impatient with the conventional medical program of constant antibiotics, cough medicines, and pain pills she tried homeopathy and some natural medicines without noticing any relief or change. She was another desperate mother who had come to me as a last resort.

With testing, I discovered that Michael was allergic to all the basic allergens except iron as well as to wheat, yeast, some vegetables and fruits (especially avocado), oranges, carrots, string beans, bananas, apples, and pears, many bacteria, viruses, and bronchial asthma tissue. I began to treat Michael with NAET for the basic allergies. He showed some improvement with the eggs and the calcium/dairy mix. The treatment for Vitamin C cleared his sensitivity to the vegetables and fruit. Then we began to treat for the B vitamins, an important precursor to the treatments for sugars, yeast, and grains. These treatments, in turn, can be the cornerstones of eliminating an asthmatic condition or any respiratory problem.

Michael was so allergic to the B vitamins that he needed separate treatments for each one along with several combinations. Mom became discouraged because his coughing hadn't subsided. I asked her to treat Michael for the B vitamins at home with the acupressure points twice a day for one week. By mistake, Michael slept with the B vitamin vial one night and his coughing decreased significantly. When he came into my office for the next visit, he had completely cleared his allergy to B vitamins. Now Mom and Dad were feeling hopeful.

I then proceeded to complete the basics. Although Michael was now only coughing occasionally on three out of seven nights, I still was not satisfied. I wanted him to be symptom-free. I decided to treat him for bronchial asthma in combination with the bronchi and lung tissues. This treatment is meant to free up a genetic predisposition to the disease. I have seen patients come out of an asthma attack by treating for asthma when they show a muscle reflex response to the bronchial asthma vial. Since this treatment, Michael has slept soundly and has not coughed once at night.

Even more dramatic for Michael than the treatment for bronchial asthma were the NAET treatments for bacteria. During three different visits I tested him for all the bacteria and treated him for the ones to which he was allergic. After clearing these allergies a year ago, he has not had a single ear infection or cold. This case illustrates the axiom that nothing is normal except good health all the time. Allergy elimination can help make this possible.

COMBINATION TREATMENT

Sometimes I do a combination treatment of saliva (containing a possible pathogen such as a virus or a bacteria) with a food or an environmental substance if I feel they are connected with the symptoms a patient is experiencing.

CASE VI

My daughter Gabrielle, who was five years old at the time, woke up one morning with a slight runny nose. Before she went to preschool, I did some reflex testing and found that she was reacting both to the food coloring in the jelly beans she had eaten the day before and to a virus. The food coloring had apparently weakened her immune system and made her susceptible to the virus she must have been carrying in her system. I decided to treat her with NAET for the food coloring and her saliva. Her runny nose stopped instantly and she went off to school. In the evening I tested her for her saliva and she was very strong. I also gave her high doses of protease enzyme, a natural antibiotic completely harmless to children of any age.

POOR DIGESTION: SUGAR AND PROTEIN INTOLERANCES

People who are intolerant to protein are unable to digest it, which leads to a deficiency of amino acids and an inability to make the sugars that are needed to fuel the brain and energize the body.

CASE VII

Sarah, a fifty-four-year-old woman with a lifelong history of asthma and chronic sinusitis had tried every therapy, including ones I had never heard of, to help her control her asthma attacks. For eight years she had experienced a series of sinus, ear, and respiratory infections that required she take a course of antibiotics every other month. She also suffered from acute food cravings, especially sugars, commenting that she always wanted to have something sweet in her mouth but restrained herself. Much to her dismay, she was also unable to taste the foods she ate. She was severely underweight, chronically fatigued, and depressed about her condition. Referred to me by someone at work whose food cravings, chronic colds, and flu had improved with the use of enzymes, she chose to try yet another approach to see if it would help restore her health. Although she wasn't hopeful, she wasn't ready to give up either.

A thorough enzyme examination and nutritional evaluation revealed that Sarah was intolerant to sugars and protein. No wonder Sarah craved sugars. But every time she ate them they caused a buildup of mucus. I immediately put her on enzymes to help her digest sugars and protein and I gave her high doses of protease enzymes as a natural antibiotic to destroy the bacteria she had been chronically fighting for many years. Her recommended diet consisted of a minimal intake of breads, fruits, and sugars of all kinds and the complete elimination of refined carbohydrates. I recommended that she eat no more than one six-ounce serving of animal protein per day but unlimited servings of vegetable protein (refer to the low sugar and carbohydrate diet in Part VI). Since starting this diet and enzyme regimen, she has not had one asthma attack or chronic cough. Her craving for sugars, chronic sinusitis, and acute allergy symptoms continued, however, until we cleared her allergies with NAET.

FOOD COLORING AND ADDITIVES

Food coloring is another potential irritant that can bring on asthma attacks.

CASE VIII

Emily, a seventy-five-year-old woman, came to my office one day with labored breathing and wheezing. Since we had already cleared her on the foods she was currently eating, she couldn't understand what had caused such a strong reaction. We reviewed her diet at least three times when suddenly she remembered that she had begun to cough right after someone had given her a butterscotch candy. When I treated her for food coloring, her labored breathing ceased.

The message here is that we should never underestimate any potential food allergen. Even the taste of something one is allergic to can cause an asthma attack, a migraine, dizziness, eczema, or other allergic symptoms. I see it every day in my office. As a matter of fact, some recent scientific research indicates that an individual can react to the cooking steam of an allergic food. I now recommend that my patients have no tactile or sensory contact with a food for twenty-five hours after being treated for it with NAET. Even the smell of fresh coffee brewing or the whiff of a certain spice can nullify a treatment.

CASE IX

A young patient named Allan who had already been treated with NAET for some basic food allergies such as eggs, milk, and sugars came to me complaining of wheezing and chest congestion. His mother wasn't sure what had brought on his asthma attack. When I asked what Allan had eaten the day before, she mentioned that he had ordered a salad at a salad bar restaurant but had avoided the sugared dressings. I know from experience that such restaurants tend to use a variety of food additives and preservatives such as hydrolyzed vegetable protein, MSG, sodium nitrate, nitrite, sulfur dioxide, BHT, and BHA, all of which can trigger an asthma attack.

When I muscle response tested Allan for food additives in relation to the lung and respiratory meridians, his muscles weakened significantly, indicating a definite allergy. Because I didn't know which additive was the culprit, however, I treated him for all of them. Immediately after the treatment his wheezing stopped. I suggested to his parents that if he started to wheeze at all during the next twenty-five hours, they should put the food additives vial in his hand and perform acupressure related to the lungs for fifteen minutes to reinforce the treatment and prevent him from losing its effects. After being cleared for this allergy, Allan no longer had to avoid food additives.

MEDICATIONS

Drugs are other potential triggers that can bring on an asthma attack as well as coughing and congestion. I usually ask my asthma patients to bring the medications (inhalers, steroids, cough syrup) they use on a regular basis with them. I can't tell you how many asthmatics, especially children, are allergic to their medications. Many of the cough medicines used on a daily basis for weeks or even months are filled with sugars and food colorings, both of which can be dramatic inducers of asthma. I always treat my patients with NAET for any allergies to drugs (such as inhalers) that cannot be eliminated right away. However, NAET treatments to drugs never seem to be permanent, so I periodically recheck to see if the treatment is needed again. Whenever possible, I eliminate the need for these drugs by using natural enzymes that alleviate some of the symptoms until all the allergens are cleared.

CASE X

A four-year-old girl named Kelly would wake up every night with severe wheezing. Her mother medicated her so she could return to sleep but she would wake up four hours later needing another dose. After we treated for the steroids (albuterol) and cough medicine she had been taking during the night, she never woke with wheezing again.

INHALANTS: DUST

Allergy treatments for dust and mold are extremely important for asthma sufferers. Although both are hardly visible, they can be life threatening and most asthma patients need to be treated for them.

CASE XI

Gabrielle, my daughter, always had trouble breathing through her nose and was a mouth-breather for the first two years of her life. She also had excess mucus in her throat that would cause occasional wheezing, sore throats, coughing, and accumulation of fluid in her middle ear. I became concerned because this fluid accumulation seemed to be causing hearing difficulties. Gabrielle had been taking enzymes since infancy and had never had an infection or needed antibiotics. I took her to a homeopathic pediatrician who experimented with many remedies that did not help her. Then I took her to a pediatric ear, nose, and throat specialist (ENT) who, after a five-minute examination, recommended placing tubes in her middle ear as well as a tonsillectomy and an adenoidectomy. Although I listened with an open mind, I decided to seek one more opinion before signing her up for surgery. The pediatrician we consulted this time said, "Your daughter has allergies!" She also said that her hearing was not impaired nor did she require surgery. I had just started using NAET in my practice, and I decided to treat Gabrielle myself. First I treated her for eggs that she craved, usually a sure indication that someone is allergic to a particular food. Her craving stopped immediately. Then I treated her for a mixture of Vitamin C and strawberries, citrus, and some vegetables. Her mucus production diminished considerably but she continued to snore. After I treated her for all the basics, she did not need to clear her throat anymore. Next I treated her for viruses, yeast, and Candida. Her hearing was now normal and she no longer had fluid in her ears. But she still snored! What could it be? I was baffled.

Early one Sunday morning, Gabrielle and I were playing in her room. I opened the blinds and noticed dust flying around the room. I had not yet treated her for dust which I was allergic to myself as a child. After cleaning her room thoroughly, I treated her for dust with NAET. That was nearly four years ago and she has not snored, wheezed, or coughed since.

CASE XII

At fifteen, my son Aaron was supposed to clean his own room and do his own laundry. But, being a typical teenager, he would put it off for days, weeks, or even longer. One night he woke up wheezing and complained that he couldn't breathe very well. Because he had spent the day in his room doing his homework, I thought it had to be something there that triggered the attack. When I suggested it might be the mattress dust, he confessed he hadn't washed his sheets for some time. I didn't want to know how long! I stripped his bed, vacuumed his mattress, and dusted and cleaned his room. He slept well that night. The next day, I treated him with NAET for the mattress dust I had saved from the vacuum cleaner. Since then, Aaron has never had any problems with wheezing or coughing. And I don't think he will ever put off washing his sheets again!

INHALANTS: CHEMICALS AND CAT AND ANIMAL DANDER

CASE XIII

Susan, a forty-one-year-old woman, came to see me with severe allergies that had caused eye tearing, fatigue, and asthma since childhood. In addition to being seasonal, her asthma attacks seemed to be triggered by foods and other environmental allergens. In particular, she suspected that chemical allergies were causing her eyes to tear. I did a complete workup including allergy testing and an enzyme evaluation. Then I treated her for the basic substances she was allergic to such as eggs, sugars, minerals, salt, and chloride. After being treated for B vitamins, she felt a significant positive change in her health. She has not had any asthma or labored breathing since.

Our next major accomplishment was treating Susan's chronically reddened, teary eyes, not improved by the basic allergy treatments. After being treated for some environmental allergies such as perfumes, chemicals, hair products, and makeup (eye shadow, mascara, blush) her eye symptoms almost entirely disappeared. However, it was not until the NAET treatment for cat and animal dander that these symptoms were completely eliminated.

INHALANTS: POLLENS, CHEMICALS, PERFUME, AND SMOKE

CASE XIV

Remember Sarah, about whom I talked earlier, who had a complete reversal of her asthma symptoms with enzyme therapy and dietary changes but still suffered chronic sinus congestion, an inability to taste foods, and some chronic eye irritation? When I tested her for environmental allergies, I found she still was allergic to grasses, trees, flowers, pollens over different seasons (which need to be treated with NAET during those seasons), perfume, cosmetics, tobacco smoke, and certain chemicals including chlorine. With these specific treatments, her sinus congestion greatly diminished and her taste began to return, a dramatic and welcome change for her.

INHALANTS: WALLPAPER FUMES

CASE XV

Rachel, a nineteen-year-old woman, grew up with asthma and used an inhaler for most of her life. Fortunately, she had never been hospitalized for a severe asthma attack but she did notice her symptoms worsening as she got older. Overweight and fatigued most of the time, she had poor digestion and reported that she always had congestion in her lungs and woke up in the morning coughing as though she were a smoker, which she had never been. Every other month she seemed to come down with a cold, the flu, or bronchitis. Rachel had worked in many different environments including a hair salon, a nightclub, and her mother's real estate business.

I immediately put her on enzymes to help her breathing and enhance her immune response. Testing indicated that her poor digestion was due to an intolerance to fats. I encouraged her to eat a diet low in fat (a diet low in animal protein, as it tends to contain large amounts of fat). I prescribed enzymes to help with the digestion of fat and to protect her against bacteria and viruses. At the same time, I began to treat her for all the basic allergies with NAET. Subsequent treatments included artificial sweeteners, dust, smog, exhaust, gas heat, radiation, paint, hair and nail chemicals, cosmetics, soaps, fabrics, formaldehyde, and carpets as well as trees, flowers, and pollens (over a two-month period).

Rachel improved in some ways but still experienced asthma attacks every night. We couldn't figure out what the trigger might be. Before I went to her house to check, I asked her, "Is there anything at all in your bedroom that you might have overlooked?" She went home and checked every inch of her room to find out what could be triggering her asthma. When she returned to my office, she was carrying a piece of grass cloth wallpaper, the only thing we had not tested. As it turned out, she was definitely allergic to it and she even felt her chest tighten up when she held it. After I treated her for the wallpaper using NAET, she noticed immediate results with instantaneous relief in her chest. She has not had another asthma attack since this treatment four years ago.

VITAMIN DEFICIENCY AND ANTIOXIDANTS

Antioxidants are essential tools for the detoxification of free radicals, which, if not detoxified, can result in severe damage to body tissues.

CASE XVI

Carey, a thirty-two-year-old woman, came to see me complaining of chronic sinus infection, postnasal drip, and a recurring cough. She was quite aware that some allergens (perfumes, chemicals, formaldehyde and certain foods) made her health worse. After an extensive workup, I found her to be allergic to all the basic allergens, the most severe of which was Vitamin C and the bioflavinoids. An abdominal palpation and twenty-four hour urinalysis pointed to liver and bowel toxicity. I started her on some enzymes for digestion and liver detoxification and repair and simultaneously began to treat her with NAET for her basic allergies.

After the treatment for Vitamin C and supplementation of her diet with Vitamin C and other antioxidants including enzymes, pau d'arco, garlic, and grape seed extract, Carey experienced dramatic positive changes in her health, including freedom from sinus congestion and coughing. She also remarked that her lifelong food cravings had diminished. Her energy increased significantly and she was all smiles each time I saw her in the following weeks.

It is important to supplement a patient's diet with a vitamin or mineral after the desensitization to that nutrient has occurred because the patient probably has been deficient for a long time, perhaps even from the day he or she was born. Symptoms change rather quickly when supplementation takes place. Some diets need long-term vitamin supplementation, others only short-term. Each person is different, and there are several testing procedures that can be done to evaluate the need for supplementation. These include hair analysis, blood analysis, urinalysis, the abdominal reflex exam, and muscle response testing. I also make use of liver and bowel cleansers, often an essential part of the healing and detoxification process for patients who have cleared many allergies.

ENZYME DEFICIENCIES

People who are allergic to oxalic acid and also sometimes to calcium tend to eat foods high in oxalic acid, causing a buildup of calcium oxalate crystals which are common constituents of kidney stones. For a complete list of foods high in oxalic acid, refer to Part VI.

CASE XVII

Years ago, before I started to practice NAET, Betty came to see me with symptoms of heartburn, severe bloating, swelling of her abdomen, and an inability to digest anything she ate. She also noted that for the last two years, she had suffered from a chronic cough and periods of shortness of breath. At sixty-six, she was slim and healthy in every other way and did not take any medication, unusual for a woman her age. In addition, her diet was impeccably well balanced and she watched her intake of fat and sugar. Her complexion and her coloring were excellent. She walked a mile every day and did hatha yoga two or three times a week.

When I performed a complete urinalysis and a thorough investigation of her diet in conjunction with a fasting and non-fasting abdominal palpation, I found her pH to be at 6. (highly acidic) and her sediment level, the precipitate of her food intake during the twenty-four-hour test period included a higher than normal calcium oxalate. This gave me certain clues about her food intake. Betty's calcium oxalate level was higher than normal and was very low in calcium on her urinalysis. This made me suspect that she might be allergic to calcium. Her palpation examination produced a positive reflex (discomfort) when I pressed or palpated her gastric reflex below her xiphoid process. She was also extremely bloated.

After prescribing a gastric enzyme to help neutralize her acidic stomach, I spent time with her reviewing her diet. Although she consumed no coffee, it turned out she adored chocolate, a food high in oxalic acid, and could not let a day go by without having some. She also mentioned that on her friends' recommendation, she had increased her calcium intake (through both calcium supplements and dairy products) to avoid the onset of osteoporosis. She remembered having trouble digesting milk as a child but thought she had outgrown it. Examination indicated that she was suffering from reflux and gastritis as well as foods high in oxalic acid such as chocolate, dairy, and calcium and seemed to be contributing to her digestive problems that could worsen over time. I advised her to stop eating chocolate, temporarily eliminate her calcium intake, and avoid foods high in oxalic acid. The combination of the diet change and the enzymes prompted her to call me two weeks later to say that her coughing was almost completely gone and she had not felt this good in years. I reminded her that she could also take her enzymes after meals, as needed, to eliminate the coughing which she did with success.

FOODS: CHOCOLATE

Three years later Betty came to see me again after hearing that I was now using a unique allergy elimination technique. She remembered my comment that she was possibly allergic to calcium and oxalates and wondered if she might also be allergic to chocolate. She wasn't able to eliminate it from her diet for long and continued to crave it. She noted that her bloating had returned but that her coughing and shortness of breath had never returned. She was also concerned about calcium deficiency and its long-term effects such as arthritis, osteoporosis, insomnia, and nervousness. She had recently begun to experience cramping and some shaking in her legs that could have been the result of a calcium deficiency.

I began by testing her on an expanded group of basic allergies. As I suspected, I found she was allergic to calcium, sugars, Vitamin C, chocolate, and protease. Repeating a thorough enzyme evaluation and urinalysis, I found her pH to be normal at 6.5 and her calcium oxalate level still to be high, although lower than her previous test. I also found her gastric reflex to be positive, as before. She admitted that she had taken her enzymes for one year and then discontinued them because she was feeling better. However, she had kept to her gastritis diet except for the chocolate, her mad love.

This time I treated her with NAET for calcium, dairy, sugars, oxalic acid, and a few other allergens over the course of a few weeks. She resumed her calcium supplements with no deleterious effect and began eating dairy products again with no bloating. She was also able to end her love affair with chocolate for the first time in her life. "Dr. Ellen," she said, "this is the first time I can walk past a Sees Candy store and not fulfill the urge to have some chocolate." After treating her for protease, I was able to put her on a wider range of enzymes that helped her digest protein. She noticed immediately that she slept better, her legs stopped shaking, and the joint pain she had been experiencing lessened. Good protein digestion helps the absorption of calcium. Her urinalysis over a two-month period showed normal oxalate and calcium levels.

BASICS

In the category of basic allergies I include ten groups: 1) eggs, chicken, tetracycline, and feathers; 2) calcium and dairy; 3) Vitamin C, fruits and vegetables; 4) B-complex; 5) sugars; 6) iron and meat products; 7) Vitamin A, fish, and shellfish; 8) mineral mix; 9) salt; and 10) chlorides.

CASE XVIII

Michael, a thirty-one-year-old music producer, was referred to my office by another of my patients. He had suffered from severe asthma since birth and could not go anywhere without his inhaler or drugs. He came to me hoping that he might be able to eliminate his medication. He already was aware that he was allergic to house dust, cats, dogs, feathers, cigarette smoke, perfume, pollens, grasses, and certain climactic changes that aggravated his asthma.

I explained to him that I needed to test and treat him on the "basic allergies" before treating him for some of the more obvious ones. He proved to be allergic to the first group. I always suspect this when someone has an allergy to feathers as well as to calcium and dairy, B-complex, sugars, and salt. All of these are common allergies for asthmatics.

Next I performed an in-depth nutritional analysis consisting of a urinalysis, abdominal palpation, food evaluation, and enzyme diagnostic test. I found him to be highly intolerant of proteins and sugars and unable to absorb certain nutrients. These intolerances caused not only his respiratory problems, but also his hypoglycemia, bloating, low adrenal function, fatigue, attention deficit problems, and low energy level. He began to take enzymes that helped digest the proteins and sugars. At the same time, I started to treat him with NAET for the ten basic allergy groups. When I treated him for the first group, I warned him that he could have a strong allergic reaction if he ate or came in contact with any of the allergens he was being treated for during the twenty-five-hour clearing period. When he failed to follow my instructions, he suffered a severe asthma attack and flu-like symptoms. When I repeated the treatment, he was able to clear his allergy to eggs, chicken, feathers, and tetracycline.

After two months on the road, Michael called to tell me he had not had another asthma attack or used his medication since the treatment for the first group. This was the longest span between attacks since he was six years old. After I finished treating him for the basic allergies, I retested him for his known allergies to cats, dogs, pollens, and house dust and found that he was no longer allergic to any of them. When I spoke to Michael recently, he couldn't remember the last time he had coughed, let alone wheezed or used his inhaler. He said he is truly a different person.

BASICS: SUGAR

CASE XIX

My son Aaron is a healthy young man who has grown up on good nutrition and enzymes for proper digestion. He has never been on a prescription antibiotic because I always prescribed enzymes as natural antibiotics. When he was two years old, I took him to a pediatrician, who, for no apparent reason, said his breathing sounded like that of an asthmatic. I was alarmed but found it hard to believe because neither my husband nor I had ever been diagnosed with asthma. Aaron had a slight cold at the time and I decided to disregard the pediatrician's comment. I never really thought about it again.

The year Aaron turned fourteen he developed a chronic cough that commenced in January and lasted until his birthday in the beginning of March. The cough recurred each year when the weather was damp, during basketball season (my son's obsession). He is an excellent basketball player but is quite hard on himself, creating a stressful situation that can compromise the immune system.

One evening I was talking on the telephone with my ninety-five-year-old grandmother. She overheard my son coughing and said: "Ellen, you used to have the same cough when you were fourteen years old." Maybe, I thought, I would have been diagnosed as an asthmatic if physicians then had been as quick to diagnose asthma as they are today. Around the age of thirteen or fourteen I had been diagnosed with allergies and treated with allergy shots. This memory was significant because I knew that hereditary factors play a key role in children's allergies. Although knowing this, I had never made the connection between my childhood allergies and those of my children. My discovery of my son's allergies corresponded to the introduction of NAET into my practice and I began to test and treat Aaron for his basic allergies. One thing I noticed was that Aaron would cough whenever he ate sugar, even though it was rare. He loved natural sodas, however, which contain large quantities of high fructose corn syrup. This sweetener is high in sugar and can often be a trigger for asthmatics. After I treated him for sugars, his coughing and wheezing completely disappeared.

FOODS: WHEAT

CASE XX

A little boy named Eric, who was not quite two, was brought to me with a chronic cough and regular, labored breathing. His mother, who traveled often for her work, had become afraid to leave him because of the special care and attention he needed. She was also concerned that the antibiotics and steroids he was regularly prescribed were actually making him more susceptible to ear and upper respiratory infections. In my clinic, I have seen people of all ages negatively affected by corticosteroids that inhibit the immune system.

Eric was tested and treated with NAET for the basic food allergies. Calcium proved to be an extremely important treatment for him because his mother had him on soy formula, high in calcium. He was also allergic to soy. Since the sugar treatment, Eric has not had one ear infection or any need for antibiotics. But the most dramatic allergens in relationship to his coughing and labored breathing were salt and wheat.

Many asthma attacks are triggered by salt, an allergen that occurs naturally in many foods such as celery, cucumbers, citrus, and water. Wheat is another key allergen for asthmatics and the treatment for it was a turning point for Eric. Sometimes, wheat can be desensitized with the clearing of B vitamins and maltose but it can be such a long-term, inherited allergy that often it has to be treated separately. I have even found different varieties of wheat to be a problem. Frequently, I have people bring the different wheat products they like to eat to ensure all the wheats are cleared as potential asthma triggers. Once Eric was cleared of all the wheats with NAET, his coughing, congestion, and labored breathing were eliminated. He is now able to eat wheat, soy, and dairy products without any problem.

ENVIRONMENT: SICK BUILDING

CASE XXI

Lisa, a woman in her forties, had severe eczema, breathing difficulties, and sinus congestion. Her many physicians lost hope of restoring her health. I proceeded to try to clear some of her symptoms with NAET and enzyme therapy. She was put on a multiple enzyme formula to help her digest protein and carbohydrates as well as an enzyme formula high in amylase to help reduce inflammation. After a few weeks, I put her on some liver detoxifying enzymes, antioxidants, and bowel cleansers. A month later she still showed absolutely no improvement. Then I began to do some detective work. She told me that she had noticed a dramatic worsening of her symptoms after she began working in her current office building. Many of her fellow employees, she said, were chronically sick with flus, sore throats, and breathing problems and she wondered about her working environment which was located on a floor without any windows.

During the energy crisis, I explained to her, we began to insulate and seal our buildings more thoroughly. This saved energy but caused pollutants to be trapped indoors, possibly creating havoc in the human body. After some thought, I decided to treat Lisa first for chemicals and then for the air in her office that she collected in an open jar left in the office overnight. After the first treatment her eczema improved dramatically and after the second her breathing cleared up completely. Today Lisa is a healthy young woman.

SMOKE

CASE XXII

After being symptom-free for three years, Susan (Case XIII) recently came to see me with red and irritated eyes. She thought perhaps it was some new makeup she had begun to use. Using certain reflex techniques, we discovered that her areas of blockage were the spleen and kidney meridians, related to the allergens tobacco smoke and solar radiation.

At first she couldn't remember coming into contact with smoke and she avoided exposing herself to the sun. As we talked, however, she recalled that she had been staying with someone who was a smoker and had actually smoked a few cigarettes herself. When I first tested her three years before, I found her extremely allergic to smoke of all kinds and wasn't surprised to see her react so dramatically now. What was surprising was that she had not had an asthma attack since our last visit despite the exposure to smoke.

I treated her for smoke that day and cautioned her to avoid smoke or items previously exposed to smoke such as clothing or furniture that could nullify the treatment and possibly cause a severe allergic reaction for twenty-five hours. Susan has been fine ever since.

CONTACTANTS: FEATHERS

How many people do you know who use down blankets and pillows? Many are probably allergic to them and wake up coughing and sneezing. Asthmatics should not use down accessories or pillows until they are treated for feathers with NAET.

CASE **XXIII**

A woman in her late twenties named Kelly came to see me for chronic sinusitis, a chronic cough, constant fatigue, and occasional asthma. She was overweight and had seen me years ago for chiropractic care on her lower back. Recently she heard I was treating allergies and was hopeful I could help her.

Testing indicated that she was allergic to eggs, chicken, feathers, B vitamins, sugars, and minerals and I began to treat her for these basic allergens. Feathers were a particularly important allergy to clear because Kelly slept with a down pillow, used a down comforter, and owned a down couch. The day after her treatment for chicken, eggs, and feathers she came in to see me to make sure she had been cleared. When she tested strong for the allergens, she hugged and kissed me, explaining that this was the first morning she could ever remember having awakened without a runny nose and congestion. She was ecstatic.

I then treated her for the other basic allergies. After the treatment for yeast and Candida, her fatigue diminished and her craving for bread disappeared. She began to lose weight after the treatments for yeast, wheat, and dairy. Since the first treatment, she has not had a problem with her sinuses and her asthma and coughing are nonexistent.

EMOTIONAL

CASE XXIV

A nine-year-old girl who constantly bit her nails turned out to have an emotional problem with her father. She recalled an incident when he insisted she accompany him somewhere she didn't want to go, and she had been angry at him for days. When we treated for the anger with NAET, she stopped biting her nails.

CASE XXV

Another patient, a man in his mid-forties, had been suffering severe lower back spasms for about a week but he did not know the origin of his pain. He came to see me after having had some chiropractic care with only temporary relief. After some reflex testing and some investigative work, I discovered it was an emotional problem related to alcohol. He watched his mother drink herself to death and his back problem erupted immediately after visiting his mother's sister, also an alcoholic. Although he rarely drinks himself, he had a drink with her. Shortly thereafter his lower back started to ache and became progressively worse.

The NAET treatment I performed was alcohol in combination with sorrow of his mother's passing. While treating him, I asked him to feel his sorrow. His back pain immediately dissipated and has not returned since. It was a remarkable treatment, one that I will never forget. He had been so disturbed by his mother's death that alcohol had become a poison for him on many levels.

HORMONES

CASE XXVI

One of my patients, a sixty-seven-year-old woman with chronic emphysema and asthma, had tried everything for her breathing difficulties that she had experienced for years. She lived a healthy life, ate a balanced diet of all organic foods, never used any alcohol, and never smoked. Her mother had died of emphysema and she was frightened that she might be destined for the same fate.

I was treating her with NAET for many allergies including foods, environmentals, drugs, and organs that had helped curtail her bouts of coughing. But nothing had any effect on her breathing problems or her lung capacity. Understandably, these symptoms frightened her the most. One day I treated her for thyroid tissue and thyroxine. The response was remarkable. Almost immediately her lung capacity expanded significantly and the change has been long lasting. We were all excited by the results. We cannot underestimate the power of an allergy and the suppression it can cause to the body. Every day at my office I witness some new miracle and learn something new.

ORGANS AND GLANDS

As I have indicated several times, I have consistently positive results treating patients with NAET using vials of different organ tissue. For example, I have treated chronic fatigue patients with thyroid and adrenal tissue and I have used pituitary tissue for depressed individuals. I have treated women with endometriosis and fibroids with uterine tissue, diabetics with brain, nerve, and pancreatic tissue, and eczema sufferers with spleen tissue. I have treated patients with colitis with large intestine tissue, migraine and fatigue sufferers with liver tissue, ulcer patients with gallbladder and stomach tissue, and individuals with chronic bladder incontinence and prostate inflammation with prostate and bladder tissue. All these treatments have yielded dramatic results. But the most obvious have been the asthma sufferers I have treated with lung and bronchial tissue.

CASE XXVII

Jane came to see me about a year ago with asthma, chronic bloating, and obesity. After a series of treatments with NAET for

PART V: *Case Studies*

foods, infectants (including bacteria, viruses, fungi, and parasites), environmental contactants, emotional incidents, and several organs her asthma is a thing of the past. She experiences only occasional bloating and she has lost forty pounds. Her NAET treatments, diet change, and enzyme therapy have all contributed to this remarkable weight loss.

Recently we treated Jane for her lungs using lung tissue. When treating with NAET for the lungs or any other organ or gland, we treat for a weakness, resistance, or hypersensitivity to the tissue of that organ or gland, causing it to function abnormally or become imbalanced. The treatment changes the relationship by desensitizing the person to the organ or gland and creates homeostasis, strength, and healing, if needed. After we treated Jane for lungs, she came in the next week and described a freedom in her breathing that she had never experienced. She went biking and was able to go beyond her normal limits with complete lung capacity as if she had been given new lungs and new air to breathe. She was ecstatic! I have seen this happen repeatedly. The treatment results usually occur shortly after the treatment and remain consistent over time.

VI | RESOURCE GUIDE

NAET Treatment Rules
Twenty-Five Hour NAET Restrictions
Foods and Materials Containing Key Allergens
Specific Diets Related To Dietary Stress
Foods high in Oxalates, Uric Acid, Alkaline,
    and Acid Foods
Most Common Infectants for Asthmatics
Spondylotherapy and Hiatal Hernia
Eye Movement Desensitization and Reprocessing
    (EMDR)
NAET Practitioners
Miscellaneous Resources
Bibliography
References
Glossary

15 | RESOURCES

NAET TREATMENT RULES

Treatment failures are a result of:

- *breaking the NAET Treatment Rules*
- *not following the NAET twenty-five hour restrictions*
- *coming within four to five feet of the treated allergens*

1. Do not wear any perfume, perfumed powder, strong-smelling deodorant, or aftershave lotion when you have a treatment or in the clinic where the treatment occurs.

2. Do not smoke before the treatment. It's important that one's clothes and hair do not smell of smoke.

3. Wash your hands before and after the treatment.

4. Do not expose yourself to extreme hot or cold temperatures after the treatment.

5. Take a shower before coming for a treatment. Do not shower or bathe for 6 hours after the treatment.

6. Do not eat, chew gum, or smoke during treatment.

7. Do not cross your hands or feet during the treatment.

8. Do not read or touch other objects for twenty minutes following the treatment.

9. Check the previous treatment with the doctor to ensure that treatment passed before proceeding to the next treatment. Do this after the twenty-five hours, and within one week, or no later than two weeks.

10. Do not expose yourself nutritionally or physically to the allergen for which you are being treated for twenty-five hours. Stay four to five feet away or the treatment could fail immediately, sometime in the future, and symptoms could reoccur. *Be careful and prepare for each treatment ahead of time.*

11. Maintain your own treatment record.

12. Wear plastic gloves and masks when being treated for environmental allergens. These allergens include metals, pollen, grasses, leather, chemicals, smog, and so forth.

13. Eat a healthy meal prior to the treatment unless other instructions are given by your doctor because many treatments require restricted diets.

14. Do not eat heavy meals immediately after allergy treatments. Do not eat anything to which you are allergic for twenty-five hours after treatment.

15. Drink plenty of water after the treatment. Distilled water is preferable unless otherwise instructed.

16. NAET treatments do not conflict with any medications and it is not necessary to stop taking them unless advised otherwise by your doctor. Asthmatics should continue taking their medications unless other recommendations are given by their physicians. Additionally, NAET treatments do not interfere with other treatments you might be receiving.

17. Check the ingredients of any supplements (vitamins, enzymes, and so on) you are taking to ensure they do not contain the allergen for which you are being treated (brewer's yeast, mint, parsley, etc.).

TWENTY-FIVE HOUR NAET RESTRICTIONS

The following section contains a list of NAET restrictions divided into two parts. The first part entitled Basic Allergens is organized in the order in which they are treated. The second part, Other Allergens, lists them in alphabetical order. These lists cover the allergens most common for asthmatics and individuals with chronic health problems. These dietary and physical restrictions should be followed strictly for a twenty-five hour period after the NAET treatment. They were developed after several years of clinical research at my clinic and are responsible for the high rate of success I have in treating allergies.

I have found it is important to both physically and nutritionally avoid the allergen for the entire twenty-five hours. A four- to five-foot distance should be maintained from the allergen. If that distance cannot be maintained, I recommend wearing gloves and in certain cases, a mask as well. One of the easiest ways to fail is to smell an allergen (from hot or cooking foods, for example). Again, I recommend wearing a mask when cooking to avoid losing the treatment. If you expose yourself in any way, you not only lose the treatment but also could experience severe symptoms immediately such as an acute asthma attack, fainting, migraine, and so forth. Or, symptoms might recur over time.

The fingertips are the most sensitive part of the body and you should wear gloves whenever your hands come closer than four to five feet from an allergen. With many of the allergens (calcium, minerals, bacteria, parasites), you should use distilled water. If you have to use distilled water, we recommend no showers or baths and do not wash your hands in anything but distilled water. Use caution when attending to toilet needs. We recommend wearing gloves because the allergen could be present in the water. It is important to prepare for every treatment in order to avoid having to go into grocery or convenience stores to purchase foods or other items after the treatment. It is virtually impossible to avoid many of the allergens when going into a store or restaurant. Again, when you are undergoing treatment and have to prepare food for your children or pet, wear plastic gloves and a mask because the steam from food could cause the treatment to fail. Avoid going into a restaurant during the twenty-five hours after treatment.

The dietary and physical restrictions included in the following pages give a most complete list. In creating this list, I made sure there was not a trace of the particular allergen. In certain cases (Vitamin B, for example), I had to list foods such as Jell-O® that I would not normally recommend because they have no nutritional value. Whenever possible I recommend that my patients eat fresh organic produce, grains, poultry, fish, and meats.

If you have any doubt about a particular food or substance, don't eat or touch it. The golden rule is "when in doubt, abstain!" Many people ask me if they can have black coffee or tea. If it is free of the allergen, I include it. When I was in doubt, I excluded it. If a food or beverage is not included, I recommend avoiding it. It is so easy to drink or eat something that contains the allergen when you consume prepared, processed, or restaurant food. Therefore, I prefer that my patients prepare meals from scratch for themselves or eat foods in their original form. In all cases I recommend abstaining from alcohol consumption for the twenty-five hours following the treatment.

Children eight years old or younger only need to avoid the allergen for six hours after the NAET treatment. The diet and every other rule applies. When treating an infant for breast milk and formula, it might be difficult to avoid milk for six hours. Try for two to three hours. The allergy might need to be treated two or three times but eventually it will completely clear.

To be successful be careful, read the rules over and over again, and prepare for each treatment by reading the restrictions ahead of time. It is always better to have a game plan than to risk failing a treatment by handling a forbidden substance. If you must handle a product that might contain the allergen, minimize the risks of failing the treatment by wearing gloves and a mask.

ADDITION TO THE NAET SELF-TREATMENT

In severe cases of asthma, I recommend that a spouse or parent learn how to perform NAET treatment to help clear the many allergens from which the asthmatic individual suffers. In addition to emergency self-treatment, I teach individuals how to do the full NAET treatment including muscle response testing and treatment along the spine. This expedites allergy elimination and accelerates healing. I do this only after a person has cleared their basic allergies because that is critical to clearing other allergens and establishing the foundation of their immune strength and support. After the basics are finished, I do extensive testing to see what allergens remain. I then work closely with each individual to see what allergens are to be cleared next and work out a plan. I educate and teach the spouse or parent and supply them with certain allergen vials for four to five treatments. I tell them emphatically they must see me every two weeks to see if they passed the treatments or if any combinations exist. Self-treatments should only be done under a *doctor's supervision*. I feel it is up to each individual doctor and patient to decide if self-treatment is the road upon which they want to embark. Many parents are delighted with this opportunity to treat their child because it allows them to participate in the healing process and when they see the progress, they are ecstatic.

Supervision by a doctor is mandatory; therefore, I do not describe the treatment in this book. If a doctor does recommend these home treatments, he or she should teach NAET to the patient and family member.

BASIC ALLERGENS

EGG MIX egg yolks, egg whites, chicken, feathers, tetracycline
Eat only: Steamed rice (white or brown), pasta (without eggs), vegetables, fruits, dairy, oils, beef, pork, fish.
Drink only: Coffee, tea, juice, water, soft drinks.
Do not eat or touch: Eggs or products containing eggs, chicken or products containing chicken (READ LABELS!) feather pillows, shampoo, or other such products containing eggs (refer to the listing of "Foods and Materials Containing Eggs" in Part VI).

CALCIUM MIX Cal-Carbonate, Cal-Gluconate, Cal-ascorbate, raw milk, cow's milk, goat's milk, milk-casein, milk-albumin
Eat only: White basmati rice, olive oil, salt, rice cakes (made with white rice only).
Drink only: Distilled water, (not mineral or spring), black tea made with distilled water (no milk).
Wash only: With distilled water.

VITAMIN C MIX ascorbic acid, chlorophyll, rose hips, rutin, hesperidin, or bioflavonoids; oxalic acid; citrus (oranges, lemons, grapefruits); berry mix (strawberry, cranberry, boysenberry, raspberry); fruit (bananas, papayas, apples, grapes, peaches, nectarines); vegetable mix (green beans, cauliflower, broccoli, brussel sprouts, cabbage, asparagus); vinegar mix (white vinegar, apple cider, rice vinegar)
Eat only: Steamed rice (white, brown, wild), eggs, baked chicken, white breads, tofu (plain), miso, shitake mushrooms, red meat (not processed), boiled beans (white, black, or lima), rice cakes, salt.
Drink only: Water, black tea, black coffee, plain soy milk.

B-COMPLEX MIX B_1, B_2, B_3, B_5, B_6, B_{12}, B_{13}, B_{15}, B_{17}, biotin, choline, inositol, folic acid, PABA
Eat only: Minute Tapioca® (cooked in water only), Jell-O® gelatin (all flavors except those with natural fruit juice), Cool Whip® topping, imitation sour cream.
Drink only: Water, Crystal Light® berry blend drink (from powder).

SUGAR MIX   maltose, glucose, dextrose, lactose, brown sugar, honey, corn sugar, raw sugar, molasses
Eat only: Eggs, red meat, poultry, oils.
Drink only: Water.
Do not eat or touch: Alcohol, milk products, toothpaste (refer to "Foods and Materials Containing Hidden Sugars" in Part VI).

IRON MIX   ferrous sulfate, ferrous gluconate, beef, pork, lamb, gelatin
Eat only: White basmati rice (no iron), salt, peanut oil.
Drink only: Distilled water (not mineral or spring).
Wash only: With distilled water. READ ALL LABELS!

VITAMIN A MIX   fish, shellfish, betacarotene
Eat only: Steamed rice (white, brown, wild), pearl barley, millet, boiled white beans, boiled turnips, boiled parsnips, boiled red kidney or lima beans, onions, mushrooms, fresh ginger root, fresh garlic, salt, tamari, plain dry almonds or almond butter (pure), plain dry roasted peanuts or peanut butter (pure), cooked spaghetti or macaroni.
Drink only: Water, black tea (no milk).

MINERAL MIX   antimony, barium, boron, beryllium, bromide, cesium, chlorine, cobalt, copper, europium, fluorine, gadolinium, gallium, germanium, gold, holmium, iodine, lanthanum, lithium, manganese, molybdenum, neodymium, nickel, niobium, palladium, rubidium, ruthenium, samarium, scandium, selenium, silver, strontium, thulium, thorium, tin, titanium, tungsten, uranium, vanadium, yttrium, zinc, zirconium

Eat only: Jello-O® gelatin pops without any natural fruit juice (1 mg. of potassium), tapioca made with distilled water (2 mg. potassium, 1 mg. phosphorus).

Drink only: Distilled water (not mineral or spring).

Wash only: With distilled water.

NOTE: *Rice has large amounts of potassium and phosphorus.*

SALT MIX, CHLORIDES sea salt, rock salt, table salt, iodized salt, sodium, chloride

Eat only: Rice (brown, white), nonsodium rice cakes (READ LABELS to ensure there is no salt) olive oil, sugar, chives, raspberries, plums, peaches, nectarines, apples without skin, fresh cherries, blackberries.

Drink only: Distilled water (not mineral or spring).

Wash only: With distilled water.

Wear: Mask and gloves when outside if one lives near the ocean.

OTHER ALLERGENS

CORN MIX   blue corn, yellow corn, white corn, cornstarch, corn silk, corn syrup

Eat only: Steamed vegetables, steamed rice, chicken, meat, fish.

Drink only: Water, black tea, black coffee.

Do not eat or touch: Blue corn, yellow corn, white corn, cornstarch, corn oats, corn syrup, corn oil, baking soda, baking powder, starched clothing (shirts, linen), ointments, powders or talcums, lozenges, supplements or other products that contain corn.

Read labels: Soft drinks, breads, toothpaste, shampoos, deodorant (refer to the listing of "Foods and Materials Containing Corn" in Part VI).

ACID

Eat only: Steamed or raw vegetables, cooked dried beans, fruits (refer to the listing of "Alkaline-Forming Foods" in Part VI).

Drink only: Water, milk.

Do not eat, drink or touch: Starches, grains, meat, coffee.

Avoid: Acid-forming foods (refer to the listing of "Acid-Forming Foods" in Part VI).

ALCOHOLS   beer, hops, red wine, white wine, champagne, rubbing alcohol, plant alcohols

Eat only: Cooked or steamed (not raw) vegetables, meat, fish, eggs, chicken.

Drink only: Water, black tea, or coffee (no milk).

Do not eat or touch: Fruits, grains, alcoholic beverages, vanilla extract, sugar, starches, foods prepared with wine, medicines containing alcohol (cough syrup), shampoos, hair products, cosmetics, makeup containing alcohol, any extract with alcohol, any homeopathic or herb preparation containing alcohol. READ ALL LABELS!

Avoid: Eating in restaurants or eating catered foods during the twenty-five hour period.

AMINO ACID 1   lysine, leucine, threonine, valine, tryptophan, isoleucine, phenylalanine
Eat only: Lettuce.
Drink only: Water.
Do not touch: Protein products for external use.

AMINO ACID 2   alanine, arginine, aspartic acid, carnitine, citrulline, cysteine, cystine, glutathione, glutamic acid, glycine, histidine, ornithine, proline, serine, taurine, glutamine, tyrosine
Eat only: Lettuce.
Drink only: Water.
Do not touch: Protein products for external use.

ANIMAL EPITHELIALS and DANDERS
Do not touch: Animals, their saliva, hair, dander, and any other products made from animals or used by animals. If you have a pet, make arrangements to stay away from him or her for twenty-five hours.

ANIMAL FATS   butter, lard, pork or pork fat, beef or beef fat, chicken or chicken fat, lamb or lamb fat, fish or fish oil
Do not eat or touch: The above items and any foods fried with or containing animal fat, refried beans, chili beans, skin lotions made with animal fat, pet food.

ARTIFICIAL SWEETENERS
Do not eat or touch: Saccharine, Equal®, Sweet'N Low®, NutraSweet®, aspartame, sorbitol, or any products containing artificial sweeteners.
Read all labels: Soft drinks, sweet relish, pickles, cookies, toothpaste.

ASPARTAME
Eat only: Grains, vegetables, fruits, meat, poultry, fish, dairy, and beans.
Do not drink or eat: Soft drinks, sweet relish, pickles, cookies, toothpaste. READ ALL LABELS!

VITAMIN B$_1$ thiamine, thiamine mononitrate, thiamine hydrochloride

Eat only: Rice cakes, mozzarella cheese, Muenster cheese, Neufchatel cheese, egg whites, oysters, angel food cake, gingersnap cookies, black olives, radishes, pickles (dill, bread and butter, kosher, and rennin only), tapioca, dried apples, lychees, butter, corn margarine, carob powder, aspartame powder.

Drink only: Water, apple juice, Hawaiian Punch® brand fruit juices (Hawaiian Punch® Fruit Punch^K Fruit Juicy, apple, cherry, grape), Kool-Aid® (sugar powder and sugar free), Country Time® (sugar and sugar free), Crystal Lite® (powder only), Tang™, black coffee.

Do not eat, drink, or touch: Dried yeast, pork, most vegetables, bran, milk, brewer's yeast, wheat germ, wheat bran, rice polishings, most whole grain cereals, milk products, leafy green vegetables, meat, liver, nuts, legumes, potatoes.

VITAMIN B$_2$ riboflavin, Vitamin G

Eat only: Baked, broiled, or poached snapper, oysters, butter, corn margarine, shallots, black olives, pickles (dill, bread and butter, rennin only), fruit leather rolls, Cool Whip®, Dream Whip®, gingersnap cookies, tapioca.

Drink only: Water, Hawaiian Punch® brand fruit juices (Fruit Juicy, apple, cherry, grape), Kool-Aid® (sugar powder and sugar Free), Country Time® (sugar and sugar free), Crystal Lite® (powder only), black coffee, Coffee Mate® nondairy creamer.

Do not eat, drink, or touch: Milk, cheese, whole grains, brewer's yeast, wheat germ, almonds, sunflower seeds, liver, leafy vegetables, kidney, fish, and eggs.

VITAMIN B$_3$ niacin, nicotinic acid, niacinamide

Eat only: The following cheeses: cheddar, Colby, cream, Edam, Gouda, Gruyere, mozzarella, Muenster, Neufchatel, Parmesan, provolone, Romano, Swiss; processed American or Swiss cheese. Eggs, fruit leather rolls, shallots, watercress, black olives, pickles (dill, bread and butter, rennin only), tapioca, gingersnap cookies, Cool Whip®, butter, corn margarine, aspartame powder.

Drink only: Water, lemon and lime juice, Hawaiian Punch® (Fruit Juicy, apple, cherry), Kool-Aid®, Country Time®, Crystal Lite®, Coffee Mate® nondairy creamer.

Do not eat or touch: Lean meat, fish, eggs, roasted peanuts, brewer's yeast, wheat germ, rice bran, rice polishings, nuts, sunflower seeds, whole wheat products, brown rice, green vegetables, liver, white meat of poultry, avocados, dates, figs, prunes.

VITAMIN B$_5$ pantothenic acid, calcium pantothenate

Eat only: Ham, Aunt Jemima® plain or whole wheat pancakes, corn tortilla, instant maple and brown sugar oatmeal, mozzarella cheese, Parmesan cheese, eggplant, kale, green peppers, chili peppers, red peppers, radishes, raw spinach, pickled herring, air-popped popcorn, almond butter, corn margarine, cocoa powder, aspartame powder, tapioca, soybean protein powder, Coffee Mate® nondairy creamer, Cool Whip®, Dream Whip®, honey.

Drink only: Water, lemon or lime juice, Kool-Aid®, Country Time®, Crystal Lite®, black coffee, Tang™.

Do not eat or touch: Brewer's yeast, wheat germ, wheat bran, whole grain breads and cereals, green vegetables, peas and beans, liver, egg yolks, crude molasses, dried lima beans, raisins, meat, cantaloupes, kidneys, hearts, nuts, chicken.

VITAMIN B$_6$ pyridoxine, pyridoxal, pyridoxamine

Eat only: Black olives, tapioca, egg whites, butter, corn margarine, Arrowroot™ baby cookies, infant oatmeal, Coffee Mate® nondairy creamer, aspartame powder, Cool Whip®, Dream Whip®.

Drink only: Water, Kool-Aid® (sugar powder and sugar Free), Country Time® (sugar and sugar free), Crystal Lite® (powder only), honey, black coffee.

PART VI: *Resource Guide*

Do not eat or touch: Brewer's yeast, bananas, avocados, wheat germ, wheat bran, soybeans, milk, egg yolks, liver, green leafy vegetables, green peppers, organ meat, legumes, kidneys, heart, cantaloupes, cabbage, molasses, beef.

VITAMIN B$_{12}$ cobalamin, cyanocobalamin
Eat only: Fruits, vegetables, beans (except refried), nuts, seeds, cracked wheat, Aunt Jemima® whole wheat pancakes, instant oatmeal, instant maple and brown sugar oatmeal, banana chips, corn chips, corn nuts, fruit leather rolls, air-popped popcorn, caramel/peanut popcorn, potato chips, pretzels, rice cakes, plain tortilla chips, tapioca, cheese soup, onion soup, tomato or tomato rice soup (no cream tomato soup), gelatin consomme, minestrone soup, vegetarian vegetable soup, gazpacho soup, defatted peanut flour, soy flour, soybean protein powder, canned spaghetti or tomato sauce, tomato paste, tamari soy sauce, vinegar, Arrowroot™ baby cookies, baking powder, aspartame powder, dry cocoa powder, fruit pectin, Coffee Mate® nondairy creamer, Cool Whip®.
Drink only: Apricot nectar, cranberry juice cocktail, grape juice, peach nectar, pear nectar, pineapple juice, prune juice, tangerine juice, carrot juice, Kool-Aid® (sugar powder and sugar Free), Country Time® (sugar and sugar free), Crystal Lite® (powder only), black coffee, Postum®, Tang.™
Do not eat, drink, or touch: Milk, eggs, aged cheese, liver, meat, pollen, pork, kidneys.

VITAMIN B$_{13}$ orotic acid
Do not eat or touch: Milk whey (the liquid portion of soured or curdled milk; READ LABELS for all dairy products), root vegetables.

VITAMIN B$_{15}$ pangamic acid, calcium pangamate
Do not eat or touch: Whole grains, seeds, nuts, whole brown rice, brewer's yeast, pumpkin seeds, sesame seeds.

VITAMIN B$_{17}$ nitrilosides, amygdalin, laetrile
Do not eat, drink, or touch: Fruits with seeds, vegetables, raspberries, cranberries, blackberries, blueberries, mung beans, lima beans, flaxseeds.

BACTERIA MIX
Do not eat, drink, or touch: Uncooked foods, sugar, any water or beverages except distilled water.

BAKING POWDER
Eat only: Fresh fruits, vegetables, meat, chicken, fish, fats.
Drink only: Water, black coffee, black tea.
Do not eat or touch: Baking powder, baking soda, baked goods, medications, toothpastes, deodorants and antiperspirants, talcum powders, soaps. READ ALL LABELS!

BAKING SODA
Eat only: Fresh fruits, vegetables, meat, chicken, fish, fats.
Drink only: Water, black coffee, black tea.
Do not eat or touch: Baking powder, baking soda, baked goods, medications, toothpastes, deodorants and antiperspirants, talcum powders, soaps. READ ALL LABELS!

BASE
Eat only: Starches, breads, meat, poultry, fish, all dairy products except milk and yogurt, and any of the foods on the list of "Acid-Forming Foods" in Part VI.
Do not eat, drink, or touch: Vegetables, beans, milk, fruit.
Avoid: Alkaline-forming foods (refer to the listing of the "Alkaline-Forming Foods" in Part VI).

BEET SUGAR
Avoid: Beets and any products containing beet sugar; READ ALL LABELS!

BERRY MIX   Strawberries, blueberries, blackberries, raspberries, loganberries, cranberries, wild berries, gooseberries
Eat only: Vegetables, grains, meat, breads, poultry, fish, dairy products.
Do not eat, drink, or touch: Berries, jams, fruits, and fruit juices made from berries.

BIOFLAVANOIDS   citrin, hesperidin, rutin
Eat only: Meat, grains, poultry, vegetables, beans, dairy products.
Do not eat, drink, or touch: Garlic, onions, lemons, limes, grapes, plums, black currants, grapefruits, apricots, buckwheat, cherries, blackberries, rose hips, and oranges.

BIOTIN   vitamin H, coenzyme R
Do not eat, drink, or touch: Brewer's yeast, unpolished rice, soybeans, liver, kidneys, milk, molasses, nuts, fruits, beef, yolks.

BROWN SUGAR
Eat only: Grains, meat, vegetables, fruits, poultry, fish.
Do not eat or touch: Anything that contains brown sugar. READ ALL LABELS!

CAFFEINE   coffee, tea, tannic acid
Eat or drink: Anything that contains no caffeine or chocolate.
Do not eat, drink, or touch: Coffee, tea, chocolate, caffeinated drinks, leather goods, tannic acid. (Do not even smell coffee brewing.)

CANDIDA MIX
Eat only: All protein (poultry, fish, meat, eggs, cooked or steamed vegetables), oils, tofu and beans for vegetarians.
Do not eat, drink, or touch: Simple sugars, grains,

fruits, dairy, yeast products (breads, beer, wine), vinegar, hops, malts, peanuts, mushrooms, condiments (soy sauce, catsup) (refer to the listing "Foods and Materials Containing Yeast" in Part VI).

Prior to treatment: Buy new clothes, socks, underwear, toothbrush, hairbrush, sheets, towels, etc. Anything you put on your body should be new and never worn before. Scrub shower stalls and bathtubs and remove mold from house. Shower and wash hair.

After treatment: Change into new clothes, socks, and shoes. No skin-to-skin contact or sexual contact. Wear mask and gloves for twenty-five hours. Do not touch animals or makeup. Wear gloves when attending to personal hygiene following toilet use. Start the 10-day Candida yeast avoidance diet listed in Part VI.

CANE SUGAR
Eat only: Fruits, meat, poultry, fish, vegetables.
Do not eat, drink, or touch: Anything with cane sugar. READ ALL LABELS!

CAULIFLOWER
Eat only: Fruits, meat, poultry, vegetables, fish, grains, beans.
Do not eat, drink, or touch: anything with cauliflower (for example, vegetable juice).

CELERY MIX
Eat only: Grains, meat, fruits, vegetables, poultry, beans, dairy products, salt, pepper.
Do not eat or touch: Anything with celery and celery salt such as sauces, dressings, vegetable juices, spice mixes, seasonings, and so forth.

CHEESE MIX   American, cheddar, jack, Parmesan, mozzarella, cottage, and the like.
Eat only: Grains, vegetables, poultry, fruits, beans.
Do not eat, drink, or touch: Anything made from dairy products.

CHEMICALS
Do not eat or drink: Water or any foods cooked in tap water.
Do not touch: Soaps, detergents, cleaning chemicals, chlorine, bleach. If your water supply is chlorinated (city water), do not wash with tap water. Use spring or distilled water.

CHICKEN   white/dark meat chicken, chicken feathers
Eat only: Vegetables, meat, fish, fruits, dairy products, beans.
Do not eat or touch: Chicken, eggs, chicken feathers, anything with eggs, egg whites, egg yolks, or feathers.
Avoid: Down pillows or cushions, down comforter, down couches, down coats. Do not go into a linen, furniture, or clothing store for twenty-five hours following the treatment.

CHOCOLATE MIX   cocoa, cocoa butter, chocolate, carob
Eat or drink only: Anything that has no caffeine or chocolate.
Do not eat, drink, or touch: Coffee, tannic acid tea, chocolate, caffeinated drinks, leather goods.

CHOLINE
Eat only: Fruits, dairy products, vegetables (except peas and green leafy vegetables), fish, poultry, meat.
Do not eat or touch: Brewer's yeast, wheat germ, egg yolks, liver, green leafy vegetables, legumes, peas, beans, brains, heart, lecithin.

CHROMIUM
Eat only: White rice, pastas, cauliflower, potatoes, fruits, salt.
Drink only: Water, black coffee, black tea (no milk).
Do not eat, drink, or touch: Meat, chicken, liver, whole grains, wheat germ, corn oil, brewer's yeast, mushrooms, sugar, shellfish, clams.

CITRUS MIX   grapefruits, lemons, limes, oranges (all types), tangerines, pineapples
Eat only: Meat, poultry, fish, fruits other than citrus, beans, grains, dairy.
Do not eat, drink, or touch: Grapefruits, lemons, oranges and orange juice, pineapples, tangerines, mandarin oranges, and limes.

COBALT
Eat only: White rice, pastas, cauliflowers, potatoes, fruits, noniodized salt.
Drink only: Water.
Do not eat, drink, or touch: Green leafy vegetables, meat, liver, kidneys, figs, buckwheat, oysters, clams, dairy products.

COFFEE MIX   coffee, tea, tannic acid, caffeine
Eat or drink only: Anything that has no caffeine or chocolate.
Do not eat, drink, touch, or smell: Coffee, tea, chocolate, caffeinated drinks, leather goods, tannic acid.

COPPER
Eat only: White rice, pastas, cauliflower, potatoes, fruits, noniodized salt.
Do not eat, drink, or touch: Tap water, almonds, green beans, peas, green leafy vegetables, whole grains, whole wheat, prunes, raisins, dried beans, liver, seafood.
NOTE: *Use only distilled water for cooking or steaming foods and for washing.*

CORN SUGAR
Eat only: Vegetables other than corn, grains other than corn, dairy products, fruits, beans, meat, poultry, fish.
Drink only: Water, coffee, tea, fresh squeezed juices.
Do not eat, drink, or touch: Corn sugar or anything with corn sugar. READ ALL LABELS! Foods can contain

corn sugar in processed, store prepared foods, or restaurant foods such as soups, sauces, stews, and so forth.

CRUDE OIL
Do not touch or smell: Gasoline or crude oil products, products made of plastics such as computer key boards, telephones, pens, vinyl chairs, book covers, toothbrush, hairbrush, and the like.
Wear: Cotton or leather gloves; wear mask when outdoors.

CUCUMBER MIX
Do not eat or touch: Fresh cucumbers, pickles, soups, salad dressings, skin products that contain cucumber.

VITAMIN D
Eat only: Poultry, meat, fruits.
Drink only: Water, black tea, black coffee (no milk).
Do not eat, drink, or touch: Egg yolks, dairy products, fish or fish oil, sprouted seeds, mushrooms, sunflower seeds or oil.

DEXTROSE
Eat only: Poultry, meat, fish. Follow same diet as sugars mix.
Do not eat or touch: Vegetables, fruits, dairy products, grains. Follow same diet as sugar mix.

DNA
Eat only: Lettuce.
Drink only: Water, black coffee, black tea.
Do not eat or touch: Proteins such as meat, fish, poultry, dairy products, grains, vegetables, fruits.

DRIED BEAN MIX   blackeyed peas, black beans, white beans, pinto beans, soybeans, peas, red beans, mung beans, kidney beans, lima beans, lentils, garbanzo beans, navy beans

Eat or drink only: Anything that does not contain beans, peas, or bean oil including rice, fruits, meat, chicken, fish, and fresh vegetables.

Do not eat or touch: Chips, crackers, baked goods, and mayonnaise made with soybean oil.

DUST MIX AND DUST MITES

Avoid: Dusty areas. Clean up the living and sleeping areas before the treatment and do not come in contact or touch dusty areas.

Wear: A mask and plastic gloves for twenty-five hours.

VITAMIN E

Eat only: Fresh fruits, carrots, potatoes, poultry, meat.

Drink only: Water, black coffee, black tea.

Do not eat or touch: Wheat germ or wheat germ oil, vegetable oils, soybeans or soybean oil, green vegetables, flours, grains, eggs, nuts, raw or sprouted seeds, fish.

EGG WHITE/EGG YOLKS follow the same restrictions for eggs listed under Basic Allergens

EQUAL®

Avoid: All products which contain Equal®. READ ALL LABELS! Soft drinks, sweet relish, pickles, cookies, toothpaste, and so forth.

VITAMIN F (fatty acids)

Do not eat or touch: Vegetable oils, wheat germ oils, linseed oils, sunflower oils, safflower oils, soybean oils, peanuts or other nuts, peanut oils, flax seeds or oil, evening primrose oils, breast milk.

FABRIC MIX

Avoid contact: With the fabrics that are being treated. Do not touch home furnishings such as couches, upholstered furniture, curtains, towels, sheets, and so on. Be careful to wear socks and/or shoes if you walk on rugs.

Do not go into stores or be in close proximity to others who might be wearing the fabrics being treated.

Wear: Gloves if in proximity to the treated fabrics (closer than four to five feet).

NOTE: *Treat one kind of fabric first. Then wear the allergy-cleared item when treating for the fabric mix.*

FISH MIX   crappie, red snapper, cod, tuna, sardine, catfish, anchovies, sea bass, halibut, petroli, orange roughy, shark, mahi mahi, salmon

Do not eat or touch: Any fish products or any oils made from fish. Do not lick or touch stamps and envelopes. Wear plastic gloves to handle pet food.

FLUORIDE

Eat only: Fruits, yellow vegetables, potatoes, cauliflower, meat, chicken, white rice.

Drink only: Distilled water (not mineral or spring), fresh squeezed juices, black coffee or black tea made with distilled water only.

Wash only: With distilled water.

Do not eat, drink, or touch: Tap water, gelatin, sunflower seeds or oil, milk, cheese, garlic, almonds, green vegetables, carrots, fish.

NOTE: *Use only distilled water for cooking or steaming foods.*

FLOWER MIX

Avoid: Flowers, pollen, and perfumes.

Wear: A mask outdoors.

FOLIC ACID   pteroylglutamic acid, folate, folacin

Eat only: Bagels, ham, salami (beef or pork), concord grapes, shredded coconut, Chex party mix, pork rinds, Chinese cabbage, iceberg lettuce, pickled herring, butter, corn margarine, tapioca, Coffee Mate®, Cool Whip®, Dream Whip.®

Drink only: Water, hot chocolate (from a mix, with

water), Kool-Aid® (sugar powder and sugar Free), Country Time® (sugar and sugar free), Crystal Lite® (powder only), black coffee, apple or cherry juice.

Do not eat, drink, or touch: Dark green leafy vegetables, broccoli, asparagus, lima beans, Irish potatoes, brewer's yeast, wheat germ, mushrooms, nuts, liver, carrots, tortula, yeast, egg yolks, cantaloupes, apricots, pumpkin, avocados, beans, whole wheat and dark rye flour, dairy products.

FOOD ADDITIVES   calcium sulfate, calcium phosphate, sodium sulfate, sodium nitrate

Eat only: Fresh vegetables or fruits, freshly cooked grains, eggs, fresh fish, chicken; READ ALL LABELS!

Drink only: Water, milk, home-squeezed juices.

Do not eat, drink, or touch: Any store-prepared, processed, frozen or restaurant foods such as hot dogs, sausages, prepacked meat, soups, crackers, candies, cookies, salad dressings, sauces, premixed powdered spice, ice cream, chewing gum, soft drinks.

FOOD COLORING

Eat only: Fresh vegetables or fruits, rice, white pasta, eggs, chicken, fish.

Drink only: Water, milk, home-squeezed juices.

Do not eat, drink, or touch: Any store prepared, processed, frozen, or restaurant foods such as hot dogs, sausages, prepacked meat, soups, crackers, candies, cookies, salad dressings, sauces, premixed powdered spices, ice cream, chewing gum, soft drinks (refer to the listing of "Foods and Materials Containing Artifical Colors" in Part VI).

FORMALDEHYDE

Avoid: New buildings or buildings with recent remodeling, new clothing, newspapers, paints, pressed woods (refer to the listing of "Foods and Materials Containing Formaldehyde" in Part VI).

Wear: A mask and cotton gloves for twenty-five hours.

FREON
Avoid: Air-conditioned areas, supermarkets, soft plastic products, refrigerator and freezer.
Wear: A mask and gloves if you must take food in and out of the the refrigerator and freezer.

FRUCTOSE
Eat only: Grains, vegetables, dairy, poultry, meat, fish.
Do not eat, drink, or touch: Fruits, or anything containing fructose, for example, high fructose corn syrup in drinks and sugared foods. READ ALL LABELS!

FRUIT MIX   bananas, papayas, apples, grapes, peaches, nectarines
Eat only: Grains, vegetables, fish, poultry, meat.
Do not eat, drink or touch: Fruits or anything containing fruits.

FUNGUS   see entry for Candida and follow the same guidelines

GELATIN
Eat only: Vegetables, rice, grains.
Drink only: Water, black coffee, black tea.
Do not eat or touch: Chicken, meat, apple skins, hard skin of other fruits, pectin (READ LABELS for jam), Jell-O®, gelatin capsules, puddings with gelatin, sticky candy, dairy products.

GERMANIUM
Eat only: Fruits, vegetables, vegetable oils, dairy, poultry, meat.
Do not eat or touch: Whole grains, sprouts, breads.

GLUCOSE   follow the sugar mix restrictions

GLUTEN
Avoid: Gluten-containing grains such as barley, buckwheat, oats, rye, and wheat.

Eat only: Corn flour, corn meal, corn starch, gluten-free wheat starch, lima bean flour, potato flour, rice, rice flour, soy flour.

GOLD

Do not touch: Gold jewelry and gold fillings in your teeth. Use plastic gloves when eating or brushing teeth to avoid touching fingertips to the gold fillings.

GRAIN MIX   wheat, millet, oats, rye, rice, wheat bran, oat bran, wild rice

Eat only: Meat, chicken, raw or cooked vegetables, and fruits.
Drink only: Water, milk, black coffee, black tea.

GRASS MIX

Avoid: Being outdoors or in contact with grass products.
Wear: A mask and gloves outdoors.

GUM MIX

Eat only: Rice, pastas, vegetables, fruits without skin, meat, chicken, eggs, fish.
Do not eat, drink, or touch: Soft drinks or carbonated drinks, chewing gum, cream cheese, glues (do not lick stamps or envelopes). READ ALL LABELS!

HISTAMINE

Do not eat, drink, or touch: Meat, poultry, fish, shell-fish, black beans, cow's milk or milk products, goat's milk, breast milk, wines.

HONEY

Eat only: Vegetables, fruits, meat, poultry, fish, grains, beans.
Do not eat, drink, or touch: Anything with honey. READ ALL LABELS!

HORMONES

Do not eat or touch: Meat, poultry, dairy products, eggs, hormone supplements.

INOSITOL
Do not eat or touch: Brewer's yeast, wheat germ, lecithin, unprocessed whole grains, nuts, milk, citrus fruits, liver, lima beans, beef, brains, heart, raisins, cantaloupes, unrefined molasses, peanuts, cabbages.

INSECT MIX   bees, ants, spiders, fleas
Avoid: Touching any insects.

IODINE
Eat only: White rice, pastas, cauliflowers, potatoes, fruits, noniodized salt.
Drink only: Water.
Do not eat or touch: Kelp, seafood, iodized salt, onions.

VITAMIN K
Eat only: Fruits, rice, potatoes, poultry, meat.
Do not eat or touch: Green vegetables, kelp, alfalfa, soybean oils, safflower oils, egg yolks, cow's milk, yogurt, liver.

LACTOSE (milk sugar)
Eat only: Grains, vegetables, meat, poultry, fish, fruits, beans.
Do not eat, drink, or touch: Anything with dairy products such as milk, cheese, yogurt, kefir. READ ALL LABELS! Lactose is often used as a preservative in ketchup and sauces.

LEAD
Eat only: White rice, pastas, cauliflowers, potatoes, fruits, noniodized salt.
Drink only: Distilled water (not mineral or spring).
Do not eat, drink, or touch: Tap water, almonds, green beans, peas, green leafy vegetables, whole grains, whole wheat, prunes, raisins, dried beans, liver, seafood, any products that may contain lead.
Avoid: Old buildings that might have lead paint.
NOTE: *Use only distilled water to cook or steam food.*

LECITHIN
Eat only: White rice, cauliflowers, potatoes, fish, poultry, meat, fruits, vegetables.
Drink only: Water, black tea, black coffee.
Do not eat or touch: Lecithin products, cookies, candy bars, vitamin supplements.

MAGNESIUM
Eat only: White rice, potatoes, cauliflowers, eggs, chicken, meat, fruits.
Drink only: Water, fresh-squeezed juices.
Do not eat or touch: Nuts or seeds, soybeans, green leafy vegetables, whole grains.

MALATHION (see also PESTICIDES)
Eat only: Cooked grains, cooked organic vegetables, cooked fruits.
Drink only: Water.
Do not eat or touch: Fresh vegetables, fruits, meat, poultry, insecticides, herbicides, spices, and herbs.

MALTOSE   grain sugar
Eat only: Fruits, vegetables, meat, poultry, fish and beans, dairy products.
Drink only: Water, fresh fruit juices, black coffee, black tea.
Do not eat or touch: Grains, breads, cereals, pastas, avoid malt and malt products.

MANGANESE
Eat only: White rice, pastas, cauliflowers, potatoes, fruits, noniodized salt.
Drink only: Water.
Do not eat or touch: Green leafy vegetables, beets, blueberries, oranges, grapefruits, apricots, nuts and grain bran, peas, kelp, raw egg yolks.

MAPLE SUGAR
Eat Only: Fruits, grains, poultry, meat, fish, vegetables, beans.

Do not eat or touch: Anything with maple sugar. Keep away from maple trees or wood.

MEAT MIX   red meat, beef, lamb, veal, liver
Eat only: Fish, vegetable, fruits, beans, grains, breads, poultry.
Do not eat or touch: Red meat or anything with meat in it. READ ALL LABELS and ask chefs how their soups, stocks, and sauces are made.

MELON MIX   crenshaws, watermelons, cantaloupes, honeydews
Eat only: Grains, vegetables, poultry, meat, fish, beans, and dairy.
Do not eat or touch: All types of melons.

MERCURY AMALGAMS
Do not eat or touch: Fish and fish products, mercury products. USE GLOVES when eating or brushing teeth to avoid close contact with mercury in the mouth from tooth fillings.

MILK MIX   cow's milk, goat's milk, breast milk
Eat only: Vegetables, grains, poultry, meat, fruits, fish, and beans.
Do not eat or touch: All milk products including yogurt, cheese, and kefir. READ ALL LABELS! Watch out for milk solids (refer to the listing of "Foods and Materials Containing Milk" later in Part VI).

MODIFIED STARCH
Eat only: Vegetables, meat, eggs, beans, fish, poultry.
Drink only: Water, fresh fruit juices, black coffee, black tea.
Do not eat or touch: Table salt, refined grain products, sauces, vitamin supplements, prescription drugs, starch products including starched shirts or garments. READ ALL LABELS!

MOLD MIX   see entry for Candida and follow the same guidelines

MOLYBDENUM
Eat only: White rice, pastas, cauliflowers, potatoes, fresh fruits, noniodized salt.
Drink only: Water.
Do not eat or touch: Whole grains, brown rice, brewer's yeast, legumes, dark green leafy vegetables.

MSG, HVP, NF, and other food additives
Eat only: Follow same restrictions as food additives.
NOTE: *MSG can be added to food under different names: HVP (hydrolyzed vegetable protein), autolyzed yeast, NF (natural flavors), sodium caseinate, calcium caseinate, hydrolyzed milk protein. READ ALL LABELS!*

NEWSPAPER
Do not touch: Any newspapers or magazines.

NEWSPAPER INK
Do not touch: Newspapers or magazines.

NUT MIX 1   peanuts, black walnuts, English walnuts
Do not eat or touch: The above and oils or butters made from them.

NUT MIX 2   cashews, almonds, pecans, brazil nuts, hazelnuts, macadamias, pistachios, sunflower seeds
Do not eat or touch: The above and oils or butters made from them.

ONION MIX   brown, red, white, green onions
Eat only: Fruits, vegetables, grains, meat, poultry, fish, dairy products, and beans.
Do not eat or touch: Onions and products made with onions.

VITAMIN P
Do not eat or touch: Citrus fruits, green peppers, grapes, apricots, strawberries, black currants, cherries, prunes, rose hips, buckwheat.

PABA MIX   para-aminobenzoic acid
Do not eat, drink, or touch: Brewer's yeast, whole grain products, milk, eggs, yogurt, wheat germ, molasses, liver, kidneys, whole grains, rice, bran, sunscreen products containing PABA.

PARASITES MIX
Drink only: Boiled water or beverages made with boiling water.
Do not eat or touch: Uncooked or raw food, plain tap water. Wear gloves when attending to personal hygiene following toilet use.

PEPPER MIX   red, green, black, yellow, Mexican, Italian, Indian peppers
Eat only: Vegetables, poultry, meat, grains, fish, dairy products, fruits, and beans.
Do not eat or touch: All peppers and any foods made with peppers.

PERFUME MIX
Avoid: Perfumed soaps, makeup products, hair products, flowers. You may have to wear a mask to avoid the scent. When being treated, wear shower cap so hair doesn't smell like perfume and change into new clothes after treatment.

PESTICIDES
Eat only: Cooked organically grown grains, cooked organic vegetables, organic fruits, organically raised meat or poultry.
Do not eat, drink, or touch: Meat, uncooked foods, insecticides, coffee, tea.
Wear: A mask outdoors if the temperature is above freezing.

PHOSPHORUS
Eat only: White rice, potatoes, cauliflowers, fresh fruits, fresh vegetables, vegetable oils.
Drink only: Water.

Do not eat or touch: Whole grains, seeds, nuts, legumes, dairy products, egg yolks, fish, corn, dried fruits, poultry, meat.

PHENOLICS following are the phenolics to which asthmatics are commonly allergic:

Cinnamic acid

Eat only: Fish, vegetables other than lettuce and tomatoes, meat, chicken, turkey, rice.

Drink only: Water.

Do not eat, drink, or touch: Fruits, cheese, lettuce, tomatoes, strawberries, vanilla, oil of cinnamon, coca beans, cow's milk, albumin, apples, apricots, avocados, bananas, beets, beet sugar, blackberries, blueberries, boysenberries, cherries, cloves, coconut, dates, grapes, grapefruits, honey, horseradish, lemons, limes, mangoes, goat milk, human milk, olives, peaches, pears, plums, prunes, quinces, raisins, rhubarb, spearmint, watermelons, yeast.

Coumarin

Eat only: vegetables and fruits other than those mentioned below.

Drink only: Water.

Do not eat or touch: Wheat, rice, barley, corn, soy, cheese, beef, eggs, lavender oil, sweet clover, cow's milk, albumin, apples, bananas, barley, beer, beets, beet sugar, celery, chicken, cinnamon, cocoa, corn, egg yolks, lemons, lettuce, limes, goat's milk, human milk, mutton, oat, blackeyed peas, green peas, peanuts, black pepper, sweet potatoes, sage, tomatoes, tuna fish, turkey, vanilla, wheat bran, whole wheat, cow's milk whey, yeast, plants.

Dopamine

Eat only: meat, fish, chicken, vegetables, nuts, beans, grains.

Drink only: Water.

Do not eat or touch: Pineapples, bananas, plantains, avocados.

Gallic acid
Eat only: vegetables other than mentioned below, turkey, meat
Drink only: Water.
Do not eat or touch: Food coloring, cream of tartar, maple syrup, beer, tea, trees, sumac, tannins, apples, apricots, bananas, barley, basil, bay leaf, lima beans, navy beans, pinto beans, red beans, soybeans, string beans, blackberries, blueberries, brussel sprouts, cantaloupes, cow's milk casein, cashew nuts, chicken, cocoa, coconuts, crabmeat, cucumbers, eggs, garlic, ginger, grapes, hops, olives, papayas, peaches, peanuts, pears, pineapples, plums, potatoes, sweet potatoes, prunes, pumpkins, quinces, raisins, rhubarb, rice, strawberries, tea, tomatoes, vanilla, walnuts, watermelons, whole wheat, yeast.

Histamine   Refer to restrictions under main listing

Indole
Eat only: Fruits, vegetables other than the greens, rice, all grains, nuts, beans, sugars.
Drink only: Water.
Do not eat, drink, or touch: Vegetable greens, milk, meat, chicken, fish, turkey, eggs.

Malvin
Eat only: Rice, meat, fish, barley, grains.
Drink only: Water.
Do not eat, drink, or touch: Chicken, corn, eggs, soy, fruits, vegetables, dairy products, nuts, spices, honey, mustard seeds, blackeyed peas, green peas, tomatoes, walnuts, watermelons.

Phenylisothiocyanate
Eat only: White rice, fish, vegetables other than those mentioned below, fruits.
Drink only: Water.
Do not eat or touch: Chicken, eggs, beef, blackeyed peas, soybeans, cheese, lamb, peanuts, mustard, green

peas, black pepper, radishes, cocoa, horseradish, cow's milk, onions, mutton, cocoa, milk albumin, milk casein, lima beans, navy beans, pinto beans, soybeans, broccoli, brussel sprouts.

   Rutin   follow list of restrictions for bioflavanoids.

   Uric Acid

Avoid: Foods high in uric acid (refer to the listing later in Part VI).

Drink only: Water.

PLASTICS

Avoid: Crude oil and plastic products such as computers, telephones, pens, toothbrushes, hairbrushes.

Wear: Cotton or leather gloves.

POLLEN MIX

Avoid: Being outdoors; use a mask and gloves outdoors.

POTASSIUM

Eat only: White rice, pastas, cauliflowers, chicken, meat, eggs.

Do not eat or touch: Vegetables, oranges, bananas, cantaloupes, tomatoes, mint leaves, watercress, potatoes, whole grains, seeds, nuts, cream of tartar.

POTATO MIX   russet, white, red, sweet, yam

Eat Only: Vegetables except potatoes, fruits, meat, poultry, fish, dairy products, grains, and beans.

Do not eat or touch: All types of potatoes and the products made from potatoes.

RADIATION

Avoid: Sun, television, microwave, X rays, computers. Treat on a rainy day or at night and stay indoors.

RED WINE   follow list of restrictions for alcohol

RNA

Eat only: Lettuce.

Drink only: Water.

Do not eat or touch: Proteins such as meat, poultry, fish, nuts.

RICE SUGAR
Eat only: Fruits, vegetables, poultry, meat, dairy products, fish, beans, cane sugar.
Drink only: Water, black coffee, tea.
Do not eat or touch: Rice, or anything with rice sugar.

SACCHARINE
Eat Only: Grains, fruits, poultry, meat, vegetables, fish, cane sugar, dairy products and beans. READ ALL LABELS!
Drink only: Water, tea, coffee.
Do not eat, drink, or touch: Products with sacchrine, soft drinks, sweet relish, pickles, cookies, toothpastes.

SELENIUM
Eat only: White rice, pastas, cauliflowers, potatoes, chicken, fruits, salt.
Drink only: Water.
Do not eat, drink or touch: Seafood, milk, eggs, whole grains, beef, beans, bran, onions, tomatoes, broccoli, garlic, mushrooms, brewer's yeast, wheat germ, kelp, sea water, sea salt.

SEROTONIN
Eat only: Grains, chicken, meat, rice, cauliflowers, eggs, apples.
Do not eat, drink or touch: Dairy products, oranges, turkey, potatoes, soy, yeast, avocados, bananas, cocoa, pineapples, plums, tomatoes.

SHELLFISH MIX   shrimp, crabs, lobster, crayfish, abalone, clams, oysters, mussels
Do not eat or touch: Any of the shellfish listed above.

SILVER
Do not eat or touch: Fish, fish by-products, items containing silver (jewelry, coins, pens, flatware) and mercury. USE GLOVES.

SMOKING
Avoid: Smoke from cigarettes, clothes, and substances that have been in contact with cigarette smoke. Wear a mask for twenty-five hours if necessary. Treat with a shower cap and change into new clothes after treatment.

SORBITOL
Eat only: Fruits, meat, poultry, fish, vegetables, cane sugar, dairy products, grains, and beans.
Drink only: Water, tea, coffee.
Do not eat, drink, or touch: Products containing sorbitol such as soft drinks, sweet relish, pickles, cookies, toothpastes. READ ALL LABELS!

SOYBEAN
Eat only: Dairy products, vegetables, meat, poultry, fish, fruits
Do not eat, drink or touch: Tofu, soy milk, soy oil, soy lecithin, any soy product; (refer to detailed listing "Foods and Materials Containing Soybeans" in Part VI).

SPICE MIX 1   ginger, cardamom, cinnamon, cloves, nutmeg, garlic, cumin, fennel, coriander, turmeric, saffron, mint
Do not eat or touch the above: READ ALL LABELS! Also included are toothpastes, massage oils, and toiletries.

SPICE MIX 2   black pepper, red pepper, green peppers, 20 different peppers, jalapenoes, onions, oregano, chives, chervil, mace, marjoram, rosemary, anise seeds, caraway seeds, basil, bay leaf, fenugreek, cream of tartar, dill, horseradish, MSG, mustard, paprika, poppy seeds, parsley, sage, sumac, vinegar
Do not eat or touch the above: READ ALL LABELS! Also included are toothpastes, massage oils, and toiletries.

SULFUR
Eat only: White rice, pastas, cauliflowers, potatoes, fruits, noniodized salt.

Drink only: Water.
Do not eat or touch: Meat, fish, eggs, dried beans, cabbages, soybeans, watercress, string beans, celery, onions, turnips, radishes.

SWEET'N LOW®
Eat only: Fruits, vegetables, meat, poultry, grains, cane sugar, dairy products, fish, and beans.
Drink only: Water, coffee, tea.
Do not eat, drink, or touch: Products that contain Sweet'N Low® such as soft drinks, sweet relish, pickles, cookies, toothpastes. READ ALL LABELS!

VITAMIN T
Do not eat or touch: Sesame seeds, egg yolks, vegetable oils.

TOMATO MIX   green, yellow, and red tomatoes
Eat only: Vegetables other than tomatoes, meat, fruits, dairy products, fish, poultry, grains, and beans.
Do not eat or touch: Tomatoes of all kinds and products made from tomatoes such as soups, sauses, and stews.

TREE MIX
Avoid: Being outdoors.
Wear: Mask, gloves, socks, and shoes outdoors.

TURKEY   turkey, milk products, tryptophan, Vitamin B_1, B_3, B_6
Do not eat, drink, or touch: Turkey, milk products, tryptophan, and all items that contain the B vitamins listed above (refer to the detailed listing of foods under Vitamin B_1, B_3, and B_6 earlier in Part VI)

VANADIUM
Do not eat or touch: Fish, seafood.

VEGETABLE FAT   almond oil, palm oil, flax seed oil, canola oil, cottonseed oil, safflower oil, sesame oil, super-heated vegetable fats, olive oil, corn oil, Crisco Oil, coconut oil, peanut oil, linseed oil, sunflower oil, mustard oil

Eat only: Steamed vegetables, steamed rice, meat, eggs, chicken, butter, animal fats, fruits.

Do not eat or touch: The oils listed above or products containing them, products for external use containing these oils.

VEGETABLE MIX   green beans, cauliflowers, broccoli, brussel sprouts, cabbages, asparagus

Eat only: Fruits, meat, dairy, fish, poultry, beans, grains.

Do not eat or touch: Vegetables of any kind.

VINEGAR MIX   white vinegar, apple cider vinegar, rice vinegar

Eat only: Grains, vegetables, meat, poultry, fish, and dairy products.

Do not eat, drink, or touch: Vinegar, rice, apples, salad dressings with vinegar, condiments such as mustard, mayonnaise, and ketchup. READ ALL LABELS!

VIRUS MIX

Avoid: Contact with sick or infected persons for twenty-five hours. Wear a mask to be safe.

WEED MIX

Avoid: Being outdoors.

Wear: A mask and gloves outdoors.

WHEAT MIX   red, white, buckwheat

Eat only: Rice, vegetables, fruits, poultry, meat, fish, dairy products, and beans.

Do not eat or touch: All wheat products, (refer to the listing "Foods and Materials Containing Wheat" later in Part VI).

WHEY

Eat only: Rice, vegetables, fruits, meat, poultry, fish.

Do not eat, drink, or touch: Dairy products, or products containing whey. READ LABELS! Also included are crackers and french breads.

WHITE WINE   follow restrictions for alcohol

WHITEN ALL   sulfites
Eat only: Cooked vegetables, pastas, rice, meat, fish, chicken, eggs.
Do not eat or touch: Uncooked or frozen vegetables, canned foods, potato salads, fruit salads, potatoes any style (baked, french fried, or the like), sauces, dips, condiments, wines, wine vinegar, fruits (especially grapes), restaurant prepared or catered foods, foods from salad bars.

WOOD MIX
Avoid: Contact with woods and items made with woods.
Wear: Gloves.

WOOL
Avoid: Wool.
Wear: Gloves and cotton socks when walking on a wool rug.

YEAST MIX   baker's yeast, brewer's yeast, tortula yeast
Eat only: Vegetables, chicken, fish, extra virgin olive oil, canola oil, sesame oil.
Do not eat or touch: Dairy products, yeast products (breads, beer, wine), vinegar, hops, malts, peanuts, mushrooms, simple sugars, condiments (soy sauce, catsup), fruits (refer to the listing "Foods and Materials Containing Yeast" in Part VI).

YOGURT   yogurt, cheese; products from whey, yogurt, or cheese
Eat only: Rice, vegetables, fruits, meat, poultry, fish.
Do not eat, drink, or touch: Dairy products such as yogurt or cheese and products containing whey as well as dairy.

ZINC

Eat only: White rice, pastas, cauliflowers, potatoes, chicken, salt.

Drink only: Water.

Do not eat or touch: Green leafy vegetables, pork, beef, lamb, fish, brown rice, eggs, milk, brewer's yeast, mushrooms, onions, peas, dried beans, seeds, wheat bran, wheat germ, herring, oysters, mustard.

FOODS AND MATERIALS CONTAINING KEY ALLERGENS
Foods Containing Artificial Colors and Flavors

TO BE AVOIDED

Bakery Goods:
All manufactured cakes, cookies, sweet rolls, pastries, doughnuts
Frozen baked goods
Many packaged baking mixes
Pie crusts

Beverages:
All instant-breakfast drinks
All quick-mix powdered drinks
Beer
Cider
Diet drinks
Prepared chocolate milk
Soft drinks
Tea, hot or cold
Wine

Candies:
All manufactured types, hard or soft

Cereals:
All cereals with artificial colors and flavors
All instant-breakfast preparations

Desserts:
All dessert mixes
All powdered puddings
Flavored yogurt
Manufactured ice creams unless the label specifies no synthetic coloring or flavoring

PERMITTED

Bakery Goods:
All commercial breads except egg bread and whole wheat (usually dyed)
All flours
Any products without artificial color or flavor; most bakery items should be prepared at home

Beverages:
Grapefruit juice
Guava nectar
Homemade lemonade or limeade from fresh lemons or limes
Milk
Pear nectar
Pineapple juice
Seven-Up®

Candies:
Homemade candies, without almonds

Cereals:
Any cereals without artifical colors or flavors, dry or cooked

Desserts:
Commercial ice cream stating no artificial flavor or color
Homemade custards and puddings
Homemade gelatins from pure gelatins with any permitted natural fruit or fruit juices
Homemade ice cream without artificial coloring or flavoring
Plain yogurt

TO BE AVOIDED

Desserts: (continued)

Fish:
Fish sticks that are
  dyed or flavored
Frozen fish fillets that are dyed
  or flavored

Luncheon meats:
Bologna
Frankfurters
Ham, bacon, pork*
Meat loaf
Salami
Sausages*

Miscellaneous Items:
All mint-flavored items
Barbecue-flavored potato chips
Catsup
Chili sauce
Cider vinegar
Cloves
Colored butter
Colored cheeses
Commercial chocolate syrup
Margarine
Mustard
Soy sauce, if flavored or colored
Wine vinegar

Poultry:
All barbecued types
All turkeys with prepared
  basting (self-basting)
Prepared stuffing

Sundry Items:
All cough drops
All mouthwashes
All pediatric medications and
  vitamins that contain artificial
  color and flavors. When

PERMITTED

Desserts: (continued)
Tapioca

Fish:
All fresh fish

Luncheon meats:
All fresh meat

Miscellaneous Items:
All cooking oils and fats
All natural (white) cheeses
Distilled white vinegar
Homemade chocolate syrup for all
  purposes
Homemade mayonnaise
Jams or jellies made from
  permitted fruits and not artificially
  colored or flavored
Mustard prepared at home from
  pure powder and distilled vinegar
Sweet butter, not colored or flavored

Poultry:
All poultry except stuffed

TO BE AVOIDED

Sundry Items: (continued)
medications are required, a
physician should be consulted.
Most over-the-counter medications
contain aspirin as well as artificial
flavors and colors (Aspirin,
Bufferin®, Excedrin®, Alka-Seltzer®,
Empirin®, Empirin Compound®,
Anacin®)
All throat lozenges
All toothpastes and toothpowders†
Antacid tablets
Perfumes

*If a product is colored or flavored, it is usually indicated on the
package

†A salt and soda mixture can be used for cleaning teeth; Neutrogena®
soap (unscented) can be substituted for toothpaste or powder

Foods and Materials Containing Corn

Adhesives
Ale
American brandies
 apple
 grape
Aspirin and other tablets

Bacon
Baking Mixes
 Aunt Jemima® Pancake Mix
 Bisquick®
 Complete Pancake Mix®
 Doughnuts
Baking Powders
Batters for frying meat, fish, fowl
Beers
Beets, Harvard
Beverages, carbonated
Bleached wheat flours
Bourbon and other whiskies
Breads and pastries

Cakes
Candy
 Box candies, all grades
 Candy bars
 Commercial candies
Carbonated beverages
Catsups
Cheerios®
Cheeses
Chili
Chop suey
Coffee, Instant
Confectioner's sugar
Cookies
Corn
 flakes
 flour
 meal
 oil (Mazola®)
 parched
 popped

soya
starch
sugars
  cerelose
  dextrose
  dyno
unripe
  canned
  fresh
  fritters
  frozen
  roasting ears
  succotash
Cough syrups
Cream pies
Cream puffs
Cups, paper

Dates, confection
Deep fat frying mixtures
Dentifrices

Excipients or diluents in:
  capsules
  suppositories
  tablets
  vitamins

Flour, bleached
Foods, fried
French dressing
Fritos®
Frostings
Fruits
Frying fats

Gelatin capsules
Gelatin dessert
Gin
Glucose products
Graham crackers
Grape juice
Gravies

Grits
Gum on envelopes, stickers,
  stamps, tapes, labels
Gums, chewing
Gummed papers

Ham, cured or tenderized
Harvard beets
Holiday-type stickers
Hominy

Ice creams
Ices
Inhalants
  bath powders
  body powders
  cooking fumes from fresh corn

Jams
Jellies
Jell-O®

Kremel

Leavening agents
  baking powders
  yeasts
Liquors
  ale
  beer
  gin
  whiskey
Lozenges

Margarine
Meat
  bacon
  bologna
  cooked, with gravies
  frankfurters
  ham, cured or tenderized
  lunch ham
  sausages, cooked

weiners
Milk, in paper cartons
Monosodium glutamate
Mull-Soy

Nescafe®™

Ointments

Pablum
Paper containers
  boxes
  cups
  plates
(Only when foods come in
  contact with these containers)
Pastries
  cakes
  cup cakes
Peanut butters
Peas, canned
Pies, creamed
Plastic food wrappers (the inner
  surfaces may be coated with
  corn starch)
Powdered sugar
Preserves
Puddings
  blanc mange
  custards
  Royal pudding

Rice, coated

Salad dressings
Salt
  salt cellars in restaurants
Sandwich spreads
Sauces
  sundaes
  meats
  fish
  vegetables

Seasoned salt
Sherberts
Similac®
String beans
  canned
  frozen
Soups
  creamed
  thickened
  vegetable
Soybean milks
Starch
Starch fumes while ironing
  clothes
Sugar, powdered
Syrups, commercially prepared
  glucose
  Karo®

Talcums
Teas, instant
Toothpaste (some)
Tortillas

Vanillin
Vegetables
  canned
  creamed
  frozen
Vinegar, distilled
Vitamins

Whiskies
  bourbon
  scotch
Wines, American*
  dessert
  fortified
  sparkling

*Some brands are corn-free

Foods Containing Eggs

Baking powder
Batters for french frying
Bavarian cream
Boiled dressings
Bouillon
Bread
Breaded foods
Cake flour
Cakes
French toast
Fritters
Frosting
Glazed rolls
Griddle cakes
Hamburger mix
Hollandaise sauce
Ice cream
Ices
Icings
Macaroni
Macaroons
Malted cocoa drinks
  Ovaltine®
Marshmallows
Meat jellies
Meat loaf

Meat molds
Meat patties
Meringues
Noodles
Pancake flour
Pancakes
Pastes
Pretzels
Pudding
Salad dressing
Sauces
Sausages
Sherberts
Souffles
Soups
  consommes
  mock turtle
  noodle
Spaghetti
Spanish creams
Tartar sauce
Timbales
Waffle mixes
Waffles
Wines

Foods and Materials Containing Formaldehyde

Formaldehyde is a formic aldehyde, a powerful disinfectant gas produced by the oxidation of methyl alcohol. The aqueous solution is a colorless, volatile fluid used as a surgical and general antiseptic as well as a preservative. It is also utilized as a reagent, a substance used in the detection or analysis of another substance by chemical, microscopic, or other means.

Common Uses of Formaldehyde Include:

Intermediates in the synthesis of
  alcohols, acids, and chemicals
Tanning agent
A rodent poison

The formulation of slow-release
  nitrogen fertilizers and in destroying micro-organisms responsible for plant disease

An added agent to make concrete, plaster, and related products impermeable to liquids

Antiperspirants and antiseptics in dentifrices, mouthwashes, and germicidal and detergent soaps

Hair-setting lotions, shampoos, and detergent soaps

Air deodorant in public places and in industrial environments

Destroying bacteria, fungi, molds, and yeasts

Disinfecting equipment in the fermentation industry and the manufacture of antibiotics

Disinfecting sickrooms and surgical instruments

Synthesis of dyes, stripping agents, and various specialty chemicals in the dye industry

The manufacture of embalming fluids when combined with alcohol, glycerol, and phenol

Preserving products such as waxes, polishes, adhesives, fats, oils, and anatomical specimens

The synthesis of explosives

Preparing fireproofing compositions to apply to fabrics in conjunction with other chemicals

Insecticidal solutions for killing flies, mosquitoes, and moths

The synthesis of Vitamin A and to improve the activity of Vitamin E preparations

Improving set strength and water resistance in paper products

Preserving and accelerating photographic developing solutions

Making natural and synthetic fibers crease-resistant, wrinkle-resistant, crushproof, water-repellent, dye-fast, flame-resistant, water-resistant, shrink-proof, moth-proof (wool), and more elastic (wool)

Making synthetic resins, wood veneer (for wall paper) and artificial aging, and reduction of shrinkage in wood preservation

One of the component parts of wallboard in construction of houses and apartments

Resin in nail polish and undercoating of nail polish

*Formaldehyde accounts for about fifty percent of the estimated total aldehydes in polluted air. The major sources of aldehyde pollution are in the incomplete combustions of hydrocarbons in gasoline and diesel engines, burning of fuels, and incineration waste. Formaldehyde is believed to be the principal agent responsible for burning of the eyes in smog. Aldehydes can also react further to form additional products such as ozone.

Foods and Materials Containing Hydrocarbons

Hydrocarbons are organic compounds comprised of hydrogen and carbon. If the geological concept that conifer forests are the precursors of the original sources of the hydrocarbons—coal, oil, gas—is valid, then we should consider these materials as well. Such an interpretation is indicated by the similar clinical effects of pine and its combustion products with those of coal, oil, and gas and their combustion products and derivatives.

Common Uses of Hydrocarbons Include:

Alcohol

Artificially colored foods and drugs

Burning green wood containing considerable oil and resin

Cements and other adhesives

Cleaning fluids and lighter fluids

Creosote impregnated wood

Evaporating oil from mechanical devices

Evaporating paints, varnish, and other solvents

Foods exposed to gas for ripening, roasting, or clarifying through bone char that is reactivated in gas-fired ovens

Fuel: coal, oil, gas, diesel and nondiesel, and their combustion

Garage odors fouling the air of living quarters

Industrial and agricultural chemicals contaminating water supplies

Insecticides

Mineral oil

Miscellaneous odors: detergents, soaps containing naphtha, ammonia, bleach, cleansing powders containing bleach, window washing compounds, certain silver and brass polishing materials, and deodorants and disinfectants (especially pine-scented)

Newsprint

Oil-soluble food sprays that permeate the cooking surface to which they are applied and cannot be removed by washing, peeling, soaking in water or vinegar, or by cooking

Paraffins used in coating and scaling, in candles, in rubber compounding, in pharmaceuticals, and in cosmetics

Pine exposure

Plastics

Plastics produced by chemical condensations

Refrigerants (freon) and spray containers

Roofing and road construction compounds

Sponge rubber

Foods Containing Milk

Baker's bread

Baking powder biscuits

Bavarian cream

Bisques

Blancmange

Boiled salad dressings

Butter
Buttermilk
Butter sauces
Cakes
Candies
Cheeses
Chocolate
Chowders
Cocoa drinks, mixtures
Cookies
Cream
Creamed foods
Cream sauces
Curds
Custards
Doughnuts
Eggs, scrambled
Flour mixtures
Foods fried in butter (fish, poultry, beef, pork)
Foods prepared au gratin
Fritters
Gravies
Hamburgers
Hard sauces
Hash
Hot cakes
Ice creams

Junket®
Malted milk
Margarine
Mashed potatoes
Meat loaf
Milk Chocolate
Omelets
Ovaltine
Pie crust (some)
Prepared mixes
  biscuits
  cakes
  cookies
  doughnuts
  muffins
  pancakes
  pie crust
  waffles
Rarebits
Salad dressings
Sausages, cooked
Scalloped dishes
Sherberts
Soda crackers
Souffles
Soups
Whey
Zwieback

Foods and Materials Containing Soybeans

Foods Containing Soybeans or Made from Soybeans:

Automobile Parts: Some automobile manufacturers are using soybeans to make a plastic from which window frames, steering wheels, gear shift knobs, distributors, and other parts are made. They also make an upholstery fabric from soybeans.

Bakery goods: Soybean flour containing only one percent oil is now used by many bakers in their dough mixtures for breads, cakes, rolls, and pastries. This keeps baked goods moist and salable several days longer. The roasted nuts are used in place of peanuts on breakfast rolls. Biscuits and several crisp crackers have soybean flour in them.

Candies: Soy flours are used in hard candies, fudge, nut candies, custards, and caramels. Lecithin is invariably derived from soybeans for use in candies, particularly chocolate, to prevent drying out and to emulsify the fats.

Cereals

Industrial and Other Contacts: Soy products are used in varnish, paints, enamels, printing ink, massage creams, candles, celluloid, linoleum, adhesives, paper finishes, blankets, cloth, nitroglycerine, urease, pet food, soaps, fertilizers, and automobile parts. It is also used for fodder, textile dressing, glycerine, coffee substitutes and to make lubricating and illuminating oil. Soybeans are used to make rubber substitutes and its lecithin is used as a stabilizer in leaded gasoline.

Meats: Pork link sausage and lunch meats can contain soybeans. The allergic individual should buy only pure meat products.

Milk Substitutes: Some bakeries use soy milk instead of cow's milk in recipes.

Miscellaneous: Soy products are used in some ice creams and in many soups. Fresh green soy sprouts are served as a vegetable, especially in Chinese dishes. Soybeans are roasted, salted, and used in place of peanuts. They are also used to make soy noodles, macaroons, and spaghetti. Some seasonings contain soy, as do a number of frying fats and shortenings. Oleomargarines and butter substitutes contain the oil and bean products. It is also present in many cookies, crackers, and snacks.

Salad Dressings: Many salad dressings and mayonnaises contain soy oil but only show on the label that they contain vegetable oil. When using a particular brand of dressing or mayonnaise, inquire as to the contents.

Sauces

NOTE: *Keep in mind that soybeans and their products are used as flour, oil, milk, and nuts. We are living in an era of expanding uses for soybeans, and the allergy sufferer should anticipate the many possible contacts. Additionally, as new food combinations become popular, many new contacts can be expected. When undergoing an NAET treatment for soybeans, eat only foods in their original form. Avoid baked, processed, and packaged foods. Wear cotton or leather gloves and a mask when handling or coming in close proximity (less than four feet) with the products on the above list.*

Foods Containing "Hidden Sugars"

Beverages:
Cola drinks
Cordials
Ginger ale
Orange ade
Root beer
Seven-Up®
Soda pop
Sweet cider
Whiskey sour

Cakes and Cookies:
Angel food
Applesauce cake
Banana cake
Brownies (plain)
Cheese cake
Chocolate cake (iced)
Chocolate cake (plain)
Chocolate cookies
Chocolate eclairs
Coffee cake
Cream puff
Cup cake (iced)
Donuts (glazed)
Donuts (plain)
Fig Newtons
Fruit cake
Gingersnaps
Jelly roll
Macaroons
Nut cookies
Oatmeal cookies
Orange cake
Pound cake
Sponge cake
Strawberry shortcake
Sugar Cookies

Candies
Chewing gum
Chocolate (cream filling)
Chocolate mints
Fudge
Hard candy
Hershey's® bar
Lifesavers®
Peanut brittle

Canned Fruits and Juices:
Apricots
Apricot syrup
Fruit cocktail
Fruit juice (sweetened)
Fruit syrup
Peaches
Stewed fruits

Dairy Products:
Ice cream
Ice cream bar
Ice cream cone
Ice cream soda
Ice cream sundae
Milk shake

Jams, Jellies, and Desserts:
Apple butter
Apple cobbler
Custard
French pastry
Jell-O®
Jelly
Orange marmalade
Strawberry

Foods Containing Wheat

Beverages:
Beer
Cocomalt
Gin (any drink with grain-
  neutral spirits)
Malted milk
Ovaltine
Postum
Whiskey
Breads:
Biscuits
Breads
  corn
  gluten
  graham
  rye (rye products are not
    entirely free of wheat)
  soy
  wheat
Crackers
Muffins
Popovers
Pretzels
Rolls
Cereals:
All wheat cereals
Bran flakes
Corn Flakes®
Cream of Wheat®
Farina®
Grapenuts®
Other malted cereals
Puffed Wheat®
Rice Krispies®
Shredded Wheat®™
Triscuits®
Wheatena®
Flours:
Buckwheat
Corn

Gluten
Graham
Lima Bean
Patent
Rye
White
Whole wheat
Pastries and Desserts:
Cakes
Candy bars
Chocolate candy
Cookies
Doughnuts
Frozen pies
Pies
Puddings
Wheat Products:
Bread
Dumplings
Macaroni
Noodles
Rusk
Spaghetti
Vermicelli
Zweiback
Miscellaneous:
Bouillon cubes
Chocolate candy
Chocolate (except bitter cocoa
  and bitter chocolate)
Cooked mixed meat dishes
Fats that have been used for
  frying
Foods rolled in flour (including
  meat)
Gravies
Griddle cakes
Hot cakes
Ice cream cones
Matzos

Mayonnaise
Most cooked and prepared meat including sausages, wieners, bologna, liverwurst, luncheon ham, and hamburger
Pancake mixes
Sauces

Synthetic pepper
Some yeasts
Thickening in ice cream
Wheat cakes
Wheat germ
Waffles

Foods Containing Yeast

The following foods contain yeast as an additive ingredient during preparation (often called leavening):

Breads
Cake and cake mixes
Canned icebox biscuits
Cookies
Crackers
Hamburger buns
Hot dog buns

Meat fried in cracker crumbs
Milk fortified with vitamins from yeast
Pastries
Pretzels
Rolls, homemade or canned

The following substances contain yeast or yeast-like substances because of their nature or the nature of their manufacture or preparation:

Buttermilk
Cheeses of all kinds including cottage cheese
Citrus fruit juices, frozen or canned (only home-squeezed are yeast-free!)
Fermented beverages including whiskey, wine, brandy, gin, rum, vodka, and root beer.
Malted products including cereals, candy, and malted milk drinks

Mushrooms
Truffles
Vinegars (apple, pear, grape, and distilled). These may be used alone or in such foods as catsup, mayonnaise, olives, pickles, sauerkraut, condiments, horseradish, French dressing, salad dressing, Bar B-Q sauce, tomato sauce, chili peppers, mince pie, and Gerber's® Oatmeal and Barley Cereal

The following contain substances that are derived from yeast or have their source in yeast. READ ALL LABELS!

Capsules or tablets containing Vitamin B made from yeast
Multiple vitamins
Some enzyme supplements con-

taining brewer's yeast
Vitamin B capsules or tablets made from yeast

Drugs Containing NO Corn, Wheat or Milk

Acetaminophen
Accutane Capsules®
Allerest Children's Chewable
  Tablets®
Allerest Eye Drops®
Allerest Nasal Spray®
Amphojel Suspension®
Amphojel Suspension without
  Flavor®
Anaprox®
Ancef Injection®
Aspirin Uniserts

Bacitracin Sterile®
Bacitracin Topical Ointment®
Bactrim Suspension™
Bactrim Tablets™
Basaljel Suspension®
Basaljel Suspension Extra
  Strength®
Benadryl Steri-Vial®™
Berocca Plus Tablets®
Berocca Tablets®
Bisacodyl (Dulcolax)®
Brexin L. A. Capsules®

Cafergot Suppositories®
Calciferol Drops™
Castor Oil
Casufru Liquid
Cedilanid-D Injection
Cerose Compound Capsules
Cerubidine Injectable®
Chardose Powder
Chloromycetin® Cream, 1%
Chloromycetin® Opthalmic
  Ointment
Chloromycetin® Palmitate Oral
  Suspension
Chloromycetin® Sodium
  Succinate Steri-Vial

Chromagen® Capsules
Claforan® Injection
Codeine Sulfate
Cod Liver Oil
Coly-Mycin M Parenteral®
Coly-Mycin S Oral Suspension®
Comhist LA Capsules®
Compazine Syrup®
Cortenema (Hydrocortisone
  Retention Enema)®
Cortril Hydrocortisone Topical
  Ointment

Dallergy Syrup®
Dantrium Intravenous®
Debrox Drops®
DHE 45 Injection®
DiaBeta Tablets®
Diapid Nasal Spray
Dilantin–30/Pediatric
  Dilantin–125®
Dilor G Liquid and Tablets®
Dimetane Ten®
Ditropan Syrup®
Docusate Sodium Capsules®
Docusate Sodium with
  Casanthranol Capsules®
Dopram Injectable®

Elase®
Emcyt Capsules®
Endep Tablets®
Entex LA Tablets®
Entex Liquid®
Equagesic Tablets®

Festal II Digestive Aid Tablets®
Festalan Tablets®
Flagyl I.V.®
Flagyl I.V. RTU®
Flagyl Tablets®

Fluogen®
Fumerin Tablets®
Furacin Products-Topical Cream®
Furadantin Oral Suspension®
Furosemide Injection®

Gantrisin Pediatric Suspension®
Gantrisin Syrup®
Gaviscon®™

Histatapp Elixir®
Hydergine LC Liquid Capsules®
Hydergine Oral Tablets,
  Sublingual Tablets, and Liquid

Ipsatol DM®
Isordil Chewable Tablets®
Isordil Tembids Capsules®
Isordil Tembids Tablets®
Isordil Titrados Tablets®

Kie Syrup®
Klor-Con Powder®
Klor-Con 8/Klor-Con 10®
Klor-Con/25 Powder®
Klor-10%®
Klorvess Effervescent Granules®
Klorvess Effervescent Tablets®

Lactocal-F Tablets
Laraodopa Tablets®
Lasix Oral Solution®
Levsin Drops®
Levsin Elixir®
Levsin PB Drops®
Levsin PB Elixir®
Lidex (Cream, Gel, Ointment,
  Topical Solution)®
Lidex-E Cream®
Lidex Ointment®
Lidex Topical Solution®
Lithonate Capsules®
Lithotabs Tablets™

Lomotil Tablets and Liquid®

Medihaler-Epi™
Medihaler Ergotamine Aerosol™
Mestinon Syrup®
Metamucil (Powder Contains
  Dextrose)®
Methergine Injection®
Milk of Magnesia
Mineral Oil
Mycelex Troches®
Mycostatin Oral Suspension®
Mytrex Cream & Ointment®

Nitro-Bid® (IV, Ointment, 2.5
  Plateau Caps, 6.5 and 9 Plateau
  Caps)
Nitrostat Injection®
Nitrostat Ointment 2%®
Nitrostat Tablets®
Nydrazid Syrup®

Omnipen for Oral Suspension®
Omnipen Pediatric Drops®

Pamelor Solution®
Penicillin G Potassium
  for Injections®
Penicillin G Potassium Tablets®
Pen Vee K Tablets®
Pen Vee K Oral Solution®
Pfizerpen Capsules and Oral
  Suspension®
Pfizerpen-AS®
Pfizerpen VK Tablets and Oral
  Suspension®
Polymyxin B Sulfate®
Procan SR®
Prolixin Decanoate®
Prolixin Elixir®
Prolixin Enanthate®
Prompt®

Reglan Injectable®
Rid (topical)®
RMS (Suppositories) Uniserts®
Robaxin Injection®
Robinul Injectable®
Robicillin for VK Oral Solution®
Rocaltrol Tablets®
Roniscol Timespan Tablets®

Saccharin Tablets
Secobarbital Sodium Capsules®
Silvadene Cream (topical)®
Sinarest 12 Hour Nasal Spray®
SK Chloral Hydrate Capsules®
SK Potassium Chloride Oral
  Solution®
Sorbitol
Star-Otic
Stelazine Concentrate®
Stoxil Ophthalmic Ointment®
Stoxil Ophthalmic Solution®
Streptase®
Streptomycin Sulfate
Sumycin Syrup
Surmontil Capsules®
Sweeta Liquid®
Synacort Cream®
Synalgos Capsules®
Synalgos DC Capsules®
Synalar HP Cream®
Synalar Ointment®
Syntocinon Injection®
Syntocinon Nasal Spray®

Tagamet Liquid®
Terra Cortril Opthalmic
  Suspension®
Terra Cortril Topical Ointment®

Terramycin IM®
Terramycin IV®
Terramycin Ophthalmic
  Ointment®
Terramycin Topical Ointment®
Theo-Dur Sprinkle®
Theo-24 Capsules®
Theolair-Plus Liquid™
Theolair-Plus Tablets™
Theragran Liquid®
Thorazine Concentrate®
Thorazine Syrup®
Topicort Cream®
Topicort Gel®
Topicycline®
Trecator-SC Tablets®
Tuss-Ornade Liquid
Tylenol Children's Chewable
  Tablets®

Urolene Blue®
Urtex®

Vi Penta F Chewables®
Vi Penta F Drops®
Virilon®
Vistaril®

Wygesic Tablets®
Wymox Capsules®
Wymox Oral Suspension®

Yeast Tablets
Yeast X®

Zantac®
Zarontin Syrup®
Zaroxolyn Tablets®

SPECIFIC DIETS RELATED
TO DIETARY STRESS

The following diets are based on individual dietary stresses. The four different dietary stresses are sugar, complex carbohydrate, fat, and protein. People generally fall into one of these specific food intolerances. This concept was discussed throughout this book and more specifically in Chapter 13.

The determination of one's specific intolerance is based on a thorough case history, a complete abdominal diagnostic palpation examination, and a twenty-four hour urine evaluation as taught by Dr. Howard Loomis. To locate a practitioner in your area, contact 21st Century Nutrition at 1-800-614-4400.

After a complete evaluation, one of these diets will be recommended to promote optimum health, weight management, and overall good energy levels. I have also included the Candida/yeast avoidance diet and the gastric diet in this section.

For additional dietary recommendations, consult the following books:

> *Eat More, Weigh Less* by Dean Ornish, M.D.
> *The New Pritikin Program* by Robert Pritikin
> *Enter the Zone* by Barry Sears, Ph.D.

DIET FOR COMPLEX CARBOHYDRATE INTOLERANCE—LOWER LEFT QUADRANT

Individuals who are carbohydrate intolerant usually crave fatty foods and have an irritable bowel. For these individuals, I recommend a diet that includes:

- liberal quantities of protein, certain cooked vegetables (see list below), water, any type of mineral water, and selected herbal teas

- moderate quantities of lipids as well as polyunsaturated vegetable oils, plant protein, fruits, and refined carbohydrates

- minimal consumption of whole grains, nuts, seeds, raw vegetables, and vegetables with seeds

- limited intake of salt including soy sauce and spicy foods that contain large amounts of salt

- limited intake of alcohol which acts as pure sugar is high in calories, void of nutrients, and can cause cravings

- avoidance of all artificial sweeteners and caffeinated beverages

Proteins: *(3–5 servings per day)*

2 egg whites
1 egg
4 oz. fish, shellfish, poultry
2 oz. low fat cottage cheese
2 oz. skim ricotta cheese
1 oz. spirulina
3 oz. tofu

2 oz. skim mozzarella cheese
4 oz. protein soy powder
1 cup low or nonfat yogurt
4 oz. beef (3 servings or less per week)
4 oz. veal
4 oz. lamb

Carbohydrates: *Unlimited amounts of the following vegetables*

cooked cauliflower
cooked yellow squash
cooked eggplant
cooked zucchini
cooked artichoke
all types of lettuce
radishes
spinach
kale
jicama

cooked onions
cooked yellow or green beans
cooked okra
cooked mushrooms
celery
onions
endive
escarole
cabbage
bok choy

Limited amounts of the following vegetables (3–4 servings per week)

4 oz. sweet peas
4 oz. cooked carrots
4 oz. cooked corn
4 oz. potatoes

4 oz. yam
4 oz. sweet potato
4 oz. cooked pumpkin

Vegetables to avoid

tomatoes
sprouts

cucumber

Fruits: *(2 servings per day)*

1 apple
1 peach
2 apricots
½ honeydew
10 cherries

fruit juices
1 nectarine
1 pear
1 cup grapes
2 plums

1 cup berries	1 cup watermelon
½ cup fresh pineapple	½ cup cantaloupe
1 cup papaya	½ banana

Limited fruits (3–4 servings per week)

1½ dried figs	½ cup raisins
1½ dates	½ cup cranberries

Complex carbohydrates:

Legumes, grains, and grain products (1–2 servings per day)

1 slice whole grain bread	½ cup brown rice
½ cup bulgur	½ cup oatmeal
½ cup quinoa	¼ bagel
½ cup pasta	½ English muffin
⅓ cup dried beans	½ waffle
1 rice cake	½ pita bread
1 corn tortilla	½ cup spelt or kamut
½ cup white rice	

Avoid

popcorn	granola
tortilla chips	

Fats: *(1–2 servings per day)*

⅓ tsp. canola oil	½ tbsp. avocado
⅓ tsp. olive oil	½ tbsp. tahini
⅓ tsp. peanut oil	1 tsp. olive oil and vinegar dressing

Limited fats (3–4 servings per week)

1 tsp. mayonnaise	½ tsp. sesame oil
⅓ tsp. soybean oil	2 tsp. bacon bits
⅓ tsp. butter	½ tbsp. cream
1 tsp. cream cheese	½ tbsp. sour cream
⅓ tsp. lard	⅓ tsp. margarine

Avoid

nuts	seeds

DIET FOR FAT INTOLERANCE—UPPER RIGHT QUADRANT

Individuals who are fat intolerant usually have a deficiency in fatty acids and possibly an exhausted thyroid. Those individuals tend to crave sugars and often suffer from eczema, liver, and gallbladder disease. For these individuals, I recommend a diet that includes:

- liberal quantities of vegetables (raw or cooked without fat or salt—see list below), fruits, legumes, protein, water, any type of mineral water, hot grain beverages, vegetable juices, fruit juices, and selected herbal teas

- moderate quantities of higher fat protein sources such as seafood, low fat dairy, whole grains (see list below under complex carbohydrates) and starchy vegetables such as potatoes, yams, and winter squashes

- avoidance or minimal consumption of animal fats, tropical oils, hydrogenated oils, butter, cocoa butter (found in chocolate), margarine, mayonnaise, shortening, meats, whole dairy products, nuts, egg yolks, fried foods, nondairy creamers, refined grains, and grain products

- using olive oil, canola oil, avocado oil, sesame oil, peanut oil, corn oil, cottonseed oil, sunflower oil, soybean oil, safflower oil, and walnut oil sparingly (1 tsp. 1–2 times per day)

- limited intake of olives and avocados because they contain high amounts of fat

- limited intake of salt including soy sauce and spicy foods that contain large amounts of salt because fat-intolerant individuals tend to be water retentive

- limited intake of alcohol because it is irritating to the liver and the upper right quadrant, can cause cravings, acts as pure sugar, is high in calories, and is void of nutrients

- avoidance of nuts, all nut butters, cream cheese, sour cream, bacon, artificial sweeteners, and caffeinated beverages

Proteins: *(1–3 servings per day)*

2 egg white
3 oz. fish, shellfish
3 oz. lean poultry
2 oz. nonfat powdered milk
2 oz. low fat or nonfat cottage cheese
6 oz. nonfat yogurt

²/₃ cup soybeans
3 oz. tofu
3 oz. lean beef (no more than 3 times per week)
3 oz. lean lamb (no more than 3 times per week)

Carbohydrates:

Unlimited amounts of the following vegetables

beets
broccoli
cauliflower
cucumbers
endive
jicama
leeks
mushrooms
onions
radishes
sprouts
water chestnuts
green or yellow beans

bok choy
cabbage
celery
eggplant
escarole
kale
lettuce
okra
parsley
rutabagas
squash
watercress

Limited amounts of the following vegetables (3–4 servings per week)

artichokes
sweet peas
potatoes
yams

carrots
corn
sweet potatoes
pumpkins

Complex carbohydrates:

Legumes, grains, and grain products (4 servings per day)

1/3 cup dried beans
1/3 cup brown rice
1 slice whole wheat bread
1/3 cup cooked wild rice
3/4 oz. rice cakes
1/2 cup cooked grits
1/2 cup cooked noodles
1 (6-inch) corn tortilla

1/3 cup cooked lentils
1/2 bagel
1/2 (6 inch) pita bread
1/2 cup barley
1/2 cup whole wheat macaroni
1/2 cup cooked oatmeal
1/2 cup steel cut oats

Fruits: *(3 servings per day)*

1 small apple
1/2 banana
1/3 cantaloupe
1 1/2 dried figs
1/2 grapefruit
10 grapes
1/2 mango
1 cup papaya
1 small pear
2 plums
1 1/4 cups strawberries

4 medium fresh apricots
3/4 cup berries
12 cherries
2 1/2 medium dates
1/4 honeydew melon
1 orange
1 peach
3/4 cup pineapple
2 medium fresh prunes
2 small tangerines

PROTEIN INTOLERANCE—LOWER RIGHT QUADRANT

Individuals who are protein intolerant usually crave sugar and tend to experience anxiety, osteoporosis because of poor calcium absorption, and possibly hypoglycemia. For those individuals, I recommend a diet that includes:

- liberal quantities of vegetables (raw or cooked without fat or salt—see list below), fruits, water, any type of mineral water, hot grain beverages, vegetable juices, fruit juices, and selected herbal teas

- moderate quantities of whole grains (see list below) and starchy vegetables such as potatoes, yams, and winter squashes

- minimal consumption of all proteins, legumes, animal fats, tropical oils, hydrogenated vegetable oils, fried foods, whole dairy products, and nuts such as coconut and macadamia

- limited intake of salt including soy sauce and spicy foods that contain large amounts of salt

- limited intake of alcohol that acts as pure sugar, is high in calories, is void of nutrients, and can cause cravings

- avoid all artificial sweeteners and caffeinated beverages

Proteins: *(1–2 serving per day)*

2 eggs (3 servings or less per week)	3 oz. tofu
3 oz. low-fat cottage cheese	3 oz. lean poultry
2 oz. skim mozzarella cheese	4 oz. fish, shellfish
4 oz. protein powder	2 oz. skim ricotta cheese
1 cup nonfat yogurt	1 oz. spirulina
no red meat	2/3 cup soybeans

Carbohydrates:

Unlimited amounts of the following vegetables

beets	bok choy
broccoli	cabbage
cauliflower	celery
cucumber	eggplant
endive	escarole

jicama

leeks

mushrooms

onions

radishes

sprouts

water chestnuts

beans, green or yellow

kale

lettuce

okra

parsley

rutabagas

squash

watercress

Limited amounts of the following vegetables (3–4 servings per week)

artichokes

· sweet peas

potatoes

yams

carrots

corn

sweet potatoes

pumpkin

Complex carbohydrates:

Legumes, grains, and grain products (3–4 servings per day)

⅓ cup dried beans

⅓ cup brown rice

1 slice whole wheat bread

½ (6 inch) pita bread

½ cup barley

½ cup whole wheat macaroni

½ cup cooked oatmeal

½ cup steel cut oats

⅓ cup cooked lentils

½ bagel

½ cup cooked wild rice

1 rice cake

½ cup cooked grits

½ cup cooked noodles

1 (6-inch) corn tortilla

½ cup millet

Fruits: *(3 servings per day)*

1 small apple

½ banana

⅓ cantaloupe

1½ dried figs

½ grapefruit

10 grapes

½ mango

1 cup papaya

1 small pear

2 plums

1¼ cups strawberries

4 medium fresh apricots

¾ cup berries

12 cherries

2½ medium dates

¼ honeydew melon

1 orange

1 peach

¾ cup pineapple

2 medium fresh prunes

2 small tangerines

Fats: *(2 servings per day)*

7 almonds or ½ tsp. almond
  butter

⅓ tsp. canola oil

⅓ tsp. olive oil

3 olives

⅓ tsp. peanut oil

½ tbsp. avocado

½ tbsp. tahini

1 tsp. olive oil and vinegar
  dressing

½ tsp. peanut butter

6 peanuts

Limited fats (3–4 servings per week)

1 tsp. mayonnaise	½ tsp. sesame oil
⅓ tsp. soybean oil	½ tsp. walnuts
½ tsp. brazil nuts	2 tsp. bacon bits
⅓ tsp. butter	½ tbsp. cream
1 tsp. cream cheese	½ tbsp. sour cream
⅓ tsp. lard	⅓ tsp. margarine

DIET FOR SUGAR INTOLERANCE— UPPER LEFT QUADRANT

Individuals who are sugar intolerant tend to crave protein and to suffer from depression, malabsorption, bloating, hyperactivity, asthma, chronic constipation, and severe food allergies. They usually have low blood sugar and exhausted adrenal glands. For those individuals, I recommend a diet that includes:

- liberal quantities of vegetables (see list on the next page), raw or cooked

- moderate quantities of lipids (fats), polyunsaturated vegetable oils, plant protein, eggs, animal protein, and fresh vegetables

- minimal consumption of sugars, fruits, grains, and dairy products

- avoidance of refined grains, refined grain products, and sweet vegetables such as potatoes, carrots, and corn

- taking protein within an hour of having the carbohydrate to balance the intake of foods

- limited intake of salt including soy sauce and spicy foods that contain large amounts of salt

- limited intake of alcohol because it weakens and stresses the adrenal glands, acts as pure sugar, is high in calories, is void of nutrients, and can cause cravings

- avoidance of all artificial sweeteners, sugars, and caffeinated beverages

Proteins: *(3–5 servings per day)*

2 egg whites	1 egg
4 oz. fish or lean poultry	3 oz. tofu

2 oz. low-fat cottage cheese	2 oz. skim mozzarella cheese
2 oz. skim ricotta cheese	4 oz. soy protein powder
1 oz. spirulina	1 cup low or nonfat yogurt
4 oz. veal	4 oz. beef (3 or less servings per
4 oz. lamb	week)

Carbohydrates:

Unlimited amounts of the following vegetables

all types of of lettuce	bell peppers
celery	mushrooms
radishes	sprouts
onions	tomatoes
cauliflower	zucchini
yellow squash	cabbage
spinach	cucumbers
endive	jicama
beans, yellow or green	bok choy
eggplant	escarole
kale	okra

Limited amounts of the following vegetables (3–4 servings per week)

1 small artichoke	4 oz. sweet peas
4 oz. potatoes	4 oz. yam
4 oz. carrots	4 oz. corn
4 oz. sweet potatoes	4 oz. pumpkin

Fruits: *(2 servings per day)*

1 apple	1 nectarine
1 peach	1 pear
2 apricots	2 plums
½ honeydew	10 grapes
10 cherries	2 plums
1 cup berries	1 cup watermelon
½ cup fresh pineapple	½ cantaloupe

Limited amounts of the following fruits (3–4 servings per week)

½ banana	1 cup papaya
½ mango	½ cup raisins
1½ dried figs	8 oz. fruit juices
1½ dates	½ cup cranberries

Complex carbohydrates:

Legumes, grains, and grain products (2 servings per day)

1 slice whole grain bread	½ cup brown rice
½ cup bulgur	½ cup oatmeal

½ cup quinoa
½ cup cereal
½ cup pasta
½ oz. tortilla chips
1 rice cake
½ pita bread
½ cup spelt or kamut

¼ bagel
½ English muffin
½ cup granola
½ waffle
2 cup popped popcorn
1 corn tortilla
⅓ cup dried beans

Fats: *(2 servings per day)*

7 almonds or ½ tsp. almond
  butter
⅓ tsp. canola oil
⅓ tsp. olive oil
3 olives
⅓ tsp. peanut oil

½ tbsp. avocado
½ tbsp. tahini
1 tsp. olive oil and vinegar dressing
½ tbsp. peanut butter
6 peanuts

Limited amounts of the following fats (3–4 servings per week)

1 tsp. mayonnaise
⅓ tsp. soybean oil
½ tsp. brazil nuts
⅓ tsp. butter
1 tsp. cream cheese
⅓ tsp. lard

½ tsp. sesame oil
½ tsp. walnuts
2 tsp. bacon bits
½ tbsp. cream
½ tbsp. sour cream
⅓ tsp. margarine

CANDIDA YEAST AVOIDANCE DIET

After being treated with NAET for Candida and yeast, I recommend my patients follow this diet for ten days. I also prescribe a natural antifungal formula to take for eight to ten weeks.

Avoid eating the following foods:

- dairy products excluding unsweetened yogurt

- yeast products such as bread, baked goods, pastries, crackers, beer, and wine

- substitute lard, Crisco, margarine, hydrogenated vegetable oils, safflower, soybean, cottonseed, and corn oils with extra virgin olive oil, grapeseed, flax, canola, or sesame oils

- pasta, corn, and corn oils

- fruits or juices

- apple cider vinegar, hops, malts, and other fermented products

- peanuts, peanut butter, and other seeds (nuts and nut butters are permitted as long as they are roasted)

- mushrooms

- marbled meats, all processed meats, bacon, sausage, corned beef, and ham

- potato chips, other fried snack foods, and fried foods in general

- all forms of simple sugars, sucrose, fructose, malt sugar, honey, date sugar, molasses, turbinado sugar (this includes candy, soda pop, and desserts)

- condiments such as soy sauce, catsup, mayonnaise, barbecue sauce, and MSG

- leftover food in general

- rice or rice cakes

- regular coffee, instant coffee, and teas of all sorts including herbal teas

Foods you can eat:

- lean cuts of meat including beef, veal, pork, lamb, wild game, eggs, chicken, turkey, shellfish, and fish (not breaded)

- unlimited amounts of low carbohydrate vegetables, seeds, and grains (see list below)

- moderate amounts of high carbohydrate vegetables (1 serving per day)

- very limited amounts of whole grains (3–4 servings per week—see list below)

Low carbohydrate vegetables:

Asparagus	Greens such as spinach, mustard,
Beets	beets, collards, kale
Broccoli	All types of lettuce
Brussel sprouts	Okra
Cabbage	Onions
Carrots	Parsley

Cauliflower
Celery
Cucumbers
Eggplant
Green peppers

Radishes
Soybeans
String beans
Fresh tomatoes
Turnips

Nuts, seeds, and oils (unprocessed and roasted):

Almonds
Brazil nuts
Cashews

Filberts
Pecans
Pumpkin seeds

High carbohydrate vegetables:

Beans and peas (dried and
  cooked)
Lima beans
Peas

Sweet corn
Sweet potatoes
Winter squash (acorn, butternut)
White potatoes

Whole gains:

Barley
Millet

Oats

Gastritis Diet

I recommend to individuals who are suffering from epigastric irritation to avoid the following gastric irritants:

Alcohol
Aspirin
Amino acids
Bile salts
Caffeine, caffeinated tea
Calcium
Chocolate
Cloves
Coffee, decaffeinated coffee
Mustard

Niacin
Nicotine
Nutmeg
Peppermint oil
Peppers (black, red, and chili)
Progesterone
Spearmint oil
Tomatoes
Vinegar

FOODS CONTAINING OXALIC AND URIC ACID

Foods Containing High Oxalic Acid

Beans in tomato sauce
Beets
Blackberries
Black raspberries
Blueberries
Celery
Chocolate
Cocoa
Collards
Concord grapes
Dandelion greens
Eggplant
Escarole
Green gooseberries
Green peppers
Grits
Lager beer

Leeks
Lemon peel
Lime peel
Okra
Parsley
Peanuts
Pecans
Red currants
Rhubarb
Rutabagas
Soybean crackers
Spinach
Summer squash
Sweet potatoes
Swiss chard
Tea
Wheat germ

Foods Containing Low Oxalic Acid

Apple juice
Avocados
Bananas
Barley water
Bottled beer
Broccoli
Brussels sprouts
Butter
Cabbage
Cauliflower
Cheese
Cherries
Chicken noodle soup
Chives
Cider
Cocoa-Cola®
Cornflakes
Cucumbers
Dry sherry

Eggs
Fish (except sardines)
Grapefruit juice
Jelly with permitted fruit
Lemon juice
Lettuce
Lime juice
Macaroni
Mangoes
Margarine
Meats
Melons
Milk
Mushrooms
Nectarines
Oatmeal
Onions
Orange juice
Peaches

Peas
Pepsi®
Pineapples
Plums
Poultry
Radishes

Red plum jam
Rice
Seedless grapes
Turnips
White potatoes
Wine

Foods Containing High Uric Acid

Asparagus
Beef
Breads and cereals
Cauliflower
Chicken, duck, and turkey
Crab, lobster, and oysters
Eel
Fish, fresh and saltwater
Game meats
Green peas
Herring
Kidney
Lamb, pork, veal, and beef
Legumes, beans, lentils, and peas

Liverbreads and cereals
Mackerel
Meat
Meat extracts
Meat soups and broths
Mushrooms
Oatmeal
Sardines
Scallops
Spinach
Sweetbreads
Wheat germ and bran
Whole grains

Foods Containing Low Uric Acid

Cheese
Coffee, tea, and sodas
Eggs
Fats
Fruits and fruit juices
Gelatin

Milk
Nuts
Other vegetables beside the
   ones listed above
Sugars, syrups, sweets

ACID- AND ALKALINE-FORMING FOODS
Alkaline-Forming Foods

Fruits:
Apples
Apricots
Bananas
Berries
Cranberries
Currants
Grapefruit

Grapes
Lemons
Melons
Oranges
Pears
Persimmons
Pineapple
Plums

Prunes
Ripe olives
Vegetables:
Artichokes
Asparagus
Beets
Brussel sprouts
Cabbage
Carrots
Cauliflower
Celery
Cucumbers
Beans:
Dried peas
Nuts:
Almonds
Dairy:
Milk

Tangerines

Endive
Fresh peppers
Lettuce
Mushrooms
Onions
Parsley
Parsnips
Peas
Sweet potatoes

Lima beans

Fresh coconut
Roasted chestnuts
Yogurt

Acid-Forming Foods

Starches:
Barley
Bran
Cornstarch
Crackers
Dried corn
Proteins:
Bacon
Baking powder
Beef
Cheese
Chicken
Clams
Crab
Duck
Eggs
Dairy Products:
All cheese
Butter

Pastries
Rye bread
Spaghetti
White bread
White flour
Whole wheat bread

Fish
Lamb
Liver
Lobster
Oysters
Pork
Scallops
Shrimp
Veal

Ice cream
Malted milk

Neutral

Corn oil
Cottonseed oil
Olive oil

Peanut oil
Sesame oil
Soybean oil

MOST COMMON INFECTANTS FOR ASTHMATICS

Bacteria

Bacteria Morgan
Bacteria Proteus
Borrelia burgdorferi—Lyme
Brucella abortus (Bang's bacillus)
Campylobacter
Clostridium innocuum
Corynebacterium anaerobius
Enterococcinum
Hemophilus vaginal
Klebsiella
Medorrhinum
Mycoplasma pneumoniae
Peptococc./Micrococc.
Pittsburgh pneumon. agent
Propionibacterium acnes

Streptococcinum
Streptococcus abdominus
Streptococcus aureus
Streptococcus faecalis
Streptococcus pyogenes
Streptococcus viridans
Thermibact. intestinalis
Tuberculinum Avis
Tuberculinum Denys
Tuberculinum Koch
Tuberculinum Marmorek
Tuberculinum residuum
Tuberculinum Rosenbach
Ureaplasma urealytica
Yersinia enterocolitica

Fungi

Alternaria
Aspergillus fumigatus
Aspergillus niger
Candida albicans
Candida pseudotropicalis
Candida rugosa
Candida tropicalis
Cladosporium

Epicococcum
Gliocladium fimbriatum
Helminthosporium sativum
Schimmelpilz I & II
Scopulariopsis brevicaulis
Trichoderma viride
Trichophyton tonsurans
Verticillium albo-atrum

Parasites

Amoebic liver abscess
Ascaris lumbricoides
Blastocystis hominis
Dientamoeba fragilis
Endolimax nana
Entamoeba coli
Filariasis
Giardia lamblia
Onchocerca volvulus
Taenia saginata

Blood Flukes: Bilharzia
  (Schistosoma)
Intestinal Flukes: Heterophyes
  heterophyes
Liver Flukes: Opisthorchis
  felineus
Lung Flukes: Paragonimus
  yokpgawai

Viruses

Adenovirus
Coxsackievirus A_7
Coxsackievirus B_1
Coxsackievirus B_2
Coxsackievirus B_3
Coxsackievirus B_5
Coxsackievirus B_6
Cytomegalovirus (CMV)
Echovirus
Enteric R.R. virus
Epstein-Barr virus (EBV)
Hepatitis A
Hepatitis B
Hepatitis non-A non-B

Herpes simplex I
Herpes simplex II
Herpes zoster
Human papillomavirus (HPV)
Infectious mononucleosis
Morbillinum (Measles)
Newcastle disease
Poliomyelitis
Respiratory synctial
Rhinovirus
Rubeola (rubella)
Varicella
Variola
Verruca (wart)

SPONDYLOTHERAPY

When breathing is difficult, have someone perform this procedure on your back. Ask the person to place one finger on each side of the C7 vertebra. C7 corresponds to the first protruding vertebra when the head is slightly tilted forward (refer to Figure 15–1). With the fingers at a right angle, tap gently approximately eighty times at one-second intervals. Repeat the procedure two to three times or until breathing becomes easier. This procedure can be done on a young child as long as it is done gently.

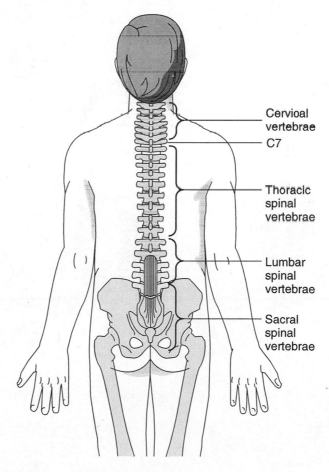

Cervioal
vertebrae

C7

Thoraclc
spinal
vertebrae

Lumbar
spinal
vertebrae

Sacral
spinal
vertebrae

Figure 15–1 Spondylotherapy Procedure

HIATAL HERNIA SOFT TISSUE PROCEDURE

Self-administer the hiatal hernia procedure whenever you have difficulty breathing after a meal. Often, acidity from the stomach area will cause undigested food to ride up, thereby creating pressure on the diaphragm and reducing the ability of the lungs to expand. Place the fingers of both hands right below where the ribs come together on the chest (refer to Figure 15–2). Simultaneously push in toward your back and down toward your feet. The movement should be consistent but gentle. This takes the pressure off the diaphragm and should ease breathing. Repeat the procedure until breathing is relieved.

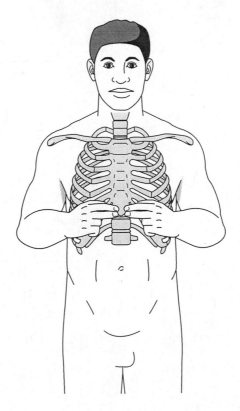

Figure 15–2   Hiatal Hernia Soft Tissue Procedure

EMDR: A NEW BREAKTHROUGH IN THERAPY

By Stephen Bodian, M.A.

What is EMDR?

EMDR (eye movement desensitization and reprocessing) is an important new psychotherapeutic technique developed by Francine Shapiro, Ph.D., a psychologist in Palo Alto. EMDR has been used with unprecedented success in the "desensitization and reprocessing" of traumatic memories.

Initially Dr. Shapiro and others had dramatic results with people suffering from the painful after-effects of rape, childhood sexual abuse, and traumatic Vietnam War experiences, a condition known as post-traumatic stress disorder (PTSD). In some cases, veterans who had suffered from nightmares and flashbacks for many years were cured of these symptoms in a few sessions. More recently, EMDR has been used successfully in treating a range of problems from phobias and free-floating anxieties to mild depression, relationship difficulties, eating disorders, low self-esteem, and grief.

How Does EMDR Work?

Dr. Shapiro discovered the technique serendipitously while noticing how she naturally processed her own unpleasant recurring memories. Although she does not claim to fully understand how it works, she offers the following tentative explanation:

> In REM (dream) sleep, we process the unpleasant experiences of the preceding day with "rapid eye movements," somehow "metabolizing" them so they do not continue to disturb us. When experiences are traumatic, however, REM sleep is insufficient to process them through. As a result, we store them in the nervous system as highly charged memories, usually associated with strong feelings and beliefs about ourselves and the world. Using eye movements similar to those of REM sleep, EMDR facilitates the reemergence and reprocessing of these memories; they no longer haunt us in the present as unwanted negative emotions and beliefs, but take their appropriate place in the perspective of the past, where they belong.

What is EMDR therapy like?

Most psychotherapists use EMDR, along with a variety of other methods, in the context of a caring, supportive, therapeutic relationship. Although it can be very effective, EMDR is not a magic elixir, and it does not seem to be equally effective with everyone.

In EMDR therapy itself, clients focus on a traumatic memory and/or a strong feeling or negative belief. If no memory is available, a feeling or belief will often be sufficient. While holding this focus, clients follow with their eyes the side-to-side motion of the therapist's fingers. After 30 or 40 such "passes," clients are asked to stop, take a deep breath, and report on what they have experienced.

Feelings may intensify (and sometimes discharge) before waning or even disappearing entirely. New memories may surface and/or old memories may become more vivid and detailed. And most significant of all, one's beliefs about oneself and the world—usually based on how one holds, or interprets, one's past experiences—may change dramatically. By the end of a session or series of sessions, painful memories and negative beliefs lose some or all of their charge, and present events no longer seem so difficult or threatening.

For each client and each problem, the approach used and the results obtained differ substantially. In many cases, EMDR ultimately roots out and reprocesses the feelings, memories, and unresolved issues that are keeping clients from moving forward in their lives.

Who can benefit from EMDR?

Clinical experience suggests that people with a range of problems can benefit from the use of EMDR. In particular, those whose difficulties are the direct result of traumatic or otherwise painful past experiences respond especially well to EMDR. If a person was physically, sexually, or emotionally mistreated as a child, experienced unresolved grief for the loss of a loved one, suffered the trauma of physical injuries or accidents, or been the victim of a natural disaster or a violent crime, EMDR is the treatment of choice. Guilt, fear, anxiety, low self-esteem, relationship difficulties, and depression have also responded well to EMDR, and continued investigation is constantly yielding new applications for the technique.

If you have any further questions about EMDR please call (415) 454-6149.

Stephan Bodian, M.A., is a psychotherapist in San Rafael, California, and an experienced practitioner of EMDR. In the context of a caring, supportive, therapeutic relationship, he has used the technique effectively for more than four years, with both men and women, in treating a range of client problems. He is the former editor of the Yoga Journal *and author of* Timeless Visions, Healing Voices.

NAET PRACTITIONERS

Names of Professionals Who Have Taken the NAET Seminars

Entries in italic type indicates those who have completed advanced NAET seminars. Look for an updated list of names on our Internat site, http://www.allergy2000.com.

ALASKA

Allen, George E.
3858 Lake Street, #20
Homer, AK 99603
907-235-7221

Azeltine, Ty Warren
P.O. Box 231366
Anchorage, AK 99503
907-563-9911

Denton, Sandra, M.D.
3201 C Street, #306,
Anchorage, AK 99503
907-563-6200

Hoch, Pamela L., C.M.T.
304 Cindy Drive
Fairbanks, AK 99701
907-456-8030

Iblen, Sandi L., R.N.
500 East Tudor
Anchorage, AK 99503
907-561-6846

Jacques, Sandra Talt, D.C.
4316 Kingston Drive
Anchorage, AK 99504
907-337-6770

Krohn, Joyce Ellen, L.Ac.
119 Second Street
Juneau, AK 99801
907-586-2577

Lamothe, Nick
4001 Lake Otis Parkway
Anchorage, AK 99508
907-346-8000

Lizer, Gerald
Mile 15½ Old Glenn Highway
Eagle River, AK 99522
907-694-9535

Miller, Marianne, D.C., P.C.
4050 Lake Otis Parkway
Anchorage, AK 99508
907-562-1062

Muller, Lela Karlene
35330 K-Beach Road, Suite 6
Soldotna, AK 99669
907-262-7977

Rowen, Robert
615 East 82nd Avenue
Anchorage, AK 99518
907-344-7775

Salzmann, Toni, R.N.
3201 C Street, #306
Anchorage, AK 99503
907-563-6200

Trekell, S.G., D.C.
7536 Lake Otis Parkway
Anchorage, AK 99523

ARIZONA

Wey, Peter, D.C.
1632 East Cottonwood Street
Cottonwood, AZ 86326
520-639-1700

CALIFORNIA

Absu, Robert, N.D., L.Ac.
25500 Rancho Niguel Road
Laguna Niguel, CA 92677
714-831-1340

Allen, Corinne
20505 Yerba Linda Boulevard 507
Yerba Linda, CA 92886

Barta, Jeanne, D.C.
5011 Clayton Road
Concord, CA 94521
510-682-4941

Beatie, Nina, D.C.
828 School Street
Napa CA 94559
707-258-0664

Bebb-Walker, Sydney, L.Ac.
5180 Sonoma Mountain Road
Santa Rosa, CA 95404
707-544-8802

Becker, Lee, L.Ac., O.M.D.
720 Haverford Avenue
Pacific Palisades, CA 90272
310-459-1194

Becker, Steven, D.C.
2001 S. Barrington Avenue
Los Angeles, CA 90025
310-479-0367

Belanger, Charles, L.Ac.
1620 Olive Avenue
Richmond, CA 94805
510-215-9525

Bledsoe, Peg, MA, OTR
12919 Alcosta Boulevard, Suite 10
San Ramon, CA 94583
510-866-1311

Bunis, Sobyl E., D.C.
34 East Sola Street
Santa Barbara, CA 93101
805-966-3003

Bush, Dave, D.C.
20631 Ventura Boulevard, #203
Woodland Hills, CA 91364
818-704-1662

Cadwallader, Claudia, L.Ac.,
    Dipl.N.B.A.O., Q.M.E.
891 Pismo Street
San Luis Obispo, CA 93401
805-541-2563

Chambreau, Marylyn, D.C.
925 North San Antonio Road
Los Altos, CA 94022
415-948-3282

Chapman, Caden, C.H.
17900 Sherman Way, #208
Reseda, CA 91335
818-757-1121

Chin, Eleanor, D.C.
50 First Street, #301
San Francisco, CA 94105
415-243-0678

Cooper, Carol, L.Ac., L.C.S.W.
32 Palm Drive
Camarillo, CA 93010
805-388-7663

Curry, Mary, L.Ac., Ph.D., O.M.D.
1502A Walnut Street
Berkeley, CA 94709
510-530-8886

Cutler, Ellen, D.C.
770 Tamalpais Drive, Suite 203
Corte Madera, CA 94925
415-924-2273

Cutler, Steven C., D.C.
770 Tamalpais Drive, Suite 203
Corte Madera, CA 94925
415-924-2273

Dickson, Martha H., D.C.
2224 Loma Vista Drive
Sacramento, CA 95825
916-974-3434

Doyle, Kathy, D.C.
5545 Claremont Avenue
Oakland, CA 94618
510-601-6325

Dubner, Allen, D.C.
10320 South De Anza Boulevard
Suite 1C
Cupertino, CA 95014
408-996-1042

Dubner, Sharon, D.C.
10320 South De Anza Boulevard
Suite 1C
Cupertino, CA 95014
408-996-1042

Eberstein, Jocelyne
10780 Santa Monica Boulevard
Los Angeles, CA 90025
310-446-1968

Elbin, Marlene
5824 Marshall Street
Oakland, CA 94608
510-601-8233

Elias, Ann, L.Ac.
214 Main Street, P.O. Box 669
Weaverville, CA 95573
916-623-2668

Esparza, Moctesuma
5618 Berkshire Drive
Los Angeles, CA 90032
310-281-3770

Fairfield, Peter, L.Ac.
364 Devon Drive
San Rafael, CA 94903
415-479-4239

Feldman, Nelson
3301 Alta Arden Suites
Sacramento, CA 95825
916-482-8600

Finkbine, Steven
22 Belle Avenue
San Anselmo, CA 94960
415-454-8008

Fitzgerald, Theresa, D.C.
2904 Rowena Avenue
Los Angeles, CA 90036
213-660-2370

Garbutt, Alfred, D.C.
1036 Sherlock Drive
Burbank, CA 91501
818-845-4678

George-Rydberg, Susan, L.Ac.
4910 Van Nuys Boulevard
Sherman Oaks, CA 91403
818-981-3440

Gold, Michelle, D.C.
2200 Range Avenue, Suite 100
Santa Rosa, CA 95403
707-579-2234

Goodkin, Valarie, L.Ac.
237 South Third Avenue
Covina, CA 91723
818-445-0326

Gordon, Arlo, D.C.
4791 Cromwell Avenue
Los Angeles, CA 90036
213-668-0711

Gorrie, David R., D.C.
17482 Irvine Boulevard, Suite C
Tustin, CA 92780
714-544-9789

Grill, John, D.D.S.
9900 Balboa Boulevard, Suite A
Northridge, CA 91325
818-701-0388

Heckard, Bruce L.
1754 Second Street, Suite A
Napa, CA 94559
707-226-8683

Herrick, Anne, L.Ac.
2214 Eunice Street
Berkeley, CA 94709
510-528-9821

Hilsdale, Karin, Ph.D., L.Ac.
301 South Fair Oaks, #102
Pasadena, CA 91105
818-585-8877

Hom, Henry, L.Ac.
1193 Valencia Street
San Francisco, CA 94110
415-647-6222

Inouye, Stanley, D.D.S.
5716 Dorset Way
Sacramento, CA 95822
916-421-2890

Johnson, Dale S., B.S.N, R.N., N.D.
230 Alder Drive
Bolinas, CA 94924
415-868-1578

Jones, Marilynn Snow, D.C.
23622 Calabasas Road, #153
Calabasas, CA 91302
818-222-2080

Josephian, Jenny, L.Ac.
1502A Walnut Street
Berkeley, CA 94709
510-548-2261

Klassy, Thomas M., I.D.E.
319 Center Street
Weaverville, CA 96093
916-623-2014

Koven, Arianne, N.D.
69115 Ramon Road, #1386
Cathedral City, CA 92234
619-328-1070

Krestan, Sandy
6016 Bernhard Avenue
Richmond, CA 94805
510-237-9952

Laborde, Leta
7589 Navigator Circle
Carlsbad, CA 92009
619-930-1949

Langer, Mark, D.C., C.C.S.P.
1928 Lombard Street
San Francisco, CA 94123
415-921-1448

Levy, Judith, L.Ac.
3001 J Street, #100
Sacramento, CA 95816
916-443-8100

Lindquist, Kirstin, L.Ac.
485 Elwood Avenue
Oakland, CA 94610
510-834-5246

Lippman, Cathie, M.D.
291 South La Cienega Boulevard
Beverly Hills, CA 90211
310-289-8430

Lydick, W. Shannon, L.Ac.
73-955 B Highway 111
Palm Desert, CA 92263
619-776-4599

Mackewicz, Stephen, L.Ac.
129 Yolo Street
Corte Madera, CA 94925
415-927-1606

Margaret, Joan, D.C.
6536 Telegraph Avenue, #A-102
Oakland, CA 94609
510-658-9066

Merlino, Kim, L.Ac.
626 Frederick Street
Santa Cruz, CA 95062
408-426-1251

Morris, Dean
555 South Sunrise Way, Suite 211
Palm Springs, CA 92264
619-322-9888

Muzychenko, John, L.Ac.
726 West Barston Avenue, #103
Fresno, CA 93704
209-479-0355

Nambudripad, Devi S., D.C. L.Ac.,
*   O.M.D., Ph.D.*
Acupuncture/Chiropractic Pain Clinic
6714 Beach Boulevard
Buena Park, CA 90621
714-523-8900/714-523-0800

Nehring, Nancy A., L.M.T.
410 West Electric Avenue, #B
La Habra, CA 90631
310-694-2486

Norton, Mary, L.Ac.
200 Broadway
Fairfax, CA 94930
415-257-4007

Pallos, Andrew, D.D.S.
30131 Town Center Drive
Laguna Niguel, CA 92677
714-495-6484

Pang, Raymond, L.Ac., N.D.
2000 Van Ness Avenue, #612
San Francisco, CA 94109
415-921-4608

Paustian, Dennis M., D.C.
2035 West Carson Street
Torrance, CA 90501
310-533-0223

Rakela, Nancy, O.M.D., L.Ac.
1802 Tenth Street
Berkeley, CA 94710
510-843-8032

Raviv, Hagit, L.Ac.
14357 Miranda Street
Van Nuys, CA 91401
818-787-8435

Rawlinson, Ian, L.Ac.
405 D Street
Petaluma, CA 94952
707-762-4309

Reuben, Carolyn, L.Ac.
4220 H Street
Sacramento, CA 95819
916-452-5887

Rose, Johanne, L.Ac.
5706 Corsa Avenue, Suite 102
Westlake Village, CA 91362
818-889-1421

Rosenblum, Nava
460 Pitt Avenue, #3
Sebastopol, CA 95472
707-823-4153

Ryf, Hope, L.Ac.
223 Thousand Oaks Boulevard, #324
Thousand Oaks, CA 91360
805-497-4074

Sage, Crystal, N.D.
616 Loretto Drive
Roseville, CA 95661
916-482-4499

Sakamoto, Jenny, L.Ac.
23441 Madison Street, #215
Torrance, CA 90505
310-373-0368

Schwartz, Robert A., D.C.
4454 Van Nuys Boulevard, #103
Sherman Oaks, CA 91403
818-990-3084

Segura, Lynn Keiko, L.Ac.
2615 Ashby Avenue
Berkeley, CA 94705
510-843-5000

Shami, Fethi, D.C.
8904 South Vermont Avenue
Los Angeles, CA 90044
213-752-3399

Shu, Steven T., O.M.D., Ph.D.
369 San Miguel Drive
Newport Beach, CA 92660
714-759-1869

Singler, Marjorie, L.Ac., M.A.
1844 San Miguel Drive
Walnut Creek, CA 94596
510-930-9422

Smillie, Jacque
147 E. Vine, Suite 10
Redlands, CA 92373
909-335-1980

Smith, Kenneth J.
4493 Triangle Road
Mariposa, CA 95338
209-966-5634

Sovola-Johnson, Shelley
838 4th Street
Crescent City, CA 95531
707-465-4114

Specht, Andrew W., D.C.
230 Second Street, #101
Encinitas, CA 92024
619-632-0098

Steele, Jan K., O.M.D., L.Ac.
5225 Wilshire Boulevard, Suite 618
Los Angeles, CA 90036
213-936-3162

Stetson, Keith, C.A.
712 Gilman Street
Berkeley, CA 94710
510-526-7125

Stout, Joanellen M., O.M.D., L.Ac.
10447 Magnolia Boulevard
North Hollywood, CA 91601
818-769-1798

Talebi, Fatima
23028 Lake Forest Drive, Suite D,
Laguna Hills, CA 92653
714-707-2877

Tamminen, Ann G., L.Ac.
7860 Brookside Avenue
Sebastopol, CA 95472
707-829-9712

1502 Walnut Street, Suite A
Berkeley, CA 94709
510-845-2094

Tatsuno, Walter T., D.C.
8950 Villa La Jolla Drive, #1100
La Jolla, CA 92037
619-457-0283

Thomas, Craig M., D.C.
1260 North Dutton Avenue, Suite 160

Santa Rosa, CA 95401
707-527-7313

Thomas, Helen M., D.C.
1260 North Dutton Avenue, Suite 160
Santa Rosa, CA 95401
707-527-7313

Valentine, Leonard
17213 Brookhurst
Fountain Valley, CA 92708
714-964-9566

Venzke, Liane, L.Ac.
124 Washington Avenue
Point Richmond, CA 94801
510-236-9403

Wagner, Carina, L.Ac.
819 Longwood Lane
Sebastopol, CA 95472
707-823-3456

Wallerstein, Dale R., D.C.
3932 Ponderosa Road
Shingle Springs, CA 95682
916-676-2233

Watkins, Alexandra, D.C.
2115 J Street, #105
Sacramento, CA 95816
916-441-2501

Whittlesey, James
7075 Redwood Boulevard, Suite E
Novato, CA 94945
707-898-0889

Wootten, Royelyn
3720 Ahl Park Court
Santa Rosa, CA 95405
707-525-1476

Zadis, Cindy, D.C.
821 Mendocino Avenue
Santa Rosa, CA 95404
707-572-7710

*Weiner, Neal K., D.V.M.
Lewiston Animal Clinic, P.O. Box 628
Lewiston, CA 96052
916-778-3109

Wolf, Barbara, L.Ac.
38 Miller Avenue, # 152
Mill Valley, CA 94941
415-838-8895
770 Tamalpais Drive, Suite 203
Corte Madera, CA 94925
415-924-2273

COLORADO

Blevins, Mary C., N.D.
5322 Pinon Valley Road
Colorado Springs, CO 80919
719-598-0373

Cortini, Cynthia M.
7030 S. Yosemite Street, Suite 220
Inglewood, CO 80112
303-721-9984

Culver, Roy A., D.C.
1316 Vivian Street
Longmont, CO 80501
303-651-1234

Melos, Linda, N.D.
280 East Bridge Street
Hotchkiss, CO 81419
970-527-6691

Mercay, Jessie, D.C.
2525 Arapahoe
Boulder, CO 80303
303-753-2544
3318 East Second Avenue
Denver, CO 80210
303-753-2543

Messer, Alan R.
829 Main Street, Suite 6
Longmont, CO 80501
303-776-6110

Owens, Beth G., O.M.D.
7661 South Ulster Court
Englewood, CO 80112
303-770-6704

Salsman, G.W.
1231 Lake Plaza
Colorado Springs, CO 80906
719-579-0180

Thomas, Jeana, D.C.
1711 South Pearl Street
Denver, CO 80210
303-744-6567

CONNECTICUT

Bailey, Richard J., D.C.
46 Mill Plain Road
Danbury, CT 06811
203-790-9563

GEORGIA

Koeppel, Heather, D.C.
1945 Cliff Valley Way, Suite 270
Atlanta, GA 30329
404-633-8255

Shin, Young S., M.D.
3850 Holcomb Bridge Road, Suite 438
Atlanta, GA 30092
770-242-0000

FLORIDA

Andely, Cynthia
100 Kings Point Drive, #1408
North Miami Beach, FL 33160
305-947-2701

Drucker, Steven, D.C.
327 Plaza Real, Suite 205
Boca Raton, FL 33432
407-392-7989

Ferrance, Paula T., A.P.
3501 Jackson Street, #206
Hollywood, FL 33021
954-986-9882

Fuller, Joseph E., D.C.
136 East Colonial
Orlando, FL 32801
407-843-1111

Kenemuth, David W.
524 First Street South
Winter Haven, FL 33880
941-294-5399

Kufe, Marita, A.P., L.Ac., O.M.D.
505 South Orange Avenue
Sarasota, FL 34232
941-366-1110

Lucarelli, Jennifer
6756 Pines Boulevard
Pembroke Pines, FL 33024
954-989-1220

Phillips, Douglas
4512 Poinsetta Avenue
West Palm Beach, FL 33407
407-848-1720

Pollak, Joseph, D.C.
1025 Forest Hill Boulevard
West Palm Beach, FL 33406
561-964-6797

Russell, Robert V.
7522 Southwest 62nd Street
Miami, FL 33143
305-667-8787

HAWAII

Amdur, Latifa, N.D.
P.O. Box 1232
Hanalei, HI 96714
808-828-1155

Christman, J. Randol, D.A.C.
3402 Keha Drive
Kihei, Maui, HI 96753
808-879-4341

Conner, Yvonne, M.D.
P.O. Box 2987
Wailuku, HI 96793
808-249-0124

Fickes, Linda A., D.C.
4400-4 Kalanianaole Highway
Honolulu, HI 96821
808-377-1811

Jones, Molly, L.Ac.
P.O. Box 658
Kapaa, HI 96746
808-822-2884

Kroll, Joni, L.Ac.
320 Uluniu Street, #2
Kailua, HI 96734
808-262-4550

Lee, Scott, R.N., L.Ac.
159 Keawe Street, Suite 5
Hilo, HI 96720
808-969-6819

Nutter, Barry J., D.C.
4614 Kilauea Avenue, #511
Honolulu, HI 96816
808-531-2015

Tan, Karen, N.D., L.Ac.
615 Piikoi St., PH-2
Honolulu, HI 96814
808-593-9445

Tavily, Farangis
P.O. Box 1487
Pahaa, HI 96778
808-334-3905

IDAHO

Cozzie, Robert, L.Ac.
P.O. Box 973
Sand Point, ID 83864
208-263-4512

Hadley, Linda, N.D., D.Sc., Ph.D.
11155 West Edna Street
Boise, ID 83713
208-322-9376

ILLINOIS

Baschleben, Jacquelyn A., D.C.
11673 Main Street
Roscoe, IL 61073
815-623-7694

Edwards, Kenneth M., D.C.
18W265–73rd Street
Darien, IL 60561
603-964-6410

Elewa, Hany, D.C.
11673 Main Street
Roscoe, IL 61073
815-623-7694

Manaligod, Librada, M.D.
104 South Michigan Avenue, #705
Chicago, IL 60603
312-372-8384

IOWA

Christensen, Laura, M.A.
414 Highland Court
Iowa City, IA 52246
319-341-0031

Frogley, Chris J.
1605 West Kimberly Road
Davenport, IA 52806
319-386-4798

KANSAS

Carver, Marcy R., N.D.
1206 South Washington
Liberal, KS 67901
316-624-9262

Christensen, James, D.O.
209 West Seventh
Coffeyville, KS 67337
316-251-1100

KENTUCKY

Konopka, Anthony
8909 Highway 329
Crestwood, KY 40014
502-241-8621

MAINE

Tsao, Fern, L.Ac.
One Roberts Road
Yarmouth, ME 04096
207-846-4433

MARYLAND

Beals, Paul V., M.D.
9101 Cherry Lane
Laurel, MD 20708
301-490-9911

Fradkin, Mark, L.Ac.
9199 Reistertown Road
Owings Mills, MD 21117
410-363-7254

Rothstein, Judy, L.Ac.
8167 Main Street, Suite 203
Ellicott City, MD 21043
410-461-6543

Stearns, Rebecca L.
6216 Montrose Road
Rockville, MD 20852
301-230-1477

MICHIGAN

Keyte, Gerald, D.
58024 Van Dyke
Washington, MI 48095
810-781-5535

Krofcheck, David L., O.M.D.
501 East Columbia Avenue
Battle Creek, MI 49015
616-962-2836

MINNESOTA

Caldwell, George S.
4379 Wilshire Boulevard, #C-312
Mound, MN 55364

NEVADA

Hetzel, David R.
2591 Windmill Parkway, #2
Henderson, NV 89014
702-260-1164

NEW JERSEY

Boals, Gordon, Ph.D.
985 Patton Street
North Brunswick, NJ 08902
908-246-1939

Huber, Scott, D.C.
2168 Millburn Avenue
Maplewood, NJ 07040
201-761-1153

NEW MEXICO

Bartnett, Beatrice, D.C., N.D., L.M.T.
1204 Mechem #10
Ruidoso, NM 88345
505-258-3046

Robinson, Robert E., D.O.M.
1502 South Saint Francis Drive
Santa Fe, NM 87505
505-983-3009

NEW YORK

Abrams, Judith, P.A., L.Ac.
342 DeWitt Boulevard
Ithaca, NY 14850
607-277-7713

Cutler, Deborah, D.C.
101 Perry Street
New York, NY 10014
212-741-6285

Medina, Isis, D.C.
115 East 23rd Street, Sixth Floor
New York, NY 10010
212-228-5600

NORTH CAROLINA

Eap, Leang, N.D.
6548 Carmel Road, Suite 124
Charlotte, NC 28226
704-544-8681

OREGON

Chiasson, Marcelle, M.D.
4055 Southwest Garden Home Road
Portland, OR 97219
503-245-3156

Dodge, Jeanette, L.Ac.
2041 Southwest 58th, Suite 207
Portland, OR 97221
503-297-7656

Gadoua, Marc, R.C.P., M.L.Ac.
1979 Southwest Fifth
Portland, OR 97201
503-295-3647

Jacobson, Rayna, L.Ac., R.N.
923 Northeast Conch Street
Portland, OR 97232
503-236-9609

Knecht, Allen, D.C.
1809 Northwest Davis
Portland, OR 97209
503-226-8010

Liggett, Laura, L.Ac., M.W.
1125 Southwest Spokane
Portland, OR 97202
503-233-9079

Lowrie, Shelley, L.Ac.
11700 Southwest Barnes Road
Portland OR 97225
503-646-5007

Martin, Debra L., N.D.
911 Country Club Road, Suite 290
Eugene, OR 97401
541-683-4071

Page, Edie, L.Ac.
4004 Southwest Kelly, Suite 100
Portland, OR 97201
503-222-2235

Peterson, Patrice, L.Ac.
1621 East 19th Avenue
Eugene, OR 97403
541-343-5004

Sheehan, Matthew, D.C.
836 East Main Street, Suite 1
Medford, OR 97504
503-773-1321

Shefi, Ellen, L.Ac., L.M.T.
2041 Southwest 58th, #207
Portland, OR 97201
503-297-7656

Taylor, Gilda, R.N.
759 Northeast Hazelton Place
Portland, OR 97232
503-238-8097

Wilson, Robert M., N.D.
2690 May Street, Suite 2,
Hood River, OR 97031
541-386-5505

PENNSYLVANIA

Bailey, Sharon
R.R. #2, Box 6640
Seven Valleys, PA 17360
717-428-1994

Frank, Cara
6333 Wayne Avenue
Philadelphia, PA 19144
215-438-2977

Hannah, Suvarna
3463 Norwood Place
Holland, PA 18966
215-579-0409

Harris, Robert D., L.Ac.
954 Montgomery Avenue, Suite 7
Narberth, PA 19072
610-668-1114

Jaffe, Carolyn, R.Ac.
309 Madison Avenue
Reading, PA 19605
610-929-0797

Materna, Gayle, R.N., M.P.H.
642 P West Brubaker Valley Road
Lititz, PA 17543
717-625-3137

Molony, David
101 Bridge Street
Catasauqua, PA 18032
610-264-2755

Nighswonger, Monte D., D.C.
1724 Yardley-Langhorne Road
Yardley, PA 19067
215-403-2683

Steinman, Sandy, M.Ac.
2416 Lititz Pike
Lancaster, PA 17601
717-581-0351

Weiss, Don M.
7805 Hasbrook Avenue
Philadelphia, PA 19111
215-728-1413

TEXAS

Baldwin, John C.
4009 Richmond Avenue
Houston, TX 77027
713-622-7777

Dore, Danny D., M.T., H.T., E.T.
2536 1/2 Times Boulevard
Houston, TX 77005
713-528-3658

Peck, Iua Lim, L.Ac., R.N.
17194 Preston Road, Suite 222
Dallas TX 75248
214-380-9070

Sprinkle, Allen, D.D.S.
1600 West College, Suite 260
Grapevine, TX 76051
817-481-6342

Wiseman, Champion, D.C., N.D.
13492 Research Boulevard
Austin, TX 78750
512-448-5042

UTAH

Anderson, Thomas, D.C.
4568 South Highland Drive, #320
Holladay, UT 84117
801-272-9989

WASHINGTON

Bentz, James, D.C.
14670 Northeast 8th Street
Bellevue, WA 98007
206-746-4045

Crinnian, Walter J., N.D.
1200 112th Avenue Northeast
Bellevue, WA 98005
206-747-9200

Gienger, Michelle, R.N.
18020 120th Avenue Southeast
Renton, WA 98058
206-271-4850

Hatfield, Lon M., M.D.
1200 East Columbia Avenue
Colville, WA 99114
509-684-3701

Heideke, Susan, L.Ac.
726 Broadway, #301
Seattle, WA 98122
206-726-0034

Levy, Divorah, M.Ac., L.Ac.
2722 Eastlake Avenue East
Seattle, WA 98103
206-324-8600

MacPherson, Steven P.
85 Northwest Alder Place, Suite C
Issaquah, WA 98027
206-391-1080

McCombs, Ann, O.O.
1545 116th Avenue Northeast
Bellevue, WA 98004
206-451-3159

McDonald, Beth, N.D.
3409 Wetmore Avenue
Everett, WA 98201
206-252-7263

Nelson, Marilee, A., R.N.
2133 28th Street Southeast
Puyallup, WA 98372
206-851-7550

Romano, Augusto, L.Ac.
4141 California Avenue Southwest
Seattle, WA 98116
206-938-1393

Ruppert, Patricia, R.N.
312 4th Street Southeast
Puyallup, WA 98372
206-770-5504

Sandaine, Randy, N.D.
525 South Main
Colville, WA 99114
509-684-1104

Stocker, Richard
191 Winslow Way West
Bainbridge Island, WA 98110
206-842-0405

Terry, Kevin L., D.C.
11002 Valley Avenue East
Puyallup, WA 98372
206-845-0543

Whittaker, Melanie
713 Southeast Everett Mall Way #D
Everett, WA 98208
206-290-5309

WISCONSIN

Cubbs, Marylee, D.C.
4421 N. Oakland Avenue, Suite 200
Shorewood, WI 53211
414-967-9000

Ensweiler, Mark, D.C., L.Ac.
2549 Plover Road
Plover, WI 54467
715-345-0655

Oldak, Patricia A., O.T., M.T.
205 Abbey Springs Drive
Fontance, WI 53215
414-275-6437

CANADA

Lussier, Joanne, D.D.S.
12265 Grenet, Suite 300
Montreal, Quebec H4J-2J9
514-336-6454

Shamess, Fiona P.
996 Lucas Avenue
Victoria, British Columbia V8X 4H5
250-727-9502

ISRAEL

Galfsky, Izhak
26 Herzel Street
Kfar-Saba 44204
09-765-5076

Hendler, Samuel, M.D.
18 Rainess Street
Tel Aviv
03-540-4911/03-522-6030/03-522-6166

*This veterinarian uses NAET in treating animals, more specifically dogs and cats.

MISCELLANEOUS RESOURCES

Asthma and Allergy Foundation of
America
1125 15th Street N.W., Suite 502
Washington, D.C. 20005
202-466-7643
800-878-4403

Allergy & Asthma Network
Mothers of Asthmatics, Inc.
3554 Chain Bridge Road, Suite 200
Fairfax, VA 22030-2709
703-385-4403

Allergy Control Products
96 Danbury Road.
Ridgefield, CT 06877
203-438-9580

Allergy Home Care Products
P.O. Box 2471
Silver Spring, MD 20915
800-327-4382
email ahcp@aol.com
http://www.ahcp.com

Laboratory for Loomis' 24-Hour
Urinalysis
Metabolic Research Labs, Inc.
6620 West 110th Street, Suite 102
Overland Park, KA 66211
914-345-0088

For Enzyme Therapist Referral
Contact:
Enzyme Formulations
6421 Enterprise Lane
Madison, WI 53719
800-614-4400

NESS: Nutritional Enzyme Support
System
100 N.W. Business Park Lane
Riverside, MO 64150
800-637-7893

For Catalog of Natural Household
Products Contact:
7th Generation Products for a
Healthy Planet
1 Mill Street, Suite 826
Burlington VT 05401-1545
800-456-1177

For Information on NAET Seminars
Contact:
Nambudripad's Allergy Research and
Relief Foundation
614 Beach Boulevard
Buena Park, CA 90621
714-523-8900

Great Smokies Diagnostic Laboratory
63 Zillicoa Street
Asheville, NC 28801-9801
704-253-0621

BIBLIOGRAPHY

Cichoke, Anthony J., M.A., D.C., D.A.C.B.N. 1993. *New Look At Enzyme Therapy*. Portland, OR: Seven Seas Publishing.

Crook, William G., M.D. 1986. *The Yeast Connection*. New York, NY: Vintage Books.

Dunne, Lavon J. 1990. *Nutrition Almanac, 3rd ed*. New York, NY: McGraw Hill.

Guyton, Arthur C., M.D. 1991. *Textbook of Medical Physiology*. Philadelphia, PA: W. B. Saunders Company, 8th ed.

Hannaway, Paul J., M.D. 1992. *The Asthma Self-Help Book*. Rocklin, CA: Prima Publishing.

Jwing-Ming, Yang. 1996. *Chinese Qigong Massage*. Jamaica Plain, MA: YMAA Publication Center.

Kirschmann, Gayla J., and Kirschmann, John D. 1996. *Nutrition Almanac, 4th ed*. New York, NY: McGraw-Hill.

Nambudripad, Devi S., D.C., L.Ac., Ph.D., O.M.D. 1993. *Say Goodbye To Ilness*. Buena Park, CA: Delta Publishing Co.

Ornish, Dean, M.D. 1993. *Eat More, Weigh Less*. New York, NY: Harper Collins Publishers, Inc.

Pennington, Jean, A.T. 1989. *Food Values*. New York, NY: Harper Collins Publishers.

Pritikin, Robert. 1990. *The New Pritikin Program*. New York, NY: Simon & Schuster Inc.

Sears, Barry, Ph.D. 1995. *Enter The Zone*. New York, NY: Harper Collins Publishers, Inc.

Strang, Virgil V. 1984. *Essential Principles of Chiropractic*. Davenport, IA: Palmer College of Chiropractic.

Vayda, William. 1994. *Attack Asthma*. Port Melbourne, Victoria: Thomas C. Lothian Pty. Ltd.

REFERENCES

ACAAI Calls for Action to Control Risk of Potentially Life Threatening Latex Allergy. Internet.

American Journal of Respiratory and Critical Care Medicine. 1995. 152:1182–1188.

Can Magnesium-Rich Foods Help Reduce Asthma Risk? 1995. Rodale Press, Inc. Magazine Collection 78F2164.

Cichoke, Anthony T., D.C., D.A.C.B.N. 1993. *New Look at Enzyme Therapy.* Porland, OR: Seven C's Publishing.

Guyton, Arthur C., M.D. *Textbook of Medical Physiology*, 7th Ed. Philadelphia, PA: R. Saunders.

High-Salt Diet May Aggravate Asthma in Men. 1994. California Center for Medical Consumers, Inc. Magazine Collection 73A3454.

Kahn, J. 1995. Heartburn May Be Cause of Asthma in Some Cases. *Medical Tribune News Service (Medscape).*

Kahn, J. 1995. Synthetic Pillows May Aggravate Asthma Symptoms. *Medical Tribune News Service.*

Kahn, J. 1996. Cooking with Gas May Increase Risk of Asthma Attacks in Women. *Medscape,* March 21.

Link Between Indoor Allergens and Children's Asthma. March, 1996. American College of Allergy, Asthma, and Immunology.

Luciano, Ralph J. 1978. Direct Observation and Photography of Electroconductive Points on Human Skin. *American Journal of Acupuncture* No. 4, Vol. 6, October-December.

Mann, D. 1995. Long-Term Estrogen May Double Risk of Developing Disease. *Medscape,* December 7.

Tamkins, Theresa. 1995. Adult-Onset Asthma May Be Allergic Reaction to Bacteria. *Medical Tribune (Medscape).*

Tamkins, Theresa. 1995. Work Related Asthma: A Widespread Problem. *Medical Tribune News Service.*

Vimy, Murray J. *Toxic Teeth: The Chronic Mercury Poisoning of Modern Man.* International DMAS Newsletter, Vol. V, Issue 2. Albuquerque, NM: Murlene Brake.

GLOSSARY

Allergen   Any physical, nutritional, or emotional substance that causes an allergic response in an individual. An allergen is an antigen that usually causes an IgE antibody response.

Allergy   Inappropriate or exaggerated reactions of the immune system to substances that in the majority of people cause no symptoms.

Anaphylaxis   Also known as anaphylactic shock, a severe and life-threatening allergic reaction. The reaction, which is rare, can be triggered as a reaction to a drug, insect bite, or less commonly after ingesting certain allergic foods.

Antibody   A protein, also called an immunoglobulin, manufactured by lymphocytes (types of white blood cells) to neutralize an antigen or allergen.

Antigen   A substance that can trigger an immune response, resulting in production of an antibody as part of the body's defense mechanism against allergies, infections, and disease.

Antihistamine   A drug that blocks the effects of histamine, a chemical released in body fluids during an allergic reaction.

Antioxidants   Free radical scavengers that remove dangerous free radical particles from the tissue, thereby strengthening the immune system, building up tissues, and regenerating the body.

Asthma   A chronic, inflammatory lung disease characterized by recurrent breathing problems. Asthma is often triggered by allergens, although infection, exercise, cold air, and other factors are also important triggers.

Attention Deficit Disorder   Also know as ADD, an increasingly serious disorder common in children who lose the ability to concentrate and focus on normal daily activities. They typically become hyperactive and irritable.

Autoimmune Reaction   An allergic reaction within or to one's own body or systems. Numerous autoimmune disorders exist.

B Cells   Blood cells produced by the immune system to act as warriors to defend the body against invaders of any kind including bacteria, viruses, cancer, and other medical conditions. The B cells produce antibodies or immunoglobulins.

Bronchi   Any of the larger air passages that connect the trachea (windpipe) to the lungs.

Bronchitis   An inflammation of the bronchi (lung airways), resulting in a persistent cough that produces large quantities of phlegm.

Bronchodilator Drugs A group of drugs used to expand the airways of the lungs.

Candidiasis Also known as Candida or yeast infection. A common infection in asthmatics. There are numerous symptoms including bloating, fatigue, and possible vaginal infections.

Celiac Disease A chronic nutritional disorder most common in young children caused by faulty absorption of food in the intestines and characterized by abdominal distention, diarrhea, and malnutrition.

Chlorofluorocarbons (CFCs) Chemical agents that, when released into the air, can damage the ozone layer of the earth. These are present in the propellants used in metered dose inhalants for asthmatics.

Chronic Fatigue Syndrome A syndrome of multiple symptoms most commonly associated with fatigue and low energy.

Circulating Immune Complexes (CICs) Tiny immune complexes that float freely in the blood or the lymph fluid. They are comprised of antigens and antibodies that can be eaten by the large macrophages of the immune system.

Coenzyme Q_{10} Important for the production of energy in all cells of the body. It occurs naturally in the body and has been found useful for heart and other health problems.

Contact Allergens or Contactants Any substance that when contacted physically causes an allergic reaction. These include chemicals, fabrics, plants, dyes, and others.

Corticosteroids A group of anti-inflammatory drugs commonly used for the treatment of asthma.

Crohn's Disease An intestinal disorder associated with colitis and irritable bowel syndrome. An autoimmune disease.

Desensitization To change one's reaction to an allergen or to make one less sensitive to something that is causing a reaction in the body.

Dust mites Microscopic insect-like creatures related to the spider. They live in blankets, pillows, carpets, upholstered furniture, and curtains. Their waste products are the main components of dust that causes the most problems for asthmatics.

Eczema An inflammation of the skin that causes itching. It is sometimes accompanied by crusting, scaling, or blisters. Many asthmatics have had or presently have eczema.

Eye Movement Desensitization and Reprocessing (EMDR)
A hypnotic technique used to help reveal and release emotional traumas that have an impact on illnesses such as asthma.

Enzymes   Complex proteins in the body that cause chemical changes in other substances in order to provide the labor force and energy necessary to keep us alive. They help convert food into chemical substances that can be used by cells to perform our everyday functions. They keep the immune system strong in order to fight disease and help nourish and clean the body. Life could not be sustained without enzymes.

Epinephrine   A naturally occurring hormone also called adrenaline, released by the adrenal glands. Epinephrine dilates the airways to improve breathing and narrows blood vessels in the skin and intestine so that an increased flow of blood reaches the muscles and allows them to cope with the demands of exercise. It is the drug used in the treatment of anaphylaxis.

Extrinsic Asthma   Asthma that is triggered by an allergic reaction, usually to something that is inhaled.

Fibromyalgia   An immune complex disorder causing general fatigue and muscle aches.

Free Radicals   Lone molecules that steal other molecules anywhere in the body they can find them. They are oxygen molecules that have split from their original form. In their quest for mates they cause damage to healthy tissues and cells. The results can be inflammation, cataracts, and accelerated aging.

Free Running Asthma Test (FRAST)   This test was started in 1995 to check high school students for exercise-induced asthma.

Galvanic Skin Response   A test involving the use of electronic devices to show any irritation to the electromagnetic pathways or organ systems, for example, blockages in the flow of electromagnetic energy in the body.

Gastric Reflux   A hyperacidic condition of the stomach, also known as gastritis, that irritates the mucous membranes of the stomach or small intestines. It is commonly known as heartburn.

Genetic   Passing from one generation to the next. Allergies and asthma can be genetic.

Hashimoto's Disease   An autoimmune disorder of the thyroid gland causing hypothyroidism.

HDL   A harmful form of cholesterol.

HEPA Filter   The most effective "high efficiency particulate air filter" to filter the air in the home to remove airborne allergens harmful to asthmatics.

Histamine   A chemical present in cells throughout the body that is released during an allergic reaction. It is one of the substances responsible for the symptoms of inflammation including sneezing and itching in allergic rhinitis. It also stimulates production of acid in the stomach and narrows the bronchi (airways) in the lungs.

Homeopathy   A natural system of medicine that uses minute doses of a remedy to cure an illness.

Homeostasis   A state of balance or equilibrium in the human body.

Hypersensitivity   Extreme sensitivity to physical, nutritional, or emotional substances that can cause symptoms in the body.

Hypoadrenal   A condition in the body where the adrenal glands are weak and do not function normally.

Hypothyroidism   A condition in the body where the thyroid gland is weak and does not function normally.

Immunoglobulin E (IgE)   When exposed to allergens, allergic individuals develop an excess of the IgE antibody. These antibodies react with allergens to release histamines and other chemicals from cell tissues and produce allergic symptoms.

Immune System   A collection of cells and proteins that works to protect the body from potentially harmful, infectious microorganisms such as bacteria, viruses, fungi, and other disease processes.

Immunosuppressor   Anything that suppresses the ability of the immune system to function normally.

Inflammation   Redness, swelling, heat, and pain in a tissue because of a chemical, physical injury, or infection. It is a characteristic of allergic reactions in the nose, lungs, and skin.

Intrinsic Asthma   Asthma that has no apparent external cause.

Kinesiology   A system of healing developed by George Goodheart, D.C. as a means of evaluating the human body by muscle testing and analysis. It draws upon the relationship between the muscles and organs of the body.

LDL   The good cholesterol in the body.

Lymphocytes   White blood cells of crucial importance to the adaptive part of the immune system that mounts a defense when dangerous invading organisms penetrate the body's defenses.

Muscle Response Testing   A technique based on kinesiology to test a muscle, or group of muscles, in the body in relation to allergens. The NAET system of allergy elimination uses this form of testing in its analysis.

Nambudripad Allergy Elimination Technique (NAET)   A technique to permanently eliminate allergies from the body developed by Dr. Devi Nambudripad and practiced by over 600 health practitioners worldwide. This technique is completely natural and drug-free. It has been effectively used in the treatment of asthma and allergies.

Neurotransmitters   A biochemical substance, such as norepinephrine or acetylcholine, that transmits nerve impulses from one nerve cell to another.

Pathogen   Any microorganism that can cause disease or allergies.

Peak Flow Monitor   An inexpensive and valuable tool for asthmatics. It measures the maximum speed with which air is forced out of the lungs and helps to monitor a worsening asthma condition. It is particularly helpful for young children who are not yet able to identify asthma symptoms.

pH   The acid-alkaline balance of the body that is so important to the maintenance of overall health.

Phenolics   Derivatives of benzene that are used to give flavor and color to foods and to help preserve them. There are many phenolics to which asthmatics react, and they need to be treated or desensitized to them.

RadioAllergoSorbent Test (RAST)   A laboratory test used to detect IgE antibodies to specific allergens.

Respiratory System   The group of organs responsible for carrying oxygen from the air to the bloodstream and for expelling the waste product, carbon dioxide.

Rotation Diet   A system of treating allergies whereby a person rotates the foods they eat every few days, never eating any of the same foods more than one day in a row. It is usually a four- to five-day rotation in order to detect and eliminate food allergies.

Sick Building Syndrome Also referred to as "building related illness." This term is used when one or more occupants of a building develops similar symptoms apparently related to some indoor pollutant(s). Many of these symptoms involve hypersensitivity of the lungs and respiratory system.

Superoxide Dismutase (SOD) A copper/zinc enzyme found in all body cells that is a primary defender against free radicals. SOD eliminates destructive superoxide molecules, a common free radical produced in the body, and soaks up free radical oxygen molecules in the bloodstream that would otherwise destroy healthy tissue. Some people are deficient in this enzyme and need to take it in supplemental form. SOD is found in green vegetables, yeast, sprouted seeds, and grains.

ABOUT THE AUTHOR

Ellen W. Cutler, D.C., is a well-established NAET Practitioner, Enzyme Therapist, Chiropractor, and Nutritionist who brings a wealth of expertise to the areas of allergies, asthma, women and children's health, nutrition, weight loss, immune disorders and chronic diseases. She has been practicing chiropractic and nutrition for 18 years, and has more than ten years of clinical experience with enzyme therapy and NAET. More than ninety-eight percent of her practice is dedicated to the treatment of allergies related to a wide array of illnesses. She has developed a national reputation for her work with NAET and enzyme therapy.

Since she focused her work on the treatment of allergies, Dr. Cutler has been a regular lecturer on topics ranging from allergies, asthma, and migraines to women's health, including hormonal imbalances, thyroid dysfunction, menopause, endometriosis, and PMS. She has appeared on various radio and TV programs, including "Alternative Medicine for Total Health." Her work has been published in the "Alternative Medicine Digest" and northern California newspapers.

Dr. Cutler earned her Chiropractic degree from Western States Chiropractic College in Portland, Oregon, after completing a BA in Psychology at the University of Buffalo, New York. She went on to do post graduate work in Kinesiology, Directional Nonforce Chiropractic, Chiropractic Orthopedics, Visceral and Cranial Manipulation, Women's Health, Nutrition, Enzyme Therapy and NAET (Nambudripad Allergy Elimination Technique).

She is a member of the American Chiropractic Association, California Chiropractic Association, North Bay Chiropractic Association, Mothers of Asthmatics, and the advisory board of NAET. She founded the Tamalpais Pain Clinic in northern California, where she lives with her husband, Steven, and two children, Aaron and Gabrielle.

INDEX